ADVANCE PRAISE FOR *THE WHOLE SOY STORY*

Anyone in America who is interested in safe, healthy nutrition must come to terms with Dr. Kaayla T. Daniel's *The Whole Soy Story*. This book is a gauntlet thrown at the feet of the soy industry, whose reputation often seems based as much on self-promotion as science. Well-written, authoritative and accessible to the layperson, this is science writing at its best.

Larry Dossey, MD
Author of *Healing Beyond the Body*,
Reinventing Medicine and *Healing Words*

This is the most important nutritional book of the decade. Every concerned American should read this brilliant and entertaining exposé. It goes a long way toward explaining some of the psychosocial perturbations that have alarmed and puzzled us.

William Campbell Douglass, II, MD
Author of *The Milk Book*
and editor of *Real Health Breakthroughs*

After being a vegetarian for nine years and eating a lot of soy, I went back to eating meat on the insistence of my doctor. I had become hypothyroid and I soon learned why. Once I started taking a thyroid supplement, I found the pills would become deactivated if I ate a soy protein bar at the same time. Soy is hardly a health food, and in the highly processed form used in most products, it's hardly natural, either. Bravo to Kaayla for digging up the whole story on soy and telling the truth.

Debra Lynn Dadd
Author of *Home Safe Home*
and ringmaster of greenring.biz

Kaayla Daniel exposes soy for what it is, a substance that, when processed, packaged and marketed by unscrupulous companies—not to mention overconsumed by the public—becomes a hormone-disrupting drug capable of causing a host of health problems, including thyroid conditions. In *The Whole Soy Story*, Kaayla Daniel dismantles the marketing mythology that sells soy as a health food, replacing it with the fascinating, well-researched and fully referenced truth about soy's very real health dangers.

Mary J. Shomon
Thyroid patient advocate, author of the bestselling
Living Well With Hypothyroidism: What Your Doctor Doesn't Tell You. . . That You Need to Know,
and founder of the thyroid-Info website www.thyroid-info.com

Dr. Kaayla Daniel brings bedazzled consumers to their senses with her dispassionate history and straightforward analysis of the science behind soy. She tells the whole soy story, the story that the public needs to hear, the story that will burst the soy bubble and turn modern seekers of good health towards real food again, foods that soy has attempted to usurp. She also brings us a message of great urgency: the estrogenic compounds in soy are natural antifertility agents. Soy thus represents a threat not only to our health, but to that of future generations.

From the Introduction by Sally Fallon,
President, The Weston A. Price Foundation and
author of *Nourishing Traditions* and *Eat Fat Lose Fat*

Dr. Kaayla T. Daniel has provided the reader with a thoroughly comprehensive review and evaluation of the soy story. This is a "must read," not only for intelligent and concerned consumers, but especially for their children and grandchildren.

Mary G. Enig, PhD, FACN, CNS
Author of *Know Your Fats: The Complete Primer for Understanding the Nutrition of Fats, Oils, and Cholesterol* and *Eat Fat, Lose Fat*

This is a book for anybody with an enquiring mind. It not only challenges commercially motivated lies, propaganda and platitudes about soy with pertinent facts, but it sweeps you along on a voyage of life-altering discovery. It reads like a detective story, but is one where you get to be the jury and judge.

Valerie James
Founder, Soy Online Service, www.soyonlineservice.co.nz

This book will open your eyes to the whole spectrum—and specter—of soy. Packed with powerful information that has seldom been mentioned outside of medical publications, this is a book you won't want to miss.

Howard Peiper, ND
Author of *The ADD and ADHD Diet*,
The Secrets of Staying Young and *Low Carb and Beyond*

There is a disturbing number of safety issues surrounding soy that have yet to be resolved. Dr. Kaayla Daniel begins an important dialogue.

Barbara Dossey, PhD, RN, HNC, FAAN
Director, Holistic Nursing Consultants, Santa Fe, NM,
and author of *Florence Nightingale: Mystic, Visionary, Healer*
and *Holistic Nursing: A Handbook for Practice* and
Rituals of Healing

At last, a book that links soy to the epidemic of ADD/ADHD and other learning disabilities. Dr. Kaayla Daniel presents convincing evidence that soy phytoestrogens can adversely affect the brains of people of all ages and that infants on soy formula are also vulnerable to toxic levels of manganese. This is "must reading" for parents, educators and health professionals.

Samuel A. Berne, OD, FCOVD
Author of *Without Ritalin: A Natural Approach to ADD*

The Whole Soy Story is one of those books that comes along once in a generation to explode a widely held nutrition myth. When I worked with nutrition pioneer Dr. Hazel Parcells, I learned that soy was deeply suspect. Through meticulous research, Dr. Kaayla T. Daniel unmasks soy for the problematic substance it is. She writes in a familiar, nontechnical style but every statement is backed up with impressive support from solid nutrition studies. This is an important addition to the literature of nutrition. Knowing the facts about soy—"the whole story"—will impact your health enormously.

Joseph Dispenza
Author of *Live Better Longer: The Parcells Center Seven-Step Plan for Health and Longevity*

Dr. Daniel's book contains everything you ever wanted to know about soy and much, much more and will make you wonder just why our nation, our bodies and our children are not being properly protected. Soy is just one more example of risks to the public that far outweigh the greedy benefits derived by big business and politicians. It is another serious wake-up call.

Doris J. Rapp, MD
Author of *Our Toxic World, A Wake Up Call: How Chemicals Damage Our Bodies, Brains, Behavior and Sex.* www.drrapp.com

The Whole Soy Story is a devastating and authoritative indictment of the safety of soy foods and a "must read" for consumers who are under the misconception that soy foods promote health. Convincingly argued and extensively supported by the medical and scientific literature, it exposes the misleading propaganda of the soy industry in promoting the supposed benefits of this inferior food.

Kilmer McCully, MD
Author of *The Homocysteine Revolution* and *The Heart Revolution*

Since I began teaching Fertility Awareness (a natural method for preventing or achieving pregnancy), I've noticed numerous menstrual irregularities among my students including anovulation, thyroid problems and progesterone deficiency. These women are in their teens, twenties and thirties; many of them have eaten low-fat diets that contain soy products since they were children. And many of them have found that eliminating soy from their diet strengthens their gynecological health. *The Whole Soy Story* explains the hazardous link between soy products and menstrual health. For anyone who cares about their own fertility and that of their children, I highly recommend Kaayla Daniel's brilliant, essential book.

Katie Singer
Author of The Garden of Fertility:
A Guide to Charting Your Fertility Signals to Prevent
or Achieve Pregnancy – Naturally – and to Gauge
Reproductive Health

A powerful and frightening look into the dangers of soy, this superbly researched and thoroughly footnoted book by Kaayla Daniel carefully peels away the pseudo-science that shrouds the soy industry and reveals the truth behind its drive to create a soy nation. Daniel predicts that the medical community will see an even greater increase in such health anomalies as precocious puberty; infertility in both men and women, learning disorders, heavy metal toxicities and hormonal disruption in the new generation of children raised on soy infant formula. A great deal of damage has already been done by the soy industry touting their product as a universal panacea. This book is an imperative read for all people, and especially those intending to have children.

T.S. Wiley
Author of Sex, Lies and Menopause: The Shocking Truth
about Hormone Replacement Therapy

This is a well-written book, richly referenced with data showing the problems with soy formula from growth to thyroid disease. In this country, more than 25 percent of formula-fed infants are given soy. It is not possible that so many infants are allergic to cow's milk formula. Rather, the use of soy formula is the direct result of clever marketing campaigns. It is tragic that as soon as the infant food industry produces a new product for so-called sick infants, it immediately mass-produces the product and uses doctors to get their product widely used. Soy formula should only be available on prescription. I hope this book will reach mothers so they can make informed decisions and not follow the profit-motivated recommendations of drug company salespersons to doctors.

Naomi Baumslag, MD, MPH
Author of *Milk, Money and Madness*,
Mother and Child Health and *Passport to Life*

Our bodies are simply not designed or adapted to safely use and metabolize more than very small quantities of any food, including soy, which is not part of the original human diet. In *The Whole Soy Story*, Kaayla Daniel ably explains the science showing that for the best long-term health, we should consume soy and soy products sparingly, if at all.

Jonathan V. Wright, MD
Medical Director, The Tahoma Clinic, Renton, WA

Women should be more afraid of the marketing of soy products than of using low-dose bio-identical hormones. Kaayla Daniel does a thorough job in presenting the risk factors associated with high-dose supplements and soy food products. No woman should take this book lightly, especially if she is interested in maintaining her health.

Larrian Gillespie, MD
Author of *The Menopause Diet*,
The Goddess Diet and *The Gladiator Diet*

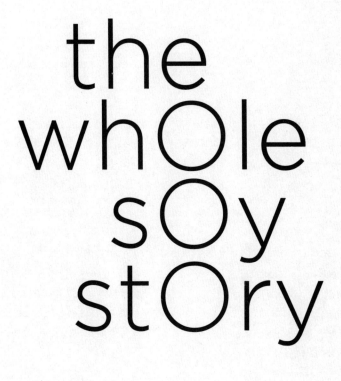

the
whOle
sOy
stOry

the whole soy story

the dark side of America's favorite health food

Kaayla T. Daniel, PhD, CCN

Introduction by Sally Fallon, author of *Nourishing Traditions*

the whole soy story
the dark side of America's favorite health food

Kaayla T. Daniel, PhD, CCN

Introduction by Sally Fallon

Text font: ITC Stone Serif Standard Medium
Title font: Gotham Light

The Whole Soy Story is intended solely for informational and educational purposes and not as personal medical advice. Please consult your health care professional if you have any questions about your health. Testimonials regarding soy published in this book have been changed in details to protect the identity of the individuals who provided them. Neither the author nor the publisher has received financial support from the beef or dairy industries.

New Trends Publishing, Inc.
Washington, DC   20007

www.NewTrendsPublishing.com   newtrends@kconline.com
US and Canadian Orders (877) 707-1776
Available to the trade through
Biblio Distribution (a division of NBN) (800) 462-6420

First Printing: 25,000

ISBN   0-9670897-5-1
PRINTED IN THE UNITED STATES OF AMERICA
Printed with soy ink, an appropriate use of soy.

To my children, Sunny and Kyrie Rose

CONTENTS

PART FOUR:
ANTINUTRIENTS IN SOYBEANS

PART FIVE:
HEAVY METALS

PART SIX:
SOY ALLERGENS: SHOCK OF THE NEW

PART SEVEN:
SOY ESTROGENS: HORMONE HAVOC

ACKNOWLEDGMENTS

This book was a team effort that could not have been accomplished without the vision, commitment and support of many people.

Sally Fallon inspired and nourished *The Whole Soy Story* from its conception, edited it with clarity, sensitivity, focus and energy and dared to publish its controversial message. A catalyst for light, truth and healing, Sally has been a good friend to me and my book.

Valerie and Richard James have boldly alerted consumers to the dangers of soy. They generously sent me professional translations of Japanese and other foreign language publications; full-text studies from hard-to-find medical and scientific journals; key correspondence with soy industry and government officials; and documents obtained at great expense and trouble using the Freedom of Information Act.

Mary G. Enig, Ph.D, recognized the dangers of soyfoods early on and was a firm supporter and careful reader of this book. As the courageous pioneer who first alerted the world to the dangers of *trans* fats and who is now proving the remarkable benefits of coconut oil, she has been an incredible role model to me.

Irvin E. Liener, Ph.D., Daniel Sheehan, Ph.D., Arpad Pusztai, Ph.D.; Retha Newbold, Ph.D.; Cliff Irvine, D.V.Sc., D.Sc., and Mike Fitzpatrick, Ph.D. have massively contributed to our knowledge of soybeans and spoken out against industry sponsored misinformation with great integrity. Special thanks to Dr. Liener, who reviewed my text with thoroughness and thoughtfulness.

Many other researchers deserve thanks for sharing key information and providing valuable feedback but asked to remain anonymous because of soy industry funding of their salaries, department budgets and laboratories.

Historian William Shurtleff of the Soyfoods Center, Lafayette, CA, has earned my respect for his monumental, unpublished history of soyfoods. Having once shared Bill's ideal of soy as a solution to world hunger, I was sad to find such overwhelming evidence of soy's damage to human health and to the environment.

Many clients and correspondents shared stories of their suffering and that of their children as a result of soyfoods or soy formula. Their urgent pleas that someone please tell the truth about soy persuaded me not to give up during the many times that the project felt overwhelming.

Peggy O'Mara, publisher, and Ashisha, editor of *Mothering*, put their readers first, resisted advertising pressures and became the first major magazine to tell the truth about soy.

Beth Salzman and Albert Robinson at St. Vincent's Hospital Medical Library provided valuable research assistance and Alice Davis of the Santa Fe Public Library, arranged for me to borrow prohibitively expensive textbooks and processing manuals through interlibrary loans.

My doctoral committee at the Union Institute and University in Cincinnati nurtured, challenged and mentored me. I wish all students could benefit from the brilliance and caring of H. Ira Fritz, Ph.D., F.A.C.N.; Mary G. Enig, Ph.D., F.A.C.N; Mitchell J. Ghen, D.O., Ph.D.; Barbara Dossey, Ph.D., R.N.; and Christina Jackson, Ph.D., R.N.

Roslyn Wallace honored me with her gift of the 2003 Aaron and Roslyn Wallace Scholarship. Her late husband's Union dissertation, with its pioneering look at healing, stress and homeostasis, informed and inspired me as I examined the diverse ways that soyfoods and soy isoflavones stress the body/mind.

Many physicians, nutritionists, writers and other colleagues offered encouragement, endorsements and/or advice, including Naomi Baumslag, M.D.; Sam Berne, O.D.; Robert Crayhon, M.S.,

C.N.S.; Francis Crinella, Ph.D.; Debra Lynn Dadd; Nancy Deville; Rebecca Ephraim, R.D., C.C.N.; Larrian Gillespie M.D.; David Goodman, Ph.D.; Winna Henry; Linda Lizotte, R.D.; Joseph Mercola D.O.; Amadea Morningstar; Leah Morton, M.D.; Howard Peiper, N.D.; Doris Rapp M.D.; Jordan Rubin, N.D.; Jack Samuels; Michael Schmidt, N.D., Ph.D.; Andreas Schuld; Mary Shomon; Katie Singer; Marcia Starck; Carol Simontacchi, C.C.N.; T.S. Wiley; William Campbell Douglass, II, M.D. and Jonathan Wright, M.D.

Marilyn McCray designed and managed my beautiful first website, www.wholesoystory.com, and has been a loyal friend for more than 20 years.

Mark Victor Hansen, Robert G. Allen, Janet Attwood and Chris Attwood of the Enlightened Millionaire Program and "The" Harv Eker mentored me and shared their "info-preneuring" knowhow.

My NY literary agent, Ashala Gabriel, believed in this project from the beginning, loyally stuck with it for more than five years and has worked tirelessly to help this book go "mainstream."

Award-winning graphic designer Kathi Dunn fulfilled my desire for an explosive cover that visually "blows the lid off nutritional dogma" and brings long-buried information to light.

Katherine Czapp made numerous important corrections and improvements with her careful reading and copyediting.

Joseph Dispenza, Kenneth Lipman, Rev. Patricia Phillips, Tom Whittier and Flora and Bern Berg encouraged and supported me and this book in more ways than I can count.

J.S. Bach's organ music never fails to heal and energize me. Without the ongoing encouragement of Mary Caskey, Michael Case, Gerald Near, Mark Childers, Gary and Connie Anderson, Dr. Stanford Lehmberg and Deacon Phyllis Orbaugh, however, I would have burned out early from all soy and no play.

My loving canine and feline companions Atma, Moksha, Mohan, Kimchi, Amba and the late Isis and Koko loved me unconditionally and never complained about their soy-free, raw-meat-and-bone diets or a house littered with soy studies.

I'm grateful to my mom, who never fed me soy burgers.

And, finally, I thank my children Sunny, 10, and Kyrie Rose, 7, for giving me joy, wisdom, humor, energy and unconditional love, as well as the perfect ending for this book: "And that's all, folks."

INTRODUCTION

Soy is the phenomenon of the times, the "healthy alternative" to meat, the "non-allergenic" dairy, the "low-cost"
protein that will feed the millions, the infant formula that
is "better than breastmilk," the "wonder food" for the New Age.
That is what the professors, the commentators, the government officials, the media and, above all, the advertisers have been telling us.
This message has fueled the growth of what has become one of the
world's largest industries—soybean production and processing.

Early soy food promotion in America aimed at two specific markets—vegetarians and the poor—soy milk and soy cereals for Seventh Day Adventists, Bac-O-Bits and meat extenders for the budget
conscious. But there was a lot of soy to sell and these markets were
limited. There was so much to sell because the market for processed
foods had experienced explosive growth since the 1950s—and most
processed foods contain soy oil. The industry found itself saddled
with a waste problem, the leftover sludge from soy-oil manufacture
which it could either dump or promote. The exigencies of corporate
life naturally chose profit-seeking over disposal and that meant ex-

1

panding the market, finding more ways to use soy ingredients in processing and convincing more people to pay money for soy-based imitation foods.

"The quickest way to gain product acceptability in the less affluent society," said a soy-industry spokesperson back in 1975, ". . . is to have the product consumed on its own merit in a more affluent society." Thus began the campaign to sell soy products to the upscale consumer, not as a cheap poverty food, but as a miracle substance that would prevent heart disease and cancer, whisk away hot flashes, build strong bones and keep us forever young. Soy funds for research enlisted the voices of university professors who haplessly demonized the competition—meat, milk, cheese, butter and eggs.

Garnering the attention of the health conscious-consumer was an important part of the strategy. Glossy magazines like *Vegetarian Times, Health* and *Self* transferred the pro-soy message from health food stores infused with the odor of vitamins to upscale markets, and a raft of books by health professionals encouraged avoidance of meat and dairy as the answer to the rising rates of disease caused by imitation foods.

The funds behind the push for soy are enormous—farmers pay a fee for every bushel of soybeans they sell and a portion of every dollar spent on Twinkies, TV dinners and the thousands of other processed foods that contain soy in one form or another, ultimately go towards the promotion of the most highly processed foods of all —imitation meat, milk, cream, cheese, yogurt, ice cream, candy bars and smoothies made from soy. Even the name of the late Robert Atkins, great defender of beef and butter, has been seconded to the cause. "Low-carb" versions of bread, pastry and pasta—the foods he warned against—are made with high-protein soy.

The push for more soy has been relentless and global in its reach. Soy protein is now found in most supermarket breads. It is being used to transform the humble tortilla, Mexico's corn-based staple food, into a protein-fortified "super-tortilla" that would "give a nutritional boost to the nearly 20 million Mexicans who live in extreme poverty." Meanwhile, Hindus in India can now buy synthetic dal and lentils made of extruded soy protein. Soybean milk processing plants are sprouting up in places like Kenya. Even China, where soy really is a poverty food and whose people want more meat, not tofu, has opted to build western-style soy factories, rather than put grazing animals on grasslands that cannot be used for growing crops.

Soy meat extenders first showed up in school lunches, although federal law once limited the levels that could be used. The USDA's NuMenu program now allows unlimited use of soy in student meals. With soy added to hamburgers, tacos and lasagna, dietitians can get the total fat content below 30 percent of calories, thereby conforming to government dictates. "With the soy-enhanced food items, students are receiving better servings of nutrients and less cholesterol and fat."

The need to create new markets for soy presented an irresistible challenge for Madison Avenue. Early advertisements for soy were primitive—a smiling farmer surrounded by musical notes and the words of a ditty for "crispy packs of nourishment"—Kellogg's variety pack, which included Corn Soya breakfast cereal; a cow's head depicted with soybean pods in a Seventh Day Adventist magazine; a small drawing of pudding topped with "frozen pure soy cream" in a 1947 *Family Circle* magazine.

During the late 1990s, ads for new-generation soy foods featured flower children riding bicycles and a not-amused mother who, according to the text, will feed her child soy foods in spite of what her elders have told her.

A survey of March 2004 health magazines reveals five-and-one-half pages of ads for products containing soy in *Alternative Medicine* (two of which promote soy as a solution to the problems of menopause); five-and-one-half pages in *Vegetarian Times*; and five pages in *Yoga Journal*. The ads that keep today's health-oriented publications afloat aim at mainstream, not alternative, culture: soy milk ads feature faces of smiling children; high-protein bars create expressions of ecstacy on upside-down models; and a hostess who serves chocolate-covered soy nuts is the toast of her party.

Open a copy of *Men's Fitness* and you will find pages and pages of full-color ads for soy-based candy bars and instant beverages promoted as a way to create the macho man with perfect abs. Sadly—ironically—most issues contain the requisite article advising these super-built Lotharios how to have great sex. Were *Men's Fitness* to warn its readers about the fact that soy lowers testosterone levels in men, advertising revenues would dry up and the magazine would fold.

Perhaps those publications devoted to startling exposés will reveal the downside of soy? We can always hope. But *Utne Reader* and *Mother Jones* often carry full-page ads for soy. Only *Mothering* magazine has published articles warning consumers about soy-based infant formula, despite full-page ads for soy.

Of all modern industries, it is advertising that keeps its finger on the pulse of public consciousness; market surveys, demographic analyses, book sale trends, focus groups, consumer polls and university research help Madison Avenue gauge the dreams and preferences of that sole arbiter of corporate profits—the American consumer. Has the industry discovered resistance to soy foods among professionals? Then soymilk is promoted as something smooth and delicious with the caption, "Don't be so stubborn!" Does soy have a weak male demographic? Then huckster soy as a prevention for prostate cancer through Michael Milken, former junk bond financier. Do shopaholics deep down desire a richer life, a commitment to something honest and real? An ad for soy-based bars and meal replacements angles the heads of two chic shoppers towards a "Supplement Facts" label: Serving Size: 1 Bar or Shake; Sense of achievement 100%; Compromise 0%. And the lonely hearts? Christiane Northrup, M.D., a well-known physician-author, tells women how to bring romance into their lives, and follows with paeans to the libido-reducing soy snacks, smoothies and chips she sells.

Do farmers need to feel good about growing soy? *The Furrow*, a magazine published in twelve languages by the John Deere tractor company, provides the requisite praise: "Just imagine you could grow the perfect food. This food not only would provide affordable nutrition, but also would be delicious and easy to prepare in a variety of ways. It would be a healthful food, with no saturated fat. In fact, you would be growing a virtual fountain of youth on your back forty. This ideal food would help prevent, and perhaps reverse, some of the world's most dreaded diseases. You could grow this miracle crop in a variety of soils and climates. Its cultivation would build up, not deplete, the land. . . this miracle food already exists. . . . It's called soy."

Health claims, of course, must appear to have scientific backing. Scientists who serve as spokespersons for the soy industry are adept at simulating claims without substance. "Each year, research on the health effects of soy and soybean components seems to increase exponentially," writes Dr. Mark Messina, organizer of five symposia on soy. "Furthermore, research is not just expanding in the primary areas under investigation, such as cancer, heart disease and osteoporosis; new findings suggest that soy has potential benefits that may be more extensive than previously thought." And this research has been generously supported by the very companies that stand to benefit.

Soy got one of its biggest boosts with a 1998 FDA ruling allowing a health claim for soy, based on research showing that soy protein could lower cholesterol levels under certain conditions. Health claims on food packages are limited to heart disease, but assertions that soy prevents cancer quickly followed in promotional literature. "In addition to protecting the heart," says a vitamin company brochure, "soy has demonstrated powerful anticancer benefits. . . the Japanese, who eat 30 times as much soy as North Americans, have a lower incidence of cancers of the breast, uterus and prostate." Claims of this sort fail to mention that the Japanese, and Asians in general, have much higher rates of other types of cancer, particularly cancer of the esophagus, stomach, pancreas and liver. The logic that links low rates of reproductive cancers to soy consumption requires attribution of high rates of thyroid and digestive cancers to the same foods, particularly as soy causes these types of cancers in laboratory animals.

Marketing costs money, especially when it needs to be bolstered with "research," but there's plenty of funds available. All soybean producers pay a mandatory assessment of one-half to one percent of the net market price of soybeans. The total—something like eighty million dollars annually—supports United Soybean's program to "strengthen the position of soybeans in the market place and maintain and expand domestic and foreign markets for uses for soybeans and soybean products." State soybean councils from Maryland, Nebraska, Delaware, Arkansas, Virginia, North Dakota, Illinois and Michigan provide another two and one-half million dollars yearly for "research." Private companies like Archer Daniels Midland also contribute their share. ADM spent $4.7 million for advertising on "Meet the Press" and $4.3 million on "Face the Nation" during the course of a year. Public relations firms help convert research projects into newspaper articles and advertising copy; law firms lobby for favorable government regulations; IMF money funds soy processing plants in foreign countries; missionaries teach indigenous peoples how to raise soybeans and make soymilk; and free trade policies keep soybean abundance flowing to overseas destinations.

Kaayla Daniel brings bedazzled consumers to their senses with her dispassionate history and straightforward analysis of the science behind soy. She tells the whole soy story, the story that the public needs to hear, the story that will burst the soy bubble and turn modern seekers of good health towards real food again, foods that soy has attempted to usurp. She also brings us a message of great urgency: the estrogenic compounds in soy are natural antifertility agents. Soy thus represents a threat not only to our health, but to our future.

Sally Fallon, President
The Weston A. Price Foundation, October, 2004

part one
A SHORT
HISTORY OF SOY

1
SOY IN THE EAST

T he ancient Chinese valued the soybean as a national trea-
sure and honored it with the name "the yellow jewel."[1]
Yes, the Chinese revered the soybean—but they did not
eat it.

The soybean is one of the "Five Sacred Grains," along with rice,
millet, barley and wheat.[2] This designation is odd in several respects.
The soybean is a legume, not really a grain, and it was not originally
used much for food. Soybeans did, however, distinguish themselves.
Farmers grew soybean plants as "green manure"—as a cover crop
plowed under to enrich the soil between plantings of food crops.
Soy plants live symbiotically with *Rhizobium*, a strain of bacteria that
forms nodules on the roots of plants in order to capture nitrogen
from the air and fix it in the soil. The Chinese written characters for
rice, barley, wheat and millet show the grains that are eaten. The
one for soy shows the powerful nitrogen-fixing roots.[3,4]

TAMING THE BEAN

Soy went from nitrogen fixer to fermented food no earlier than
about 2500 years ago.[5,6] Until then, the Chinese considered soybeans
inedible. How the ancient Chinese knew that soybeans remain toxic
after ordinary cooking remains a mystery. Anthropologists survey-
ing 50 societies in Southeast Asia, Asia and the Pacific discovered

that soybeans were perceived as a suitable food for humans only after the discovery of processing methods that could largely deactivate an antinutrient found in soybeans known as the trypsin inhibitor.[7] Although precise identification of trypsin inhibitors would have to wait until the mid-20th century, it is likely that the people in these societies concluded from personal experience that a food causing so much digestive distress, bloating and gas should not be eaten. The discovery of fermentation allowed the Chinese to tame the soybeans' undesirable, rowdier elements and domesticate them into a well-mannered food.

The ancient Chinese originally developed the technique for making *chiang*—a soupier version of the soybean paste best known by the Japanese name miso—to preserve protein-rich animal foods. Fish, shellfish, game and meat—often including blood, bones and guts—were salted and immersed in a mixture of salt and rice wine until the foods broke down into a chunky paste. Additional fermentation deepened the flavors and aromas. The process wasn't used on soybeans and grains until sometime between the second century BC and fourth century AD.[8,9] Soy sauce, originally the liquid poured off during the production of *chiang,* appeared around the same time, although it would not be widely produced for centuries.[10] *Natto*, tempeh and other fermented whole soybean products entered the food supply much later, with *natto* appearing sometime around 1000 AD and tempeh no earlier than the 1600s.[11,12]

Thus, claims that soybeans have been a major part of the Asian diet for more than 3000 years—or from "time immemorial"—are simply not true. Historian William Shurtleff of the Soyfoods Center in Lafayette, California, explains that although various legends about soybeans and soyfoods exist in texts dating back to 2838 BC, "it is now generally considered that these are a fabrication some 2,600 years later by Han Dynasty historians who, in the traditional Chinese way, wished to endow all things worthy of respect with ancient ancestry."[13]

In Japan, mythology tells us that the goddess Oketsuhime

Mikoto gave birth to fermented soybeans for the benefit of future generations.[14] History tells us that Buddhist priests followed up with the research and development. Miso probably arrived in Japan with the arrival of Chinese missionary priests sometime between 540 and 552 AD,[15] although soybean pickles and fermented sauces seem to have been invented independently in the northeastern provinces.[16] Either way, the earliest forms of Japanese miso resembled Chinese *chiang,* a product that generally contained spices, oil and often meat. In time, the Japanese developed a simpler and subtler product that they honored with the new name of "miso," which first appeared in dated 806 and 938 AD.[17] In the 12th century AD, samurai warriors took control of the country and popularized a national cuisine of simplicity and frugality, one in which grains starred as the center-piece of a meal, supported by miso soup, cooked vegetables and small amounts of fish, shellfish or tofu. It was not until this late date that a soy-and-grain-based miso began to play an important role in the Japanese diet.[18,19]

THE MEAT WITHOUT A BONE

Tofu—which is a precipitated rather than a fermented prod-uct—came about the same time as miso. Legend has it that in 164 BC, Lord Liu-An of Huai-nan, China—a renowned alchemist, medi-tator and ruler—discovered that a puree of cooked soybeans could be separated into solids and liquid using *nigari,* a form of magne-sium chloride found in seawater. The drained curds were formed into solid cakes, called tofu. Liu-An's initial reason for turning soy-bean dross into tofu gold was his desire to add a low-cost protein to the vegetarian monastic diet.[19-21] Over time, the monks may have noticed that randy behavior declined when tofu consumption went up. The aptly named "meat without a bone" soon appeared regu-larly on monastery menus as an aid to spiritual development and sexual abstinence, a dietary strategy validated by recent studies show-ing that the plant-form of estrogens (called phytoestrogens) in soy can lower testosterone levels.[22] (See Chapters 28 and 29.)

Tofu became a staple in Buddhist monasteries and was invested with spiritual powers that only the truly enlightened are likely to fully comprehend. For example, Bodhidarma, a holy man who founded the Chinese Zen school, decided to test tofu's understanding of the Buddha's way by engaging it in "dharma combat." (Dharma means the "ultimate law" or "right conduct.") What exactly Bodhidarma meant or how he accomplished this testing is less than clear, though tofu's sponge-like capacity to absorb nearly anything apparently carried the day. Tofu not only passed muster, but earned

IS SOY A STAPLE?

Proponents of soy foods often state that soy is a staple food in Asian countries. A staple is defined as a major part, element or feature, with the implication that a staple food contributes a large portion of calories to a diet.

Actually, the people of China, Korea, Vietnam, Thailand, Indonesia, Mongolia and even Japan don't eat very much soy.

Food in Chinese Culture, a collection of scholarly papers published in 1977, reports that soy foods accounted for only 1.5 percent of calories in the Chinese diet, compared with 65 percent of calories from pork.

Nutrition during Pregnancy and Lactation, published by the California Department of Health in 1975 lists soyfoods as minor sources of protein in Japan and China. Major sources of protein listed were meat including organ meats, poultry, fish and eggs.

Finally, the type of food Asians eat is very different from what is appearing on the American table. Think small amounts of old-fashioned products like miso and tempeh, not soy sausages, soy burgers, chicken-like soy patties, TVP chili, tofu cheesecake, packaged soymilk, or other of the ingenious new soy products that have infiltrated the American marketplace.

firm praise for its simplicity, honesty, straightforwardness and "lovely white robes."[23]

Consumption of tofu soon spread throughout China, Korea and Southeast Asia. By 700 AD, it was accepted as a meat or fish replacement, at least when pork, seafood and other preferred sources were unaffordable or unavailable. Except in areas of famine, tofu was served as a condiment, consumed in small amounts usually in fish broth, not as a main course.[24,25]

Tofu probably came to Japan by way of Korea with Buddhist monks and missionaries around the eighth century AD.[26] Entrepreneurial priests and cooks in the cities of Kamakara and Kyoto teamed up to open tofu shops and restaurants within the walls of the temples and monasteries. Mushrooming demand led to tofu shops throughout the cities, then on to towns and remote rural areas. By the 14th century tofu had lost its aura of "white robed" exclusivity and became a regular food for workers and peasants who could afford little meat.[27]

TEMPEH NATION

In Indonesia, tempeh is the soybean food of choice. With 41,000 tempeh shops, including some in remote rural areas, tempeh appears to be an ancient food. Yet the world's earliest reference to tempeh manufacture occurs in the *Serat Centini*, a book published in 1815 on the orders of Sunan Sugih, Crown Prince of Central Java. Soybeans probably came to Indonesia around 1000 AD with the advent of regular trade with southern China. The Indonesians had made fermented coconut press for centuries and tempeh probably resulted from the application of this technique to soybeans. After 1595, during the period of Dutch colonization, tempeh (along with other indigenous foods) became known as food for the poor, even though people of all classes continued to consume it. That perception remained after independence. Indeed, Sukarno, President of the Indonesia Republic from 1945-1967, once admonished his fellow citizens, "Don't be a tempeh nation."[28]

Cooks in China, Japan, Korea, Indonesia and other East Asian countries all developed distinct soybean cuisines, but shared a reliance on fermentation, precipitation, or both. Except in monasteries, during famines and among the very poor, Asians consumed their products only in small amounts, as condiments or seasonings, and not as substitutes for animal foods like fish or pork. They rarely—if ever—baked or boiled soybeans, ground them into flour, or roasted them to make nut-like snacks.[29,30] In all likelihood, trial and error showed that such methods performed miserably compared to the time-honored traditional techniques, and consistently left diners with a stomach ache or worse. Because most Asians did not press or crush great quantities of soybeans to extract soy oil, they never faced the challenge of finding creative ways to use massive amounts of the leftover protein. The soy oil they did extract worked fine to light lamps, and the protein served as an excellent fertilizer.[31] The exception was the northern province of Manchuria, which had a thriving soy oil export business from the 1850s until the 1920s.[32] After World War II, Americans occupied Japan and encouraged the Japanese to adopt western technology, food processing patterns and dietary customs, instigating changes that would alter the ways that soybeans are processed, marketed and consumed.

SOY IN OKINAWA

Even soy proponents now admit that the "average" consumption of soy foods in Asia is not great. So vegan John Robbins, author of *Diet for a New America, May All Be Fed* and *The Food Revolution* claims that what's important is the level of soy consumption "in those parts of Asia which demonstrate the highest levels of human health." Robbins asserts that that "there is no question about where that is. The elder population of Okinawa (a prefecture of Japan) have the best health and greatest longevity on the planet."[33]

Robbins claims that the reason the Okinawans enjoy such longevity is because they eat two servings of soy foods per day, with soy constituting 12 percent of their calories. He bases these figures on the Okinawa Centenarian Study, as reported in the best-selling books *The Okinawa Program* and *The Okinawa Diet Plan* by Bradley Willcox, D. Craig Willcox and Makoto Suzuki.[34,35]

How much soy Okinawans eat, however, is not at all clear in these books. The authors say that the Okinawans eat "60 to 120 grams per day of soy protein," which means, according to the context, soy foods eaten as a whole food protein source. But the authors also include a table that lists total legume consumption (including soy) in the amounts of about 75 grams per day for the years 1949 and 1993. On yet another page, we learn that people eat an average of three ounces of soy products per day, mostly tofu and miso. And then we read that the Okinawans eat two servings of soy, but each serving is only one ounce. As for soy making up 12 percent of the Okinawan diet, Robbins pulled that figure from a pie chart in which the 12 percent piece represents flavonoid-rich foods, not soy alone. Will the correct figures please stand up?

There are other credibility problems with the Okinawa Centenarian Study, at least as interpreted in the authors' popular books. In 2001, Dr. Suzuki reported in the *Asia Pacific Journal of Clinical Nutrition* that "monounsaturates" were the principal fatty acids in the Okinawan diet.[36] In the books, this was translated into a recommendation for canola oil, a genetically modified version of rapeseed oil developed in Canada that could not possibly have become a staple of anyone's diet before the 1980s. According to gerontologist Kazuhiko Taira, the most common cooking fat used traditionally in Okanawa is a very different monounsaturated fat— lard. Although often called a "saturated fat," lard is 50 percent monounsaturated fat (including small amounts of the health-producing antimicrobial palmitoleic acid), 40 percent saturated fat and 10 percent polyunsaturated. Taira also reports that healthy and vigorous Okinawans eat 100 grams *each* of pork and fish each day.[37] Thus, the diet of the long-lived Okinawans is actually very different from the kind of soy-rich vegan diet that Robbins recommends.

Finally, the longevity of Okinawans has been attributed to many factors besides soy consumption. Indeed the three authors of the Okinawa Centenarian Study name caloric restriction as "the key to eating the Okinawa way." And although they share the good news that diet, not genes, is the key to longevity—meaning we too can live long and well if we follow their plans—Dr. Suzuki has reported elsewhere[38] that the genes of Okinawan centenarians actually do differ from those of normal individuals and are a factor in their superior longevity.

2
SOY GOES WEST

S oy went west when traders, missionaries, botanists and other travelers brought soybeans back from China and Japan. Soy beans served as useful ballast on ships as well as culinary or horticultural curiosities. In 17th-century France, soy sauce became the "secret seasoning" used at court banquets; but other types of soy foods failed to appeal to the western palate. In 1770, Ben Franklin sent soybeans home from the continent with the enthusiastic recommendation that they be grown in America. Although his beans were planted, soybeans remained a little-known commodity in the United States for more than a century. At the 1927 meeting of the American Soybean Association, William J. Morse of the United States Department of Agriculture looked back to 1907 when "it seemed unlikely to all except a few soybean enthusiasts or 'soybean cranks' as they were then called, that the soybean would ever amount to much more." It wasn't until 1935 that the acres of soybeans grown for food oil equaled those used for crop rotation.[1-5]

In short, Europeans and Americans were slow to welcome soy into western cuisine. To use a popular Japanese expression—convincing westerners of the virtues of soy foods proved about as "futile as trying to clamp two pieces of tofu together."

BEAN CRUSADES

Soy's first American prophet was John Harvey Kellogg, M.D. (1852-1943), the breakfast cereal king, who used pamphlets, books and a bully pulpit to champion the health benefits of the bean, harangue against the evils of meat, develop some notoriously unpalatable meat substitutes, and otherwise milk soybeans for all they were worth. A 1944 advertisement for vegetable soybeans even bid us to "meet the vegetable cow." The creation of one of Dr. Kellogg's students, the ad showed the head of a cow made entirely from soybeans and with the horns, forelock and parts of eyes, nostril and mouth made of green pods.[6,7]

Another crusader was Artemy Alexis Horvath, Ph.D., who worked—more effectively, if less eccentrically—on the academic as well as the popular fronts. Born in Russia in 1886, this mystery man traveled throughout the world and worked for the United States Bureau of Mines and other government agencies. In his 1931 manifesto "Soya Flour as a National Food," Horvath insisted that soy deserved a place of honor on the American table, claiming that soy eaters would gain both physical stamina and "mental virility." He reasoned that it must have been soy that allowed the Chinese to attain a high level of culture at a time in history when Americans and Europeans were barbarians.[8,9]

Henry Ford also had grand plans for soy. In 1929, he established a laboratory in Dearborn, MI, to conduct research into the ways different plants might serve industrial uses, and in 1931 decided to focus his efforts on soy. By 1933, he had spent $1.2 million and *Fortune* magazine reported "he is as much interested in the soya bean as he is in the V-8." Ford believed that soy plastics would be the material of the future for car bodies, window frames, steering wheels, gearshift knobs, bathtubs, sinks and refrigerators. Although he never succeeded in mass producing his "Soymobile," Ford did create a solid prototype. In 1937, he called in reporters, jumped up and down on an unbending sheet of curved plastic made out of soy and exclaimed, "if that was steel, it would have caved in!" In 1940,

Ford installed a plastic trunk lid on one of his personal cars and whacked it with an axe to prove its dent resistance.[10]

Jokes ran rampant in the national media. *The Cleveland Press*, for example, wondered why Ford did not strengthen his plastic by adding spinach. Other newspapers opined that the new substance could be put to better use in battleship armor and the manufacture of coffins.[11] Though Robert Boyer, a Ford executive, drove the soy-plastic car for a few weeks, he eventually abandoned it because of "a strong odor reminiscent of a mortuary."[12]

By 1938, Ford often appeared in public sporting a tie made from soybean fiber and three years later he made a public appearance in a suit tailored out of soybean-fiber cloth. Although the *Detroit Times* reported, "He is as delighted as a boy with his first pair of long pants," the truth was another soy story. The suit was itchy when dry, smelled like a wet dog when damp, and was so prone to ripping that he could not bend over or cross his legs.[13-15]

Ford hired his boyhood friend Edsel Ruddiman, formerly dean of the School of Pharmacy at Vanderbilt University, to develop and popularize soy foods. Ruddiman accomplished the former but apparently not the latter as one of Ford's secretaries described a soybean biscuit as "the most vile thing ever put into human mouths." However, white rats found it edible and Ford professed to like it.[16] Whether excess soy consumption had anything to do with the mental lapses, irritability, anxiety and unreasonableness that marked Ford's personality later in life[17] is speculative but accords with some recent scientific findings (see Chapters 26-29).

Meanwhile in Europe, Adolf Hitler was fervently promoting soybeans, vegetarianism and natural foods.[18] In 1929, Benito Mussolini ordered the formation of the Committee for the Study of Soya, and boldly announced a plan to require soy flour as a mandatory ingredient in the Italian staple polenta.[19,20] In 1940, a vegetarian physician used the forum of the *British Medical Journal* to scold the British Ministry of Food for not following the examples of Hitler and Mussolini, which he perceived as "a great sign of the times."[21]

John Harvey Kellogg's followers in Battle Creek, Michigan agreed, noting that "the soybean has come to have a prominent place in the military dietetics of Germany."[22]

In the 1950s and 1960s, the Communist Party in the Soviet Union pushed soy protein and soy margarines as the solution to low-cost feeding of the masses and called the soybean "our young

---

A FORD IN YOUR FUTURE

Henry Ford liked to publicize his soy food experiments by summoning reporters to soybean luncheons. The most notable of these was held at the 1934 World's Fair. The menu included the following, all partially or completely made with soybeans:

Tomato juice with soy sauce
Celery stuffed with soy cheese
Soybean puree
Soybean croquettes with green soybeans
Soy bread and butter
Apple pie with soybean crust
Soy coffee
Soymilk
Soy ice cream
Soy cookies and candy.

A guest wrote, "Nothing we newsmen ate that day led us to foresee that soybeans were destined to become an ingredient in many popular food products. We accepted as reasonable the possibility that the bean might become a leading cattle feed or industrial material."

SOURCE: David L. Lewis. *The Public Image of Henry Ford* (Detroit, Wayne State University Press, 1987) 285-286.

---

revolutionary Chinese ally."[23] In Cuba, a Seventh Day Adventist company invited Fidel Castro to lunch on its products at a church school in Cuba. "Best pork chops I ever ate," said the premier as he wiped his beard. But the chops came from soybeans, not a pig. [24] In 1984 Castro obtained a "mechanical cow" from Brazil and put it promptly into operation, making soymilk and other products. Although the first soy milks produced tasted so "beany" that the Cuban people fed them to their pets, continuing shortages of dairy products led the Cuban government to persist. Since 1995, Cuba has become known as "the rising star among developing countries in the use of soyfoods"—especially of soy yogurt and drinks which are distributed free of charge to children ages 7 to 14.[25]

In the United States, soy food was widely regarded as a "poverty food" or a "hippie food." Despite the soy industry's valiant attempts at image rehabilitation, real men still didn't eat tofu. Nor did presidents. In 1973 Richard Nixon made headlines while visiting Japan when he confessed that he had never seen a soybean. [26]

BEAN COUNTING AND THE INDUSTRIAL REVOLUTION

As the ingenuity of Dr. Kellogg, Ford, Mussolini and others makes clear, Americans and Europeans have always treated soybeans very differently from the way Asians do. Soy in the West is a product of the industrial revolution—an opportunity for technologists to develop cheap meat substitutes, to find clever new ways to hide soy in familiar food products, to formulate soy-based pharmaceuticals, and to develop a plant-based, renewable resource that could replace petroleum-based plastics and fuels.

Even today, in the West, very few soybeans are sold for whole food products. Soybeans were not even seriously considered for food in the United States until World War II shortages created a demand for a cheap source of protein. To this day, the "good old soys" of Asia—miso, tempeh and *natto*—thrive only in niche markets. Although tofu sales have certainly risen during the past two decades, soy's dubious status is reflected in ongoing tofu jokes made by cartoonists and humorists, from Gary Larson to Dave Barry. Until recently, soy proponents were so much on the defensive that a writer for the *New Yorker* quoted a booster admitting, "There's something about the soybean that just seems to put a lot of people off. You know, if soybeans are in storage along with cereals rats will always eat the soybeans last. Even the rats don't like us."[27]

No matter. The soy industry knows that the big profits are not to be found in old-fashioned, funny-tasting foreign foods, but from splitting the "yellow jewel" into two golden commodities—oil and protein.

SPLITTING PROFITS

Soy oil, the bean's first—and for many years primary—profit center, has been promoted since the founding of the National Soybean Growers Association in 1920 (renamed the American Soybean Association in 1925).[28] For years, the soy protein left over from oil extraction went exclusively to animals, poultry and, more recently, fish farms. Today the industry aggressively markets soy protein as a people feed as well.

Hard-working food scientists have found so many inexpensive ways to improve or disguise the color, flavor, "bite characteristics," "mouth feel" and aftertaste of soy protein-based products that soy is now an ingredient in nearly every food sold at supermarkets and health food stores. (See Chapters 6, 7, 8 and 11.) The industry also makes a profit from other waste products, most notably soy lecithin (widely used in the food processing industry as an emulsifier), protease inhibitors (digestive distressers sold as cancer preventatives), and isoflavones (plant estrogens promoted as "safe" hormone therapy, cholesterol reducers, and cancer cures). (See Chapters 10, 13, 16, 26, 29, 30.)

PLASTICS

Nearly every soy product Henry Ford envisaged has become reality, yet bean mobiles are not rolling down the road, motorists aren't filling up their gas tanks with soy bio-diesel fuels, and industrial uses of soy have barely made a dent in the petroleum industry. In 1997, nearly 94 percent of the soybean oil produced went into food products—primarily salad and cooking oils, shortening and margarine. Only six percent went for industrial use.

That percentage may soon go up.[29] Soy-based plastics, resins, polyurethanes, paints, varnishes, inks, crayons, cosmetics, mattresses, cushions, shoe soles, carpet padding, insulation, imitation marble, construction materials, engine lubricants and bio-diesel fuel are just a few of the products coming on line. These new products are said to be more cost effective and environmentally friendly than those based on petroleum, although it would be interesting to explore precisely how much petroleum it takes to grow and process commercial soybeans.

GROSS NATIONAL PRODUCT

The possibilities for recycled soy seem endless. Biodegradable soy plastics may soon be recycled into animal feeds. And Nabil Said, Ph.D., Director of Research and Development at Insta-Pro, a processing technology company, reports that a "value added" product made of animal waste and soy protein has been transformed into an animal chow. So far chicken and pig manure have worked well as raw ingredients, though the more fibrous cow pies have failed to pan out.[30] Concerns about mad cow disease and some state regulations, however, have stopped a stampede for this particular "value added" soy product.[31] As a result, "bean turd" production for pet kibble, fish rations and livestock feed remains small.

Consumers who wonder what could possibly be next might remember the steaks made of soy mixed with ground-up human corpses served up in the 1971 sci-fi movie *Soylent Green*, starring Charleton Heston. In fact, animal, poultry and fish carcasses have been routinely converted into "useful feed ingredients" and processed with soy protein into "complete feeds" for years.[32]

DATELINE SOY

It is a myth that Asians have consumed soy foods for many thousands of years. Soy is actually a relatively recent addition to Asian cuisine. (Dates are approximate.)

200 BC: Soybean *chiang*—a soupy fermented paste and precursor of miso—originates in China. Soy sauce was a byproduct of *chiang* making.

164 BC: Tofu invented in China as a vegetarian protein source for monks living celibate life styles.

600 AD: Early forms of miso and tofu are brought to Japan with the Buddhist missionaries.

1000: *Natto* invented in Japan.

1100s: Samurai warriors in Japan popularize a national cuisine of simplicity and frugality in which grains serve as the centerpiece of a meal, supported by miso soup, cooked vegetables and small amounts of fish, shellfish or tofu.

1279-1368: Soy oil first considered an edible oil. Lard, sesame and rapeseed oil were preferred.

1600s: The earliest that tempeh could have been invented in Indonesia.

1866: The first historical reference to soymilk in China. By the 1920s soymilk was popular with the elderly and infirm. Soymilk did not become popular in Japan until the 1960s.

two: soy goes west

1928: First soy infant formula developed in China. The very first soy formula was invented by a Baltimore pediatrician in 1909.

Post World War II: American technology and marketing bring highly processed soyfoods made with soy flour, soy protein isolate, soy protein concentrate and textured vegetable protein ingredients to China, Japan and other countries.

SOURCES: For details and citations, see Chapters 1-12.

3

THE PLOY OF SOY

Historically, east was east and west was west. No longer. The soy industry has Americanized soy around the globe, running into serious opposition only when Monsanto—the "biotech bully boy"—pushed for acceptance of its genetically modified (GM) "Frankenstein" soybeans.[1-4] The problems with soy, however, go beyond the dangers of bioengineering.

Soybeans grown for export have replaced indigenous crops in many countries around the world, causing serious local food shortages and the loss of small family farms to corporate agribusinesses. High-tech soy processing plants have supplanted local cottage industries, causing loss of dietary and cultural diversity as well as fewer jobs for locals.[5] And though we often hear about the loss of Amazon rainforest to ranchers raising cattle for fast-food franchises, soybean farming has wrought even greater devastation, causing the deforestation of an area larger than the state of New Jersey in less than a year.[6] Yet the soybean is promoted as the salvation to world hunger and a "green," environmentally sound alternative to meat production.

The soy industry even claims that its modern processed soyfoods

27

are the natural heritage of people of Asia. In fact, the myth that soy is eaten in great quantity in Asia is an invention of the soy industry itself, determined to take advantage of a huge, untapped market.

The average consumption per year of dry soybeans in China, Indonesia, Korea, Japan and Taiwan comes to 3.4, 6.3, 10.9 and 13 kilograms, respectively.[7] That boils down to only 9.3 to 36 grams per day. The Organisation for Economic Co-operation and Development estimates the consumption of soybeans in Japan at a mere 18 grams per day, slightly more than one tablespoon.[8] The famous China-Cornell-Oxford Study—in which researchers headed by T. Colin Campbell of Cornell University traveled around China to survey the dietary habits of 6,500 adults in 130 rural villages—revealed an average legume consumption of only 12 grams per day, only one-third of which is soy.[9]

Although reported levels of soy consumption vary somewhat from study to study, it is abundantly clear that Asians do not eat abundantly of soy foods. Even Mark Messina, Ph.D., a spokesperson for the soy industry and the organizer of five symposia on the role of soy in the prevention and treatment of chronic disease, states that the Japanese (some of the highest consumers of soy foods) average only 8.6 grams of soy protein per day.[10] This is well under the U.S. government's recommended dose of 25 grams for protection against cardiovascular disease and a mere fraction of the amounts touted by popular authors such as Christiane Northrup, M.D. Millions of women have put their trust in this popular author who is, unfortunately, highly compromised by her role as a spokesperson for the soy product Revival.

Furthermore, the types of soy foods consumed in Asia are very different from those now appearing on the American table. Although the westernizing of China, Japan and other Asian countries has caused a slight decline in consumption of old-fashioned, whole-food soy products such as miso, tofu and tempeh, it has opened up a potentially huge market for American-style imitation products like soy milk, veggie burgers, chicken substitutes, TVP chili, tofu cheesecake,

FRANKENSOY
CRY FOR THEE, ARGENTINA

In 1997 Argentina became one of the first countries to authorize the use of genetically modified (GM) seed. Soon after, farmers began growing Monsanto's Roundup Ready strain of soybean, designed to be resistant to the herbicide glyphosate. The farmers were seduced by Monsanto's promise of increased productivity and decreased herbicide use with Roundup Ready soy.

The economic dream crop, however, soon became a nightmare. Problems with herbicide resistant "superweeds" led GM soy growers to double the amount of herbicides used by conventional farmers. Bacteria died, leaving soil so inert that dead weeds would not rot. Farmers and neighbors near GM fields have suffered health problems such as rashes and tearing eyes, while many livestock have died or given birth to deformed young.

In addition, 10,000 square miles of rainforest were leveled for soybean production and 150,000 small farmers driven off their land by big farmers eager to grow more soy. Meanwhile, the production of milk, rice, maize, potatoes, lentils and other food staples needed to feed the people of Argentina fell, replaced by soybeans grown for export to Europe and China.

Despite clear environmental and economic crises, Colin Merritt, biotechnology manager for Monsanto, says GM soy has been an "exemplary success" in South America. Similar "successes" are showing up in the U.S. and elsewhere.

SOURCES: Utton, Tim. Nightmare of the GM weeds. *Daily Mail* (UK), April 15, 2004. www.gmwatch.org; Rohter, Larry. Relentless foe of the Amazon jungle: soybeans. *NY Times*, September 17, 2003.

soy ice cream, protein shakes and energy bars. Sales of soy milk—a product rarely consumed in Asia prior to the 20th century (see Chapter 6)—are steadily increasing in Japan.[11]

Once an exporter of soybeans, China is now the world's largest importer of U.S. soybeans. China is increasingly purchasing western processed soy products for human consumption as well as soybean meal for use in its poultry, swine and fish industries. DuPont, the world's largest producer of soy protein, owns 20 joint ventures and independent investment enterprises in China, with a total investment of more than 700 million U.S. dollars.[12]

In America, soy is aggressively marketed as an upscale "health food" that can prevent heart disease and cancer, build healthy bones and stop menopausal symptoms. Despite a lack of any real proof for these claims, soy foods are one of the fastest growing sectors in the food industry with retail sales growing from $0.852 billion in 1992 to $4 billion in 2003. Retail sales grew 21.1 percent in 2000 with the strongest increases in sales of soymilk, energy bars, meat analogues and cold cereals, with an increase of 26.8 percent in mainstream supermarkets, 11.8 percent in natural product supermarkets and 5.5 percent in all other natural food stores. These figures come from studies carried out by SPINS (a company founded in 1995 that provides marketing information on the health and wellness industry) and Soyatech (a company founded in 1984 that publishes the annual *Soya & Oilseed Bluebook*, the industry's leading source of information on soy companies and products, and that runs www.soyatech.com, a business-to-business internet site for the industry).[13-15]

Formerly a poverty or "hippie" food, soy foods are now nearly as expensive as meat and pricier than dairy. As a top gun marketer hired by the soy industry recommended back in 1975, "The quickest way to gain product acceptability in the less affluent society is to have the product consumed on its own merit by a more affluent society."[16] Heightening consumer awareness of "health benefits" has done the trick, transforming the former "fringe food," sold in small natural food stores, to a mainstream item in grocery stores. Some of America's largest food companies now manufacture soy foods, including Kraft, Kellogg, ConAgra, General Mills, Heinz, Unilever-BestFoods and Dean Foods.

Who consumes these soy products? Historically, consumers were vegetarians and people trying to avoid meat or dairy. The soy industry has identified today's "new soy consumer" as a person who "looks at the goodness of soy and the positive nutrition it offers."[17] Thirteen percent of female consumers and 11 percent of males choose soy to prevent disease. Educated shoppers are more likely to buy soy products than high school graduates, according to market researchers Philip Fass and Mary Jane Mount of Archer Daniels Midland at the symposium, *Soyfoods 2001: New Technology Innovations and Effective Marketing Tactics.*[18]

The United Soybean Board's promotion strategy is to target "key influencers," including food manufacturers, chefs and dietitians.[19] And because science is a sound basis for marketing strategy, the industry has put millions into medical research, including a meta-analysis funded by Protein Technologies International to establish the FDA's cholesterol-lowering heart health claim. The United Soybean Board's "Soy Health Research Program" helps researchers prepare

POISONOUS PLANT DATABASE

While the Food and Drug Administration (FDA) has approved a heart health claim for soy protein, the agency also lists soy in its "Poisonous Plant Database." A search of the word "soy" in the database reveals 256 references, including studies that warn about goiter, growth problems, amino acid deficiencies, mineral malabsorption, endocrine disruption and carcinogenesis.

Source: http://vm.cfsan.fea.gov/-djw/pltx.cgi?QUERY=SOY

proposals submitted to the National Institutes of Health (NIH), a strategy that in its second year turned $30,000 worth of assistance into $4 million worth of tax-payer funded NIH grants.[20]

These ploys have led to industry-sponsored "checkbook" research, generously funded university departments, well-publicized symposia, advertising control of the media, the courting of journalists and aggressive lobbying in Washington, D.C. And because scientists have been unable to prove the health benefits of soy, industry efforts have also led to a mastery of the art of ambiguous health claims. As the Illinois Center for Soy Foods advises, "The presence of a short package claim on the front label generates more specific attribute-related thoughts, more inferences, and creates a more believable and positive image of the product in the consumer's mind than a long package claim."[21] It all adds up to what Brian Sansoni, Senior Manager for Public Policy at the Grocery Manufacturers of America, calls a "buzz" about soy products that "intrigues people until they want to try them."[22]

The campaign has been nothing less than brilliant. Soy hype has led to high hopes—and higher profits. Lost in the hoopla has been the whole soy story.

HIDE THE SOYLAMI!

In his Far Side Collection *Unnatural Selections*, cartoonist Gary Larson appeals to tofu haters everywhere when he depicts a hunting scene with the punch line. "In sudden disgust, the three lionesses realized they had killed a tofudebeest—one of the Serengeti's most obnoxious health antelopes." In a similar spirit, the satirical *Onion* newspaper—"America's Finest News Source"—offers up "13 of the most popular items for meat-shunning Americans," to wit:

Approximeat
Roast Almost
Prosciuttofu
Rocky Mountain Soysters
Kielbeancurdasa
Soystrami
Misteak
Fake-un Double Cheesebulghur
Nauseages
Mockwurst
I Can't Believe It's Not a Dead Animal
Tofuck You, Meat Lover
Nofu—the Tofu Substitute

LOW CARB BLUES

Dieters trying to stick to the bestselling Atkins, South Beach and Zone diets ushered in the hottest marketing trend of 2003—low-carb versions of high-carb favorites such as pasta, bread, crackers and cookies. Nearly 4,000 new products reached supermarket and health food store shelves, with most substituting soy protein for traditional flours. Although sales initially experienced double—and even triple—digit growth, the market collapsed as consumers discovered that they didn't care for the taste, aftertaste, texture or mouth feel of the higher priced goods. What's more, many gained weight either from the license to eat or from the soy itself. (Soy protein, after all, was used in Japan to fatten animals not employed in farmwork.) *The New York Times* reported that "Atkins Nutritionals took some of the biggest financial hits" and by May 2004 had written off $53 million of unsold and expired food, sending the company into a financial tailspin. Founded in 1989, the company began pushing soy with a vengeance soon after Dr. Atkins' death from a fall on ice in April 2003.

SOURCES: Warner, Melanie. Is the low-carb boom over? As sales growth slows, Atkins and others suffer. *New York Times*, December 5, 2005, Section 3, 1, 9.

Shurtleff, William, Aoyagi, Akiko. History of Soybean Crushing: Soy Oil and Soybean Meal. From *History of Soybeans and Soyfoods: Past, Present and Future*. Unpublished manuscript (Soyfoods Center, Lafayette, CA) 43.

part two
TYPES OF SOY

4
GREEN PODS, YELLOW BEANS AND BLACK EYES

Soybeans grow in fuzzy green pods, two to three round beans to a pod. The plants are bright green and grow two to three feet high. The beans are usually a yellowish tan, the size of peas, and marked with a single, distinctive black eye— nature's way of warning us, perhaps, that they can cause trouble.

BEAN THERE

Botanists classify soybeans as legumes of the genus *Glycine*. *Glycine max* refers to the cultivated soybean, *Glycine soja* to the wild one. Of the two main types of legumes—oilseeds and pulses—soybeans are the seed type, while lentils are the best known examples of pulses. Soy's closest relatives are clover, peas and alfalfa. Because of their ability to fix nitrogen, the soybean and its relatives have played an important role in maintaining nitrogen balance in the environment. Because most other plants obtain their cellular nitrogen from nitrate and ammonia in soil or water, nitrogen fixation is one of the soybean's most important agronomic characteristics.[1]

READERS' GUIDE
TO NATURALLY OCCURRING
ANTINUTRIENTS AND TOXINS IN SOY

All soybeans contain antinutritional factors (known as antinutrients) and toxins. Mother Nature puts them there to block seeds from sprouting prematurely and to harm insects and other predators that would otherwise eat too many of them. Unfortunately, they can harm us as well unless the soybeans are properly processed to neutralize them.

This brief glossary is provided to help readers more easily understand this section's discussion of types of soyfoods and the qualitative differences between old-fashioned and modern processing methods.

ALLERGENS cause allergic reactions. Soy is one of the top 8 allergens.

GOITROGENS damage the thyroid.

LECTINS cause red blood cells to clump together and may cause immune system reactions.

OLIGOSACCHARIDES are the pesky sugars that cause bloating and flatulence.

OXALATES prevent proper absorption of calcium and have been linked to kidney stones and a painful disease known as vulvodynia.

PHYTATES impair absorption of minerals such as zinc, iron and calcium.

four: green pods, yellow beans and black eyes

ISOFLAVONES are phytoestrogens (plant estrogens) that act like hormones and affect the reproductive and nervous systems. Some of the best known isoflavones are genistein and daidzein.

PROTEASE INHIBITORS, most notably TRYPSIN INHIBITORS interfere with the digestive enzymes protease and trypsin. This can lead to gastric distress, poor protein digestion and an overworked pancreas.

SAPONINS bind with bile. They may lower cholesterol and may damage the intestinal lining.

For full and detailed discussion of soy's antinutrients and toxins, See Parts Four, Five and Seven.

There are more than 300 varieties of soybeans. The larger, more expensive vegetable soybeans are preferred for making whole soy foods over the smaller, more widely available field beans, which are split into oil and meal. Food beans were bred to have a lighter seed coat, a higher protein level and a lower oil content. In the United States, all commercial beans are yellow or tan, as other colors are excluded by grading standards.[2]

Japanese manufacturers prefer large soybeans with a high protein content for tofu production, but round small beans with a soft texture for *natto*. For *edamame,* the best soybeans are large in size with a high sugar content and tender texture. Most soybeans are harvested at the dry, mature stage, with only a very small proportion at the immature vegetable stage.[3]

Since the early 1990s, the U.S. share of soybean production has declined from about 50 percent to 35.6 percent, with increased production bringing Brazil up to 29.4 percent and Argentina to 17.4

percent. China produces only 7.8 percent of the world's soybean crop. Soybeans in the United States are primarily grown in the northern Midwestern states from Ohio to Kansas and South Dakota, in southern states along the Mississippi River and in the southeastern states. In some growing areas, soybeans can be double-cropped with winter wheat, allowing farmers to get two crops per year from the same fields.[4-6]

DONE THAT: THE BIRTH OF FRANKENSOY

More than two thirds of the U.S. soybean crop now come from genetically modified (GM) soybeans patented and sold by Monsanto, known as the "Frankenstein Food Giant."[7,8] The company spent many years and millions of dollars trying to develop a soybean that would be resistant to its profitable weed killer Roundup, an organophosphate whose active ingredient is glyphosate. The goal was to make it easy for farmers to kill weeds without damaging the crops.

Although Monsanto's researchers developed several strains of glyphosate-resistant soybeans over the years, the plants withered and died because they were unable to properly synthesize the amino acids tyrosine, phenylalanine and tryptophan. The problem seemed insurmountable until scientists discovered a hardy bacterium living in the glyphosate-rich sewage of the Monsanto factory. The problem was how to insert the bacterial genes across the species barrier into the soybean. This proved no small feat, but finally resulted in a patented soybean plant with a Roundup-tolerant gene that never before existed in nature and could not have evolved naturally.[9-11] The adoption of GM crops has been the most rapid in the United States although Argentina offers the clearest lesson in environmental dangers. (See Sidebar on page 29.)

SOY SPROUTS: YOUNG AND RESTLESS

Soy sprouts are grown by germinating whole soybeans for five to seven days. Slightly larger and firmer than the more familiar mung bean sprouts, they are higher in vitamin C and beta-carotene and are usually served lightly boiled in salads or sauteed as part of a stir fry.[12]

Traditionally, soy sprouts are eaten in Korea but less often in China or Japan. They are less popular than mung beans everywhere because of their stronger, beanier flavor and tougher texture. William Morse of the United States Department of Agriculture reported on expeditions to Asia from 1929-1932, noting that soy sprouts were widely available in vegetable markets and that they were served boiled and sprinkled with salt as a side vegetable or relish throughout the winter months.[13]

The use of soy sprouts as food did not come about until the Sung Dynasty (AD 960-1127). Traditional people seem to have known intuitively that the sprouts are not as healthy as they look.[14] Science has now shown us that short-term germination increases the strength of soy's antinutrient fractions; long-term sprouting plus fermentation will decrease and nearly eliminate them (see Chapters 15-20). Either way, the plant estrogens remain present. No wonder soy sprouts are mentioned in historical accounts as useful, sometime-pharmaceuticals, not as daily food.[15]

EDAMAME: SWEET GREEN ADOLESCENCE

Edamame is the Japanese word for green vegetable soybeans. These young, sweet-tasting soybeans are harvested at the point when they are well developed but still soft and green. They contain lower levels of antinutrients and plant estrogens than adult beans. Boiled or steamed in the pod for 20 minutes or less, they are chilled, salted and removed from the pod and served as either an *hors d'oeuvre* or a green vegetable. *Edamame* is usually sold frozen, either shelled or in the pod.[16,17] Unlike mature soybeans, *edamame* do not have as much of the beany, bitter flavor; they have a higher ascorbic acid and beta-carotene content, and lower amounts of the undesirable protease inhibitors, phytates and oligosaccharides. In flavor and texture, they compare favorably with butter beans and lima beans.[18]

The main problem, as noted by an Ohio farmer named T. V.

FRANKENSOY: SAFE AS TESTED

Monsanto obtained FDA approval and rushed its new-born GM soybean plants to market in 1996 based on its claim that GM soybeans are substantially equivalent to conventional ones—hence safe.

Many scientists who have looked at Monsanto's testing methods, however, have found that the testing was not only inadequate and incomplete but rigged to reach a favorable conclusion. To wit:

- The soybeans used for analyses and animal feed tests were grown without application of the herbicide. Thus the test results were obtained by using a sample different from that which is being sold in the marketplace.

- Monsanto tested unsprayed beans and so provided no data on endocrine-disrupting estrogen sprayed onto the soybeans with the herbicide Roundup.

- The protein analysis did not come from the Roundup Ready soybean itself but from the resistant bacterium whose genes were inserted into the new plant. The two may or may not be equivalent. Tests used to verify antigenic equivalence do not prove that the amino acid sequences are the same and rearrangements are normal in the DNA sequence of a plant as it accommodates a new gene.

- In acute toxicity tests on rats, scientists used the bacterium, not the GM soybean.

* Feeding experiments conducted on rat, cow, chicken, catfish and quail were of short-term duration and did not test chronic toxicity or across generations. Even so, the data for body weights and weights of liver, kidney and testicles showed obvious adverse effects in the male rats fed GM soy.

* Lowered body weights of males fed toasted soybean were described in the data sheet as "statistically significant" but not in the conclusion, which states "no statistical significance is observed."

* Cows fed Roundup Ready soybeans produced higher levels of milk, which might be a direct consequence of higher estrogen levels in these soybeans.

* Data from an early experiment were omitted because they showed lower protein levels and significantly lower levels of the essential amino acid phenylalanine.

These and many other indications of experimental manipulation, misinterpretation, falsified conclusions and flagrant disregard of data have led to demands for independent safety assessments.

SOURCES

Monsanto genetically engineered soya has elevated hormone levels: public health threat. International scientists appeal to governments world wide. Press release. Third Meeting of the Open-ended Ad hoc Working Group on Biosafety of the UN-Convention on Biological Diversity. Montreal, October 13, 1997.

Kawata, Masaharu. Monsanto's dangerous logic as seen in the application documents submitted to the Health Ministry of Japan. Third World Biosafety Information Service, July 28, 2003. www.organicconsumers.org.

Keeler, Barbara. Lappe, Mark. Close analysis of Monsanto's data reveals key differences in its RoundUpReady™ soybeans. *Los Angeles Times*, January 7, 2001.

Peticolas back in 1855, is that green soybeans are "inconvenient" because they are "so difficult to hull." Accordingly, the first commercially canned green soybeans were not produced until the mid-1930s. Even at that late date, Dr. John Harvey Kellogg complained to the U.S. Department of Agriculture that he had not found a way to hull them fast enough so that they could be canned economically. In 1935, Henry Ford's Edison Institute solved the problem with a mechanized process.[19] Today most *edamame* are sold frozen—either with or without the pods. Many people enjoy snacking on *edamame* and removing the hulls by hand.

Tasty though they may be, historian William Shurtleff of the Soyfoods Center in Lafayette, CA, knows of no early references to green vegetable soybeans in China. An herbal guide from 1406 (Ming Dynasty) indicated that whole pods of young soybeans could be eaten or ground for use with flour, but recommended such uses *only* during times of famine.[20] Kinder words are found in a *Materia Medica* from 1620, which recommends *edamame,* but only for the medicinal purpose of killing "bad or evil chi."[21] By 1929, Morse of the USDA reported that "as early as May, small bundles of plants with full grown pods were seen on the market. At the present time the market is virtually flooded with bundles of plants with full grown pods, the seeds of which are also full grown. The pods are boiled in salt water and the beans eaten from the pods."[22]

BOILED AND BAKED SOYBEANS: OLD, TOUGH AND INCOMPARABLY RUDE

Mature beans are yellow, beige or tan, although rarer varieties come black, brown, green or bicolored. All lose color as they ripen and age into hard, dry beans with a long shelf life.[23]

People who prepare soybeans from scratch usually buy the dried beans sold in the bulk bins at health food stores. The basic flavor of plain, boiled or baked, soybeans is, well, "beany" with a "greasy mouthfeel."[24] Soybeans have a stronger taste and higher fat content than other beans—definitely not to everyone's liking. The one thing

44

most people agree on is that mature dried soybeans must be thoroughly cooked and never, ever eaten raw. ✓

Even when soaked overnight, soybeans generally require at least two hours of pressure cooking or seven to nine hours boiling on a stove top. Different varieties have different degrees of toughness. Even then, some soybeans do not become completely soft and mashable. USDA researchers discovered that soybeans remain hard and unpalatable with simmering, but that cooking at temperatures above the boiling point will break up the cellulose structure and develop a richness of flavor not otherwise obtainable.[25] Scientific journals, historical accounts and anecdotal evidence alike testify to acute digestive distress from raw or *al dente* soybeans (see Chapter 16). Thoroughly softened or not, boiled or baked soybeans have a rude reputation for gas production.

Traditionally, Asians almost *never* eat boiled or baked soybeans. The notable exception is during the winter in northern parts of China, where whole soybeans may be cooked with pork feet, salt and other spices until they become very tender. The gelatin greatly aids digestion. The dish is known as *dong gu,* meaning "frozen bone."[26]

5
THE GOOD OLD SOYS
soybeans with culture

The ancient Chinese and Japanese knew what modern food processors choose to forget—that soybeans must be soaked, cooked and fermented in order to transform them into a food both edible and healthful. When we ferment food, we enlist bacteria, fungi and other beneficial microorganisms to help break down complex proteins, starches and fats into highly digestible amino acids, simple sugars and fatty acids. The process results in a near-total biochemical transformation.[1]

Fermented soybean products enjoy high honor throughout Asia as digestive aids, potent medicines, powerful energizers, stamina builders and longevity elixirs. Treasured as more valuable than gold, the molds and cultures used to make miso, *shoyu*, *natto*, tempeh and other fermented soybean products are often heavily insured and safeguarded in fire-, flood- and burglar-proof vaults. Miso masters attempting to explain the mysteries of their craft speak reverently about interactions between the small movements of microorganisms and the great movements of the four seasons, of fostering sacred partnerships between microrganisms and macrohumans, of harmonic convergences of the micro-kingdoms and the macroworld.[2,3]

The rituals, language and mystique that have grown up around fermented soybeans appear to be quintessentially Eastern, but the benefits of fermentation are well known outside of Asia. Similar culturing processes turn milk into clabbered milk, yogurt, sour cream or cheese; grapes into wine; cabbage into sauerkraut; cucumbers into pickles; and fruits and spices into chutney. In the days before refrigeration, canning and rapid global transportation, peoples all over the world used fermentation to preserve foods and enhance their nutritive power. The ancient Greeks referred to this power to transform food as "alchemy."[4]

DROSS INTO GOLD

Of all the foods that are commonly fermented, none needs it more than the soybean. Soy protein is notoriously hard to digest unless enzymes and microorganisms go to work on it first. These tiny workers not only predigest the soybeans, but deactivate the powerful protease inhibitors (see Chapter 16) that inhibit our digestive enzymes and overwork the pancreas. A recent Japanese study showed that old-fashioned fermented soyfoods retained only a tiny percentage of trypsin inhibitor compared to that in the whole raw soybean, which on average contains 4,819u/100g. After processing, *natto* was 0.7 percent, soy sauce 0.8 percent, and miso 0.3 percent.[5]

Fermentation also helps deflate soy's flatus-producing carbohydrates, its mineral-depleting phytates, and other problem-causing antinutrients (see Chapters 15-20). Miso and other cultured soybean products are highly digestible—perhaps as high as 90 percent digestible, a significant improvement over the 60-68 percent digestibility of roasted or boiled soybeans.[6-8]

Fermented soy products rarely cause a lot of gas. Researchers testing 16 beans and bean products for gas production found that tempeh was "essentially non-flatulent." Although tempeh is fermented for only 24 to 48 hours, the processes of repeated soaking and cooking before the initial inoculation, as well as a final cooking before serving, deactivate the troublesome complex sugars known as oligosaccharides.[9,10]

B HERE NOW

Microbial activity also dramatically improves the simple soybean's nutritional profile. Although antinutrients known as phytates in most soybean products block proper absorption of calcium, iron, zinc and other minerals, fermentation produces the enzyme phytase, which reduces phytate levels substantially. Microorganisms also pump up the levels of the B vitamins riboflavin, niacin, niacinamide, B_6, pantothenic acid and folate, although they may slightly decrease levels of thiamine.[11-13] Fermentation also increases the levels of vitamin K, needed for healthy bones.[14] Strong antioxidants have been reported in tempeh.[15,16]

News stories reporting high levels of vitamin B_{12} levels in fermented soyfoods—particularly in tempeh—are not usually accurate. The most common molds used to manufacture tempeh, *Rhizopus oligosporus*, produce analogues of B_{12}, not the physiologically active forms.[17,18] These analogues actually increase the body's need for B_{12}.

Klebsiella pneumoniae and *Citrobacter freundii* bacteria, however, appear to produce genuine B_{12} and are now deliberately added by some tempeh makers to the starter. (Unfortunately, these specialized soy products are difficult to find in the U.S.) The B_{12} content of tempeh fermented with both *R. oligosporus* and *Cit. freundii* was three times higher than a control fermented with *Cit. freundii* only. Further research is needed to determine results from other fermented soy products made with the help of various bacteria and molds.[19-21]

The minerals in old-fashioned soy products are better assimilated than those found in modern soy products thanks to the deactivation of phytates.[22] However, the high salt content of miso, *natto*, and soy sauce leads many health practitioners to advise eating them "sparingly."[23]

Miso, tempeh and other old-fashioned fermented products also contain essential fatty acids (EFAs). The slow fermentation process may change the fatty acid composition of soybeans, but without damaging the beneficial omega-3 fatty acids. This vulnerable component of soy oil is lost, damaged or outright removed by the heat and pressure of modern processing methods (see Chapters 9 and 14). During tempeh making, the concentration of the EFAs (linoleic and alpha linolenic acid) decreases while the concentration of monounsaturated oleic acid increases. In the making of *natto*, there are no significant changes in fatty acid composition of the soy lipids, indicating that the enzyme lipase is not produced by the *B. natto* bacteria.[24]

Even more remarkable, the valuable fatty acid GLA (gamma linolenic acid)—a highly usable form of omega-6—may be produced by the *Rhizopus* strain of bacteria, good news indeed, given the acute shortage of readymade GLA in nearly all commonly eaten foods.[25] Other sources of GLA include borage oil, evening primrose oil and black currant oil, prescribed for a variety of conditions, including cancer, premenstrual syndrome, cystic fibrosis, irritable bowel syndrome and many skin conditions.[26,27] Asians eating fermented soy products take in this valuable fatty acid on a regular basis.

PROTEIN POWER

Despite their considerable benefits, fermented soyfoods are not ideal sources of proteins. Although their amino acids are not damaged—the sorry fate of soy proteins processed using modern methods—they are low in the vital sulfur amino acids—methionine, cystine, cysteine and taurine (see Chapter 13). However, the protein picture brightens considerably when soybeans are fermented along with rice or barley to create the most popular forms of miso and tempeh.

As Frances Moore Lappé taught us in the book *Diet for a Small Planet*, beans and grains contain complementary proteins, with the excesses of one compensating for the deficiencies of the other.[28] While Lappé's theory seems plausible, the actual practice of eating beans and grains together has left many vegetarians protein deficient. Part of the problem lies in the fast cooking methods and shortcuts taken in today's kitchens and by food processing companies. The solution is to give hungry microorganisms and enzymes first dibs so that the proteins appear at the dinner table already predigested. The protein quality of beans plus grain then improves markedly.

A look at the Net Protein Utilization (NPU) index indicates that miso scores a 72, higher than soybeans at 61, rice at 70, and barley at 60. This is due not only to the powerful grain-soybean combination, but to the reduction by fermentation to those proteins' most utilizable forms. However, not even miso comes close to milk or eggs, which have NPU scores of 82 and 94, respectively.[29]

For this reason, most Asians prefer to cover their protein bases with one more step—serving these products with fish or animal products. In Japan, miso is stirred into bonito or sardine-based soup broths nearly everywhere except at vegetarian monasteries. Chinese, Korean and Indonesians like to stir meat or seafood—if available and affordable—into the fermenting mix itself. Although tempeh averages 19.5 percent protein (close to chicken at 21 percent and beef at 20 percent), Indonesians have experimented with a fermented tempeh, fish and rice combination, which contains as much as 23.7 percent protein.[30]

DIGESTIVE AID

Predigestion is only one of the many jobs performed by the lactic acid-forming bacteria, salt-resistant yeasts, molds and other wee beasties that live in fermented soybean products. The "old salts" that survive the rigors of long-term fermentation are peculiarly well adapted to one final job—facilitating the digestion of other foods eaten at the same time. Thus old-fashioned fermented soyfoods earn their reputation as digestive aids.[31]

HORMONE REPLACEMENT

Fermented soy products contain plant estrogens in the highly absorbable aglucone and glucoside forms. Non-fermented soyfoods contain the glucoside form, which requires intestinal bacteria to break them down into the more bioavailable aglycone. Some research suggests that the aglucone forms are anticarcinogenic but that the glucoside forms are not.[32,33] Whether any form of isoflavones is a blessing is debatable, and will be discussed in depth in Part Seven. The risk of unwanted side effects from soy estrogens plugging up hormone receptor sites and perturbing pathways may be one of the reasons why Asians have traditionally eaten only small amounts of these foods. Indeed, loss of sex drive was the desired outcome when priests consumed such foods in quantity in Zen monasteries. . . and why Japanese wives may take revenge on unfaithful husbands by increasing their daily dose of tofu.[34]

DISEASE CONTROL

The microorganisms in fermented soy also help prevent disease. Of the 161 strains of aerobic bacteria isolated in miso and other fermented soybean products, almost all combat *Escherichia coli* and *Staphylococcus aureus*—two common causes of food poisoning. In Indonesia, Hong Kong and Singapore during World War II, prisoners suffering from acute dysentery recovered when rations of whole boiled soybeans were replaced with tempeh.[35] The *Rhizopus* mold seems to inhibit the growth of dysentery-causing bacteria. Researchers studying the impact of soy sauce on five strains of *E. coli* found that that no single component of traditionally fermented soy sauce could be credited for the success of anti-*E. coli* action.[36]

Traditional fermenting techniques ensure that soy products are almost never contaminated with aflatoxin, mycotoxins or dangerous molds or bacteria. Aflatoxins—a carcinogenic and toxic factor often found in moldy grains and peanuts—are not stable in soy sauce or miso.[37-39] This would seem to be true only of the old-fashioned products as aflatoxin contamination has been identified recently as a major problem in modern soy and peanut products.[40-41]

five: the good old soys

GLOW PROTECTION

Finally, the "good old soys" may protect us from radiation poisoning. After World War II, Dr. Shinichiro Akizuki noticed that healers who treated atomic bomb victims at St. Francis Hospital in Nagasaki suffered few ill effects from residual radiation if they ate miso and seaweed. Agricultural research scientist Morishita Kenichiro later discovered that miso and *natto* contain dipicolinic acid, an alkaloid capable of grabbing onto radioactive strontium so that it can be ushered safely out of the body.[42] Radioprotective effects extend to X-ray and radiation therapies used for medical diagnoses and cancer treatment, with a 2001 study showing significantly greater protection coming from misos that have undergone lengthy (rather than short or medium-term) fermentation.[43] Anecdotal evidence suggests that miso is similarly protective against electromagnetic fields and pollution from computer screens, television, microwaves, power lines, smokers and automobile exhaust.[44]

OUNCE OF PREVENTION

Even so, westerners should regard reports about the "good old soys" with a grain or two of salt. Popular news stories tend to treat all soy foods alike, but the old-fashioned traditional products bear little or no resemblance to the modern soybean products promoted by the soy industry and sold in American grocery stores. And Asians simply do not eat any soybean products in great quantity. They are used in small amounts as condiments or seasonings, not as main courses, and rarely more than once a day.[45] Even with the finest organic and perfectly prepared soybeans, the lesson is, "Less is more."

MISO: PASTE FOR LIFE

Miso is a rich, sweet, mellow or salty paste made from soybeans, grain (generally rice or barley), salt, water and *Aspergillus oryzae* culture. Colors range from the creamy beiges and sun yellows of the lighter, sweeter varieties to the red and deep browns of the earthier, saltier and "meatier" ones. Miso is used widely in Japan, Korea, Taiwan, Indonesia and China, with different regions favoring different types.

Miso is used to flavor soups, sauces, dressing, marinades and patés. The process of making miso soup can be as simple as stirring the miso paste into simmering water, but the subtleties are highly complex. Japanese women aren't considered eligible for marriage until they've mastered the fine art of miso soup-making. Four elements are involved: miso, vegetables or other solids, garnishes and a richly flavored base known as *dashi*. Outside of the vegetarian monasteries, *dashi* is prepared with dried bonito flakes or dried sardines. Similarly, Chinese cooks make miso soup with a richly flavored chicken broth and Koreans with beef.[46] Because enzymes are destroyed at temperatures above 118 degrees F, and because they lose some of their power above 105 degrees F, the miso is added at the last minute, and the soup removed from the stove as soon as the first boiling bubble appears.[47]

Three types of miso predominate in Japan: rice, barley and soybean. The first two combine soybeans with salt and the chosen grain, the last is just salt and beans. Special misos containing chopped vegetables, nuts, seeds, seafoods, seasonings and spices are generally sweet and have a fairly short shelf life. They are not used for miso soup but served as toppings for vegetables, salads, grain dishes or crackers. One type known as "finger lickin'" miso was a popular dessert or sweet before modern sugar confections came in vogue.[48]

In China, *chiang (jiang)* is the name for a dark, salty, thick and chunky soybean paste, often made with wheat and seafoods.[49]

Japanese miso production begins with soaking whole soybeans in water and cooking until tender. The beans are then dusted with a fungal starter, usually *Aspergillus oryzae,* and combined with rice or barley. These nuggets incubate until the fungus matures and turns the product white, warm and fuzzy. The mature nuggets are then mixed with salt and water and left in cedar vats to ferment for one to three years. During aging, the bean-rice or bean-barley nuggets turn to paste, while flavors and aromas develop. The process takes place at the natural temperature of its environment, slowing down in the winter and speeding up in the summer. When the miso is fully ripened, it is blended, pressed and packaged.[50]

Small-time Japanese producers of rice and barley misos produce hundreds of distinct varieties by varying the ratio of beans to grains. *Hatcho* and other grain-free soybean and salt misos come in fewer varieties. The relative lack of carbohydrates and moderate to high salt content make lengthy aging necessary, and this invariably leads to darker colors, stronger odors and flavors that many westerners consider acquired tastes. *Hatcho* miso is renowned for its strengthening effects and medicinal properties and was taken on six Japanese expeditions to the South Pole.[51]

During most of its history, miso was used to preserve meat and vegetables.[52] On a tour of Tokyo in the early 1930s, William Morse and other USDA researchers found "considerable quantities of fish preserved in white miso and in sake mash" and that nearly all food stores carried vegetables preserved in red miso. Morse said that he enjoyed a dinner of beef preserved in white miso that reminded him of "sugar-cured hams of the southern states." Of the use of miso as a preservative, he wryly observed that it would "undoubtedly prove far less harmful than some of the products (alcohol) now used in violation of the 18th amendment."[53]

During the past few decades, American miso masters have successfully made miso using peanuts, chickpeas, peas, lentils, azuki and other beans in place of soybeans; with corn, millet, wheat or buckwheat in place of the traditional rice or barley; and with kelp replacing some of the salt. Traditional miso is made only with natural whole ingredients. It is never pasteurized, an unnecessary process that destroys the enzymes that aid digestion.[54]

QUICK AND EASY

Quick misos were first produced on a large scale around 1960. These are fermented for three to 21 days in temperature-controlled, heated environments. To improve flavor, aroma and appearance, sweeteners (usually sugar or caramel syrup), bleaches, sorbic acid preservatives, food colorings and MSG are likely to be added. The products are always pasteurized.[55-57]

The most common quick misos are dehydrated instant powders and dried soup mixes. Spray-dried versions are made by mixing miso with enough water to make a slurry, then blowing it in a fine spray into the top of a 150-foot-tall tower filled with circulating hot air. The miso dries as it falls. The spray inlet temperature is a very hot 482 degrees F, which kills all the enzymes and probably a lot of the vitamins as well. Today, freeze drying is preferred. Regular miso is spread one inch thick on steel trays, slid into a large vacuum chamber and quick frozen at a very low temperature of about minus 22 degrees F. It is then dried at about 104 degrees F for 10 to 15 hours. Although this method better preserves flavor and aroma, nearly all dried misos contain MSG, sodium succinate, inosinic acid and various other flavorings, colorings and additives.[58] Those sold in American health food stores generally have a much shorter list of questionable ingredients but concerns about the loss of enzymes remain.

NATTO: THE LAST STRAW

There's nothing natty about *natto*. This soaked, boiled or steamed and then fermented, whole-soybean product is notable for its sticky coat, cheesy texture, musty taste, sliminess and pungent odor. *Natto* first appeared in northeastern Japan about 1,000 years ago. Traditionally, it smelled like straw because it was made by inoculating whole cooked soybeans with *Bacillus subtilis* or *Bacillus natto* and incubated in straw. The straw also absorbed the none-too-fragrant ammonia-like odor. Because of frequent contamination by unwanted microrganisms, natto makers abandoned the straw method in favor of inoculating the cooked beans with *B. natto*, then mixing and packing the product in wooden boxes or polyethylene bags.[59]

Natto may be served with mustard and soy sauce, or used in soups and spreads in Japanese cuisine. A little goes a long way. Children love it—not for its strong, some would say, rotten flavor—but because its glistening threads can be stretched, making it one of the all-time great play foods. As a food, *natto* is popular only in certain parts of Japan. Many restaurants that serve *natto* require patrons to sit in a private area so as not to offend other patrons with the distinctive smell.

Natto is one of the few fermented soy products in which the bacteria predominate over the fungi. It's made the news as a good source of vitamin K, which exists in only a few foods other than animal fats like butter but is vital to blood clotting and healthy bone formation and preservation.[60]

TEMPEH: BREAKING THE MOLD

Tempeh, the most popular fermented food in Indonesia, is a chunky, chewy, nutty, smoky—and moldy product. It is easy to digest and especially rich in B vitamins, minerals, omega-3 fatty acids and enzymes.[61,62]

The traditional tempeh-making process is a long one. Dry whole soybeans are boiled, drained and hulled; soaked and prefermented for 24 hours; boiled again for an hour, drained and cooled; inoculated with *Rhizopus oligosporus* or another *Rhizopus* strain; wrapped in banana leaves; and allowed to ferment at room temperature for 24 to 48 hours. In addition to the mold, numerous bacteria, yeast and other microorganisms proliferate in tempeh. Scientists studying 81 tempeh samples isolated 69 molds, 78 species of bacteria and 150 species of yeast. Tempeh can be made of soybeans alone or combined with rice, barley, wheat, seaweed, peanuts, fish or other ingredients. Fermentation of tempeh is short and simple, and it can easily be done at home. Today, the pace of tempeh-making is somewhat increased by using soybeans that have been dehulled, cracked and cooked in water with a little vinegar.[63]

Tempeh is very perishable. In America, it is generally sold as a vacuum-packed frozen slab. It can be grilled, broiled, baked or put into soups, stews, chilis, and casseroles. It is firm enough to be sliced or cubed, fried and baked, yet it tender and easy to chew and digest.

Expect to find mold on it. That mold is the very key to tempeh's healthful properties, particularly its digestibility. White is fine. So are gray or black pin holes on the surface. More black means the tempeh is stale and likely to be bitter. Strong ammonia smells or green mold carry the unmistakeable message—"Throw it out."[64]

SOY SAUCE: THE REAL McSOY

Soy sauce is the best-known flavor enhancer in Asian cooking. It's the one old-fashioned soy product used regularly by Americans—or it would be if the soy sauces sold here bore any resemblance to the original. In a recent "How America Eats" survey, *Bon Appetit* magazine reported that soy sauce enjoys a 64 percent approval rating, lagging behind only Dijon mustard at 79 percent and salsa at 75 percent. [65]

Traditional Japanese soy sauce or *shoyu* is a brown liquid made from soybeans that have undergone a long fermenting process. It's made by adding spores from an *Aspergillus* mold to a mixture of roasted soybeans and roasted, cracked wheat. The culture is grown for three days, then mixed with salt water and brewed in non-temperature controlled fermentation tanks for six to eighteen months. It took the Japanese 600 years to develop this distinct, high-quality product from the juices left over from miso manufacture.[66,67]

A similar product made only with soybeans (without the wheat) is known as *tamari.* In America *tamari* has become an all-purpose term that refers to any natural soy sauce. This inaccuracy came from the macrobiotic leader George Ohsawa, who used the word *tamari* when *shoyu* proved too difficult for westerners to pronounce or spell.

The Japanese also make a product named *shiro* using a very high ratio of wheat, fermented under conditions designed to prevent color development. It is very light yellow to tan and has a lower amino acid content.[68]

Genuine Chinese soy sauce has a stronger and saltier flavor, tends to be a homemade product, and is rarely sold in the west.[69]

When William Morse of the USDA visited Japan on his expeditions to Asia between 1928-1932, he reported that soy sauce was manufactured on a large scale and universally used by the Japanese, rich and poor. At one operation he counted 90 large vats where the mash was allowed to cure for 18 months.[70]

After World War II, American forces occupying Japan donated surplus American soybeans—but only to manufacturers who abandoned old-fashioned traditional processes in favor of newfangled, chemical hydrolysis methods using hydrochloric acid. This so disturbed traditional *shoyu* makers that Kikkoman set out to find a process that would be faster and acceptable to the Americans but would not entirely abandon Japanese tradition. In 1948, the company came up with a new method that involved the fermentation of hydrolyzed vegetable protein. The combination of speed, economy and taste so impressed American officials that Kikkoman won its full allotment of soybeans. Traditional Japanese *shoyu* producers were apparently less impressed for they reinstituted their traditional time-intensive methods soon after the occupiers went home.[71] In America, however, major soy sauce producers moved ahead with ever more automation, chemicals, preservatives, pasteurization, artificial colorings, sweeteners and flavor enhancers such as MSG.

SOYLD SAUCE

The soy sauce-like products most commonly sold in American supermarkets and used at Chinese restaurants are commonly made in two days or less. Soybean meal and often corn startches are rapidly reduced to their component amino acids using a high-tech process known as "rapid hydrolysis" or "acid hydrolysis," which involves heating defatted soy proteins with 18 percent hydrochloric acid for 8 to 12 hours, then neutralizing the brew with sodium carbonate. The result is a dark brown liquid—a chemical soy sauce. When mixed with some genuine fermented soy sauce to improve its flavor and odor, it is called a "semi-chemical" soy sauce. Sugars, caramel colorings and other flavorings are added before further refinement, pasteurization and bottling.[72-74]

The rapid hydrolysis method uses the enzyme glutamase as a reactor. This creates large amounts of an unnatural form of glutamic acid that is found in MSG. In contrast, production of genuine old - fashioned soy sauce uses the enzyme glutaminase to form glutamic acid, which imparts a delicious taste.[75] Other undesirables also appear during chemical hydrolysis —levulinic and formic acids, instead of beneficial lactic acid, and gas producers dimethyl sulfide, hydrogen sulfide and furfurol from the amino acid methionine. The hydrolysis process results in total destruction of the essential amino acid tryptophan.[76]

Modern soy sauces may also contain dangerous levels of chemicals known as chloropropanols, which are produced when soy sauce production is speeded up using acid hydrolyation methods. In Great Britain, nearly 25 percent of commercial soy sauces were found to contain dangerous levels of these chemicals, and products were recalled in 2001. New Zealand supermarket chains also withdrew soy sauces from their stores. No recalls occurred in America, but because most modern companies use some form of this method and exercise less-than-perfect quality control, the safety of commercial soy sauces cannot be assured.[77-79]

Researchers have also found furanones in soy sauce. These are mutagenic to bacteria and cause DNA damage in lab tests.[80-81] Salsolinol, a neurotoxin linked to DNA damage and chromosomal aberrations, Parkinson's disease and cancer, has been identified in soy sauce.[82] Ethyl carbamate—also linked to cancer—is found in commercial samples of soy sauce, miso and some alcoholic beverages. The maximum concentrations observed were 73 mcg per kg in soy sauce compared to the tiny amount of 7.9 mcg per kg found in miso.[83]

Soy sauce also contains a high content of the amino acid tyramine, a potent precursor of mutagens produced by nitrites.[84-91] The tyramine content makes this product unsuitable for people taking monoamine oxidase inhibitor (MAOI) drugs, which are commonly prescribed for depression, migraines and high blood pressure.[92,93] The best known tyramine-rich foods are aged cheeses, red wines, smoked and pickled herring and beer. Eating any of them—including tyramine-rich soy sauce—while taking MAOI drugs can bring on an episode of high blood pressure accompanied by severe headache, palpitations and nausea.

Recently, the Chinese Ministry of Health approved the fortification of soy sauce with iron to help prevent and treat iron-deficiency anemia, a problem affecting 12.3 percent of urban and 26.7 percent of rural Chinese schoolchildren and as much as 35 percent of women of childbearing age.[94] This special soy sauce will treat iron deficiencies caused, in part, by soy foods in the diets of the poor. Beans and grains contain high levels of phytates that cause iron and other mineral deficiencies (see Chapter 17).

NO BRAGGING RIGHTS

Bragg's Amino Acids—an unfermented liquid soy product invented by health food pioneer Paul Bragg—is a soy sauce alternative preferred by many health aficionados. Its main claim to fame has been a lower sodium content than *tamari* or *shoyu*. Lower sodium does mean low, however, and the company was warned in 1996 by the FDA that its "no salt" label was misleading and that the "healthy" claim was unwarranted given those high sodium levels. The company was also told to cease and desist using its "No MSG" claim. As a "hydrolyzed protein," Bragg's contains free glutamic acid, better known as MSG, and aspartic acid, two well-known neurotoxins.

SOURCE: Letter from Elaine Messa, Director of the FDA's District Office, Irvine, CA, to Patricia Bragg, President, Live Food Products, May 29, 1996. See Chapter 11 for a discussion of the dangers of hydrolyzed proteins.

MY SOY STORY: WIPED OUT

I am very sensitive to MSG so I always avoid foods that have it on the label. Since I avoid red meat, I am concerned about getting enough protein. One day I bought some Bragg's Amino Acids and added it to some soup that I had made—the label said "No MSG" so I thought it would be OK. Within an hour of eating the bowl of soup I had a full-blown MSG reaction—face red and swollen, heart pounding, and feeling irritated and angry at everything. I did not sleep at all that night. I was completely wiped out.

I have since learned that the hydrolyzed protein in foods like Bragg's Amino Acids always contains free glutamic acid, or MSG. Sometime later Bragg's stopped putting "No MSG" on their labels. Wish I had known at the time.

L.P., Winchester, VA

6
NOT MILK AND UNCHEESE
the udder alternatives

oy drink—popularly known as soy milk—is a lactose-free dairy substitute that is made from soybeans that have been soaked, ground, cooked and strained.

SOY BEVERAGES
LAND OF MILK AND MONEY

The food industry is now aggressively marketing soy beverages with everything short of a soy mustache campaign, selling them in gable-top cartons right next to dairy products in the refrigerated sections of grocery stores. Sales of soy milks came to nearly $600 million in 2001 and are projected to reach $1 billion by 2005.[1]

Soy milk drinkers might be startled to learn that the Chinese did not traditionally value soy milk. Soy milk was nothing more than a step in the tofu-making process. The earliest reference to soy milk as a beverage appears in 1866,[2] and by the 1920s and 1930s, soy milk was popular as an occasional drink served to the elderly and often mixed with shrimp or egg yolk.[3-5] Harry Miller, an American-born Seventh Day Adventist physician and missionary, nicknamed the "Albert Schweitzer of China," is credited with building fifteen hospitals and inventing a commercially feasible method to manufacture soy milk in China.[6-8]

It is Dr. Miller who first informs us that soy milk was not traditional in Japan. In a 1959 article for *Soybean Digest* entitled "Why Japan Needs Soy Milk," he described seven months spent as a surgeon and physician at the Tokyo Sanitarium and Hospital and how his idea of a soybean beverage and milk made from the soybean used for soups was something "altogether new." After setting up a pilot plant to make soy milk, soy cream, soy ice cream and a soy spread, he came up with the idea "of such additions to be made to the tofu plants."[9] Despite Dr. Miller's efforts, the Japanese found the flavor and odor of soymilk undesirable, and soymilk consumption did not pick up until the late 1970s when the soy industry began advertising soy milk as a "healthful, 'pick-me-up' energy drink for stressed workers and business people."[10]

Dr. Miller and his son Willis established the first soy dairy in Shanghai in 1939, but never had a chance to find out how it would succeed. Within months Japan invaded China, bombed the factory and sent the Millers packing to Mt. Vernon, Ohio, where they undertook the conversion of Americans to the virtues of soy milk.[10] Later in life, Dr. Miller continued his work in China, Taiwan and India. His medical practice included a specialty in goiter surgery,[11] an interesting choice given our current knowledge about soy's damaging effects on the thyroid gland (see Chapter 27).

It is a surprising fact that the very first soy dairy was not even founded in Asia, but northwest of Paris in 1910 by Li Yu-Ying, a Chinese citizen, biologist and engineer.[12]

SOY DRINK: MILKING THE BEAN

The old-fashioned soy milk-making process begins with a long, relaxing soak. The softened beans are then ground on a stone grinder, using massive amounts of water. The mush goes into a cloth bag, is placed under a heavy rock, and pressed and squeezed until most of the liquid runs out. The soy paste is then boiled in fresh water. Large amounts of filthy scum rise to the surface and are carefully removed.[13,14]

The modern method is faster and cheaper—and some manufacturers retain the scum.[15] Modern methods also speed up the presoaking phase with the use of an alkaline solution, skip the squeezing and skimming steps, use common tap water, and cook the soy paste in a pressure cooker. The speed comes at a cost: the high pH of the soaking solution followed by pressure cooking destroys key nutrients, including vitamins and the sulfur-containing amino acids. This processing combination also decreases the quality of the amino

UNSAFE AT ANY SPEED

Homemade soy milk would appear to be fresher, cleaner and safer than readymade packaged brews. But it's "buyer beware" when it comes to some of the speedy new machines on the market. Robert Cohen—the "Not Milk Man" who has assertively publicized the health dangers of commercial dairy products—recently put a soy milk machine known as the SoyToy on the market. Ignoring centuries of accrued wisdom, Cohen boasts that his machine makes soymilk in only 25 minutes and does not require presoaked beans. Soymilk that has not been properly soaked, skimmed and cooked at length is "all natural" all right, and guaranteed to deliver a full load of the soybean's antinutrients. For most "not milk" drinkers, that could mean digestive distress, gas and mineral malabsorption.

SOURCE: Make soymilk with SoyToy – new machine, unique process. Business Wire via NewsEdge Corporation. www.soyatech.com. Posted 6/17/2002. Detailed information about the antinutrients in soy and the importance of deactivating them through proper processing is provided in Chapters 15-20.

acid lysine and may produce a toxin, lysinoalanine.[16] Although levels of lysinoalanine in soy milk are low, there are valid safety concerns (see Chapter 11).

Taste is what most concerns the soy industry. As Peter Golbitz, President of Soyatech in Bar Harbor, Maine, puts it, "The challenge for the soy industry has been identifying and inactivating the components primarily responsible for the undesirable beany flavor, aroma and aftertaste in soymilk."[17] The guilty party in this case is the enzyme lipoxygenase, which oxidizes the polyunsaturated fatty acids in soy, causing the "beaniness" and rancidity. The industry's attempted solutions have been high heat, pressure cooking and replacement of the traditional presoaking with a fast blanch in an alkaline solution of sodium bicarbonate (baking soda). Major manufacturers have even "offed" the off flavors using a deodorizing process similar to that used in oil refining, one that involves subjecting cooked soymilk to extremely high temperatures in the presence of a strong vacuum.[18]

To cover up any "beaniness" that remains, processors pull out the sweeteners and flavorings. Almost all commercially sold soymilks contain barley malt, brown rice syrup, raw cane crystals or some other form of sugar. The higher the sugar, the higher the acceptability among consumers. Although many consumers believe that flavors such as "plain" or "original" have no sugar added, they are almost always sweetened. Even so, a panel of professional "sensory analysts" at the Arthur D. Little Company evaluated the taste, color, viscosity, balance, fullness, bitterness and aftertaste of all the leading soy beverages and found them wanting. The company helps the processed food industry "translate the voice of the consumer into product specifications."[19] The panel's verdict on soy milk was that it does not currently meet consumer standards for flavor quality and flavor consistency, and will not capture the mass market until vast improvements are made.

The worst problems were: the darker, dirty-looking color of some brands of soy milk (compared to the white of dairy milk); chalky "mouth feel;" musty or burnt protein odors; and beany and bitter aftertastes. None of the soymilks evaluated came close to matching the flavor quality of dairy milk, although vanilla-flavored soymilks fared best. While consumers perceive refrigerated soy products as fresher and better, these products did not score any higher than the shelf-stable versions in the taste tests.[20-23]

Eliminating the aftertaste is a particularly challenging task. The undesirable sour, bitter and astringent characteristics come from oxidized phospholipids (rancid lecithin), oxidized fatty acids (rancid soy oil), the antinutrients called saponins, and the soy estrogens known as isoflavones. The last are so bitter and astringent that they produce dry mouth.[24,25] This has put the soy industry into a quandary. The only way it can make its soy milk please consumers is to remove some of the very toxins that it has assiduously promoted as beneficial for preventing cancer and lowering cholesterol. The opportunity to profit from selling both the soy milk *and* bottles of isoflavone supplements will surely prevail.

WILLY WONKA'S SOYMILK FACTORY

How much sugar is needed to sweeten an eight-ounce serving of soymilk? Anywhere from 4 to 16 grams (slightly less than 1 teaspoon to slightly more than 1 tablespoon). The Center for Food Reformulation at TIAX, a collaborative product and technology development firm based in Cambridge, MA, recently compared 64 soymilks on the market and concluded that the most common way food processors meet "consumer flavor expectations is to add sugar."

SOURCE: Soymilk industry still struggling to satisfy consumer taste: study by TIAX's Center for Food Reformulation shows sugar levels in soymilk on the rise. August 13, 2003. www.thesoydaily.com.

FORTIFICATION

Most soymilks are also fortified with calcium, vitamin D and other vitamins and minerals inadequately represented in soybeans, and stabilized with emulsifiers. This has been true at least since 1931 when a Seventh Day Adventist company fortified soy milk with calcium.[26]

MY SOY STORY: RETHINKING MY RECOMMENDATION

I have experienced first-hand problems with soy milk. For many years I was one of the strong supporters of drinking soy milk. A few years ago, I was diagnosed with an endometrioma (a form of cyst) of the right ovary. It was at this time that I became aware of unpleasant side effects each time I ingested soy milk. I would experience symptoms of tiredness, irritability, abdominal bloating, flatulence and extremely tender breasts. I also noted excess fluid retention.

I have tried several times since having the endometrioma removed to drink soy milk. On each occasion the above symptoms returned. I have also recently been diagnosed with a multi-nodular goiter of the thyroid gland. The right side is the worst, containing several nodules (same side as the endometrioma).

As a natural health practitioner, it has been necessary for me to rethink my recommendation of soy milk, particularly as I specialize in infertility and cannot afford to interfere with my patients' hormone health. It has also been brought to my attention from one 33-year-old male patient who after many years of using soy milk ceased having it to find that his energy levels increased and his rather poor libido improved almost instantly and has not changed in the last six months.   R.K., Akron, Ohio

Even in health-food store soy foods, these added supplements are cheap, mass-produced products. The soy milk industry puts vitamin D_2 in soymilk, even though the dairy industry quietly stopped adding this form of the vitamin years ago. While any form of vitamin D helps people meet their RDAs (Recommended Daily Allowances), D_2 has been linked to hyperactivity, coronary heart disease and allergic reactions.[27]

Low fat—or "lite" soymilks—are made with soy protein isolate (SPI), not the full-fat soybean. To improve both color and texture, manufacturers work with a whole palette of additives. Several years ago, titanium oxide, a form of white paint, was popular. Those who did not shake the containers thoroughly often found watery soymilk with lumps of white glop at the bottom. The soy industry has now moved on to less palette-able, more palatable solutions to the color-texture problem. Because soymilk made with SPI needs at least some oil to provide creaminess, canola oil—not soy oil—is often added. The soy industry knows that its own oil is not perceived as healthy.

YOGURTS, PUDDINGS AND COTTAGE CHEESES

Soy milk-derived products such as soy puddings, ice creams, yogurts, cottage cheese and whipped creams are entering the mainstream but they still earn poor reviews from taste testers. In 2003, *Time* magazine wrote "The soy-based yogurts we tried. . . were chalky, gritty and sour, with a chemical aftertaste. You might go for them, but a typical reaction from one of our testers was 'awful.'"[28] Most soy milk-derived products contain a thickener derived from a red seaweed known as carrageenan. This water-soluble polymer or gum often serves as a fat substitute. For years food scientists assumed it to be safe, but recent studies show that carrageenan can cause ulcerations and malignancies in the gastrointestinal tract of animals.[29]

CHEDDAR AND JACK: WHO SOYLD MY CHEESE?

Soymilk is the starting point for the making of the soy cheeses for pizza, Mexican food, and pasta. Soy cheeses can be artificially flavored to resemble American cheese, mozzarella, cheddar, Monterey jack and Parmesan, and they're increasingly used by fast food operations such as Pizza Hut.

Most soy cheeses are made with some casein, a cow's milk protein that helps make the ersatz product taste more like "real" cheese. Without it, soy cheeses that are heated will soften, but not melt and stretch. The taste and texture of totally vegan soy cheese products incur the wrath of both professional reviewers and members of the public, who have described these imitation cheeses as "barely edible," "yukky," "disgusting," "plastic," "rubbery," and "smelling like old, stinky socks."[30] Even the Center for Science in the Public Interest, an organization that says it wants to recommend vegan cheeses to its constituents, criticized the soy versions of Swiss, cheddar and jack cheese for being "barely distinguishable from each other" and said "none came close to even a decent store brand of cheddar, never mind havarti or Jarlsberg."[31]

Although often promoted as "healthful" with the phrase "no cholesterol," many brands of soy cheeses contain dangerous partially hydrogenated fats—with the highest levels in the brands that taste the best. The main ingredient of Tofutti brand soy cheese, for example, is water, followed by partially hydrogenated soybean oil. Citizens for Science in the Public Interest found that "each 2/3 ounce slice contains 2 grams of artery-clogging *trans* fats."[32]

SOY HEALTHY:
WHAT IS THIS FOOD?

Water, sugar, corn oil, soy proteins, tofu, pecans, high fructose corn syrup, brown sugar, mod food starch, veg mono and diglycerides, cocoa butter, guar, locust bean and cellulose gums, carrageenan, nat. flavors, salt, caramel and annatto colors.

Answer: Tofutti non-dairy frozen dessert. Flavor: Better Pecan.

Recently Kraft Foods patented a method for preparing "natural" cheeses containing 30 percent soy protein. The new method uses enzymes to turn soybeans into soy protein hydrolyzates, basic amino acids that food chemists can fully integrate into the structure of casein. This complex is then added to milk, which is clotted with rennet to form curds and whey. Conventional cheese-making techniques turn the curds into cheese. Without the initial enzyme treatment, the soy would interfere with milk clotting and prevent the formation of a proper curd.[33] Regarding the possible dangers of hydrolyzates (see Chapter 11), the company is mum.

SOY ICE CREAM: THE BIG FREEZE

Soy ice creams have fared slightly better than soy cheeses. Indeed, Peter Golbitz of Soyatech credits Tofutti, the first commercially successful soy ice cream substitute, as having "proved to Americans that a soybean-based food product could actually taste good."[34] Calling the product "Tofutti," however, is a bit of a stretch. Indeed in the 1980s, muckraking reporters exposed the product as containing no tofu whatsoever. Today the first three ingredients in the different flavors of Tofutti are water, white sugar and corn oil, followed by soy protein isolate and sometimes tofu. Brown sugar and high fructose corn syrup make up most of the rest. The long list of ingredients is printed with abbreviated wording in tiny, hard-to-read type around the edge of the top of the carton. Newer brands of soy ice cream such as Soy Dream and Imagine contain fewer ingredients; they consist mainly of water, some form of sugar, soy and more sugar.

YUBA: IT'S A WRAP

A soymilk derivative rarely found in American markets is *yuba*, a traditional Japanese product made by boiling soymilk and lifting off the skin that forms on the surface. Dried into sheets and flakes, *yuba* is used as wrappers for rice or vegetables, or deep fried to make soy chips for snacking. The product is expensive because it is so labor intensive.[35-37]

American companies are developing instead an edible, biodegradable wrap made from soy proteins that can be coated onto the food products or used in place of plastic wrap. Plans are for these soy films to be impregnated with antimicrobial agents, and applied to foods either by wrapping them or spraying them with a liquid that dries into a coating. The industry expects that consumers will appreciate the convenience of well-wrapped foods that have nothing to remove and nothing to throw away.[38]

TOFU: ON THE BLOCK

Tofu is famous for its bland, self-effacing personality. Tofu absorbs other spices and flavors readily and comes in so many different textures that it can be easily cut, crumbled or creamed. It's the perfect food for people who think they want to eat soy, but prefer not to know it's there. Many of the tofu cookbooks on the market play to the public's essential dislike of tofu with titles like *This Can't Be Tofu!*[39]

Tofu is more digestible than other soybean products. Most of soy's unwanted components—including the infamous flatulence-producing oligosaccharides—concentrate in the soaking liquid rather than in the curd so they are reduced in quantity, but not completely eliminated. Those who don't eat too much rarely experience major gas problems unless they have soy allergy or food sensitivity (see Chapters 15 and 24).

Tofu is made by adding a curdling agent to soymilk, which then separates into curds and whey. The curds can be eaten in the fresh, soft and soupy state but they are usually pressed and firmed into the cakes and sold as tofu. The final product sold in American stores is almost never fermented, aged or ripened, so it is not accurate to refer to tofu as "soybean cheese." That's another product altogether, as discussed above.

In China, the traditional curdling agent is gypsum, a rock primarily composed of calcium sulfite, better known as Plaster of Paris. The Japanese prefer an agent taken from sea salt that they call *nigari*, which is primarily composed of magnesium chloride, better known as Epsom Salts. The choice of a curdling salt determines whether the tofu will be high in calcium or magnesium. Soybeans are not good sources of either mineral.[40,41]

To make the delicately textured form of tofu known as "silken tofu," a thick soymilk or soy yogurt is poured directly into a package along with calcium sulfate or glucono-delta-lactone. The sealed package is then heated to cause coagulation and shipped directly to the stores. Silken tofu is preferred by the Japanese. Smooth and delicate like custard, it still contains the whey. Consequently, it has more vitamins than regular tofu but also more of the unwanted antinutrients.[42,43]

Tofu is easily prepared from whole soybeans at home or in small shops. Although several American tofu chefs and cooks at The Farm (a vegan community in Summertown, Tennessee) have invented faster methods of making tofu from readymade soy flour, their methods produce a less digestible product that is higher in antinutrients. But the main reason most manufacturers still begin with well-soaked whole beans is that it's more economical.[44]

Many tofu products sold are pasteurized (which adds 30 to 60 days to the shelf life of refrigerated tofu) or aseptically packaged (which makes it possible to store them for a year or more at room temperature). Cases of microbial contamination have been reported, particularly for tofus sold in produce sections rather than out of refrigerated cases.[45]

Although tofu sales grew from $95 million in 1990 to $130 million in 1996, companies complain that tofu sales have come on "hard times" during the last few years. Apparently, consumers are rejecting it in favor of easy-to-prepare, ready-to-eat and low-fat soy meat alternatives.[46] As a result, several tofu companies have started targeting their products for particular uses, labeling them "soft for blending," "medium for mixing" or "super firm for dicing." Tofu 2 Go products are precooked and come packaged with dipping sauces for ready-to-eat lunches. Several brands also come preflavored with barbecued, curried or other seasonings. Sweeteners, MSG and natural or artificial flavorings may be present. Tofu's relatively high fat content has also led the soy industry to develop low-fat or "lite" versions of tofu.

The tofu eaten in many rural areas of China differs substantially from the familiar Japanese and American versions. In the *National Geographic* film *Faces of Asia: A Tale of Tofu*,[47] Chinese villagers are shown collecting the soymilk they have just made and then pouring it into a cauldron and boiling it for at least six more hours. According to the film's narrator, the tofu masters go to all this trouble to get rid of the "poisons" in the bean. The Chinese then curdle this milk and consume some of the curds within 24 hours. The rest is fermented for at least three months, a process that not only preserves the tofu—without refrigeration, drying or aseptic packaging— but turns it into a nutritionally dense product similar to miso, tempeh and other "good old soys."

Fermented tofu cubes—covered with white or yellowish white fungus mycelia—have a firm texture, salty taste and distinct flavor. They are consumed as an appetizer or relish by the Chinese people. In Japan, a tofu fermented in miso has a cheese-like taste and is called *sofu*.[48,49]

DOWN TO THE DREGS: OKARA

Traditionally, okara was a byproduct of the soymilk and tofu-making processes. Today it is more likely to come from soy protein isolate manufacture. It's the leftover soybean pulp—the husk, the dregs, the grinds. It looks like moist sawdust, consists of little more than fiber, has an exceptional water-absorbing capacity and is mostly indigestible. The Japanese call it "tofu's head," to distinguish it from the curd, which is known as "tofu's brain." Comprised of the carbohydrate chains found in the outer bran layers of whole grains, okara is a high fiber product that can help move the bowels.[50,51]

Okara absorbs flavors well, has a somewhat "nutty" flavor, and is used in some vegetarian burgers and soy sausages sold in frozen

OVERSEAS PROPHETS

Not content with their profits in America, where soymilk is experiencing double-digit growth, soy promoters have turned their attention to the continent of India, a nation that holds the cow sacred and that has depended on milk products for its animal protein and fat for thousands of years. Ignoring the wisdom of classic Ayurvedic medicine, medical leaders in India have started warning Indians about the dangers of milk, claiming that 50 to 90 percent of Indians are lactose intolerant! "The time to find a healthy alternative to dairy is right now," says Neal Barnard, M.D., president of the Physicians Committee for Responsible Medicine (PCRM) in Washington, DC.

An avid proponent of vegan nutrition, Dr. Barnard warns that cow's milk contains many pesticide residues and that "Parents who unknowingly purchase chemical milk may be poisoning their children." Rather than recommend the obvious solution of fresh, clean milk—the kind that has nourished the Indian people for thousands of years—Dr. Barnard proposes soy. milk as an alternative. He does not mention the fact that soy milk also contains pesticide residues, along with plant estrogens and other toxins.

One Indian doctor who was sold on the concept was the late Professor Dr. S. R. Naik, former head of the Department of Gastroenterology at the Sanjay Gandhi Post Graduate Institute of Medical Sciences. Dr. Naik stated that there was no safe age to begin drinking cow and buffalo milk and that he "would surely welcome soya milk as a superior nutritional and healthy product to replace milk for everyone." Demand for soy milk is so high that Dr. Barnard complains, "We need soya milk, but we can't get it." American soy firms to the rescue!

SOURCE: www.indiaserver.com.

PARENT WARNING:
SOY MILK AND INFANTS

Is soy milk an adequate substitute for infant formula? Health-conscious vegan parents want to know. Here's how the soy industry replied in December 1998 when the following sincere but nearly illiterate question came up on the Question and Answer forum at the INTSOY (International Soybean Program) website.

"We are interested in adequating home made soy milk for infants. Do you have a recepe to know how much fatty acids (oil) and sacarose I have to add to make more adequake for low income families that cannot buy formula and have specific problems that make breast feeding not an option?"

Karl E. Weingartner, Ph.D., passed the buck as follows: "You may want to discuss this matter with your child's pediatrician. The soymilk companies usually add vitamin A and vitamin D. However, soy-containing infant formulas contain many supplemental items including vitamins, minerals, fatty acids and more."

"*May* want to"? Soy milk is so dangerous to infants that commercial manufacturers such as WestSoy and others carry strong warnings on their cartons. Indeed, news headlines about babies severely damaged by soy milk used as a substitute for infant formula sent ripples through the health-food industry in 1990. The first news story involved a severely malnourished five-month old infant who was admitted to Arkansas Children's Hospital, Little Rock suffering from heart failure, rickets, vasculitis and neurological damage. The baby girl had been fed nothing but Soy Moo—a soy drink manufactured by Harvest Foods—since she was three days old. An analysis of Soy Moo by the Arkansas Children's Hospital revealed severe deficiencies in calcium, niacin and vitamins D, E and C. Soon after, the FDA learned of a two-month old girl in California who was taken to a physician because she had failed to gain weight or develop properly. She was suffering from severe malnutrition after receiving EdenSoy exclusively from birth upon the recommendation of a midwife.

On June 13, 1990, Stuart Nightingale, M.D., Assistant Commissioner for Health Affairs at the FDA, issued a warning about such use of soy milks saying they were "grossly lacking in the nutrients needed for infants" and asked all manufacturers, importers and private label distributors to put warning labels on soymilks so they that would not be used as formula substitutes.

SOURCES:
www.uiuc.edu/archives/experts/utilization/1998a/0746.html.

FDA Consumer Magazine, September 1990, DHHS Publication 91-2236.

food sections. It also appears in some breads and baked goods. In Indonesia, it may be inoculated with mold spores, pressed into cakes and incubated for 14 to 48 hours until it becomes bound into a fermented cake. A similar product is made in China, but fermented for 10-15 days then dried in the sun and fried.[52,53]

NOT IN NATURE

Pleasing consumers—and milking more of their dollars—remains the challenge as the soybean industry seeks effective and economical ways to improve the taste, color and texture of milk-like and cheese-like soybean products. Plain, "natural" and traditional Asian products just won't pass muster in the American marketplace, and there is nothing natural about what will actually sell. As Peter Golbitz of Soyatech put it, "Soymilk is one of those unique food products that doesn't exist naturally in nature, such as a fruit, vegetable or cow's milk—it is, and always has been, a processed food. Since there are many options available to processors today in regards to process type, variety of soybean, type of sugar and an array of flavoring and masking additives, product formulators need real guidelines to follow to create winning products."[54] For his "enormous contributions" to the cause, Golbitz won the 2004 Soyfoods Industry Leadership Award.[55]

MY SOY STORY: BONES AT RISK

I am a 56 year-old male, in excellent health. I'm a vegetarian who occasionally eats fish and eggs and I also get a lot of exercise. Several years ago, I began to consume huge quantities of soy and soy products: soy beans, soy meat substitutes, soy milk, the whole thing. This summer I had an extensive series of blood tests and was shocked to find out that my parathyroid hormone (PTH) level was 274.0 (the normal range is 12.0- 72.0). My doctor told me to stop eating soy and to take calcium supplements with vitamin D. I retested several months later and my PTH was back to normal. I can only conclude that all that soy was interfering with my calcium absorption and that my parathyroid glands were telling my body to extract calcium from my bones so that there would be enough calcium in my blood. Also, on these tests my levels of T3 and T4 were on the low end of "normal." It seems frightening that we are exposed to so much pro-soy propaganda. I certainly fell for it. If I hadn't had those blood tests, I'd still be practically living on soy, and I'd be well on my way to developing osteoporosis.　　　　　　　　　　　　J.K., Raleigh, N.C

7
ALL-AMERICAN SOY
first generation
soy products

Soy flour is a basic, low-tech product made from soybeans that have been hulled, cracked, heated and ground. It tastes so beany, goes rancid so easily and performs so poorly that not very much of it can be used in baked goods. Even so, soy flour has enjoyed a few minutes of fame. Memories of soy flour-enriched wartime rations and vegetarian fare at hippie communes die slowly. Indeed soy flour has sunk so much food over the years that public relations flacks have had to work overtime rehabbing its image.[1-3]

SOY FLOUR: NO RISING STAR

Soy flour was rarely eaten in Asia, although it was used as food during the north China famine of 1920 to 1921.[4] In America and Europe in the 1920s, it was "not yet a common commodity," although on record as a food for invalids and diabetics. The United States Department of Agriculture investigated the potential of soy flour at that time and found it could work in bread, muffins, biscuits, crackers, macaroni and pastry, so long as soy flour comprised no more than one-fourth of the total.[5]

Natural, full-fat soy flour is made from the whole soybean, and comes in both raw and toasted versions. Raw soy flour—known to the trade as "enzyme active"—is used as a bleaching agent and crumb color enhancer. The little enzyme that does the trick is lipoxygenase.[6-8] To keep it alive, the flour must remain raw, though raw flour is notoriously indigestible and even unsafe. Medical journals report hospitalizations caused by consumption of raw and incompletely cooked soy flours loaded with antinutrients, the most dangerous of which are the protease inhibitors (see Chapter 16).

Lipoxygenase has another major disadvantage—it gives soy flour its famous "beany" and "bitter" taste. Indeed in 1967 a panel of evaluators could detect raw full-fat soy flours 80 percent of the time even when the flours were diluted as much as 1:750 with wheat flour. Methanol, ethanol and steam treatments improved the flavor scores, but the bad flavors could still be detected.[9]

Toasting the soy flour helps solve the antinutrient problem, but at the expense of damaging the soy oil, which in soy flour turns rancid so easily that buyers are advised to keep it refrigerated or frozen. The term "toasting" is used in the industry to refer to moist cooking with steam, and has nothing to do with what happens with the small kitchen appliance known as a toaster. Because of the rancidity problem—not to mention the profits to be made from the sale of the oil—most soy flours are of the low-fat—or defatted—type. Although stripped of most of their oils through a hexane solvent extraction process, enough remains to contribute to the development of rancid "off flavors." Accordingly, most companies include a deodorizing step as part of the manufacturing process.[10]

The amount of fat in soy flour varies. The usual procedure is to defat soybean flakes and then add back a controlled amount of fat after the flakes have been milled. Defatted flour usually contains less than one percent fat. Low-fat flour may have some oil left in, or, more typically, contain oil added back to provide five to six percent fat. High-fat flour has soy oil added to a specified level, most often

15 percent. Full-fat flours are made from whole soybeans. Finally, there are lecithinated soybean flours containing five to 15 percent lecithin, added to serve the emulsifying needs of the food indus-try.[11,12]

Processors of soy flour rely on heat to deactivate the soybeans' anti-nutritional factors, but heat processing doesn't work all that well. So many of the protease inhibitors (that block protein diges-tion) and the oligosaccharides (that cause flatulence) remain that soy flour has an international reputation as a cause of digestive cramp-ing, bloating and gas.[13-16]

For decades, the soy industry pressed for fortification of flour with soy protein as the solution to world hunger. Breads, after all, are the number one convenience food eaten by the masses. This idea might have taken off had there not been one major obstacle: soy-fortified flours didn't just taste bad, they tasted terrible. Although the United States has donated billions of dollars of food commodi-ties containing soy protein to feeding programs in Third World coun-tries, there have been many occasions when they couldn't even give it away.[17]

Today soy flour is widely used in commercial baked goods. Though billed as a protein booster or cholesterol lowerer, soy flour is actually used to save bakers bundles of money. Many commercial recipes add soy flour as an egg substitute, using a mixture of one tablespoon of soy flour with one tablespoon of water. Soy flour is used even more often as an even cheaper replacement for the al-ready cheap nonfat milk solids.

Bakers frequently choose soy flour for its ability to moisten the final product, helping retain the illusion of freshness.[18] Most commercial breads today contain small amounts of soy flour, even though they are not labeled as soy products.

Even in baked goods marketed as containing soy, soy flour can replace no more than one-fourth to one-third of the total flour in quick breads, cakes and cookies before it adversely affects the taste, color and texture. To slip more soy flour into bread, the industry often relies on chemical leaveners such as sodium stearoyl-2-lactylate (SSL), calcium stearoyl-2-lactylate (CL) or ethoxylated monoglyerides. These help achieve acceptable loaf volume and texture. Because soy flour tends to brown more rapidly than other flours, cooks must lower the temperature or decrease the baking time. When raw "enzyme active" soy flours are used to improve color and dough handling, these low temperatures and short baking times can lead to incompletely cooked soy proteins.[19] This has caused more than the usual digestive distress and the occasional hospitalization.[20,21]

Today soy flour is being phased out in favor of more costly high-tech upstarts—soy protein concentrate and soy protein isolate (see Chapter 8). These offer superior flavor with less bitterness and beaniness, a whiter color, longer shelf life, and fewer side effects in the form of cramping and gas.[22-24]

SOY GRITS: CRACKING UP

Soy grits are whole, dry soybeans that have been lightly toasted and then cracked into little pieces. Full fat or defatted, the only difference between grits and soy flour is the particle size. Like soy flour, most grits easily become rancid and should be refrigerated, frozen or stored in a cool, dry place. Soy grits taste "beany" like whole soybeans, but cook up more quickly—a mere 45 minutes compared to the many hours needed to soften the whole beans. Because such a short cooking time does little to deactivate the soybean's harmful protease inhibitors and other antinutrients, there is every reason to believe that soy grits share the capacity of whole beans and soy flours to cause painful—and even dangerous—cramps, bloating and gas. They are used in baked products, meat substitutes and extenders.[25-28]

SOY NUTS: AIR FARE

Soy fans reach for crisp and crunchy soy nuts with brand names like Peanotz instead of real peanuts or cashews. The nuts, of course, are not nuts at all, but soybeans soaked for three or more hours, then either deep fried or oven roasted until well browned. They are likely to be salted, sugared or even coated with chocolate to cover up the basic bean flavor. The protein level is higher than peanuts.[29]

Roasted soy nuts are not thought of as a traditional food in Asia, but such nuts were widely sold there in confectionary and food shops by the early 20th century. Generally, the nuts were sugar coated and sprinkled with seaweed, making them look like mottled beans. Candied soy nuts that had been boiled in syrup were also sold.[30]

Sugary cover-ups help solve the flavor problem but have no effect on an even worse problem—flatulence.

SOYNUT BUTTER: BETTER SPREAD THINLY

Soy nut butter is ground from roasted soy nuts. It's not much different from peanut butter—*if* you can get past the texture, the aftertaste and the pumped up price. Pure soy nut butter is hard to

---

FRESH AND CONFIDENT:
THE NON-P.U. BEAN

Don't like the flavor and aroma of traditional soy foods? Do we have a bean for you! "Naturally deodorized" and "healthier," the L'STAR hybrid soybean is "only a few harvests a way from reality" and set to "revolutionize the soy market." With it, food manufacturers will be able to eliminate that embarrassing inner bean odor and put greater amounts of soy flour and soy oil into your food products. While less rancid oils are certainly a plus, health-conscious consumers concerned about soy allergens, goitrogens, estrogens, and other antinutrients and toxins might not want to embrace the non-P.U. bean.

SOURCE: Delicious, nutrient-rich, non-GM soybean to be unveiled at upcoming seminar. Posted 9/6/2004 www.soyatech.com.

give away, much less to sell. Accordingly, most products are gussied up with corn syrup, evaporated cane juice, malodextrin, salt, MSG, and other dubious additives, even most brands sold in health food stores. Soy oil and soy protein are added to improve consistency. All warnings about soy nuts apply.

MY SOY STORY: MY GIRLFRIEND ALMOST LEFT ME

I've always been a "meat and potatoes" man but my dad and uncle died of heart attacks and I don't want that to happen to me. Since my cholesterol was a tad high and soy is supposed to lower your cholesterol, I decided to start mixing soy grits into my hamburgers and to snack on energy bars and soy nuts. I did my best to eat this awful food but whenever I did I had bad stomach cramps. I blew up like a balloon and had so much gas my girlfriend almost left me. My breath and body odor weren't too good either. If this stuff is supposed to be so good for you, why did I smell so bad?

R.W., Madison, WI

8
ALL-AMERICAN SOY
second generation
soy products

American ingenuity has created a whole new era in soy foods starring ersatz products—known in the business as "analogues"—with names like Soysage, Not Dogs, Fakin' Bacon, Sham Ham, Soyloin, Veat, Wham, Tuno, Bolono, Foney Baloney, Ice Bean, Hip Whip and Tofurella. Named after—and made to look like—the familiar meat and dairy products they are meant to replace, these products cost so much that soyfoods no longer carry the stigma of "poverty food." This is partly because higher-priced, blander-tasting soy protein concentrates and isolates are replacing bad-tasting but cheap soy flours. The higher prices have led to higher profits because soy suddenly fits the image of an upscale health food.

THE GOOD, THE BAD AND THE UGLY

Not everyone agrees that the fake foods compete with the real thing. And some of them still taste pretty lousy. Staff reporters at *U.S. News and World Reports* reported an informal taste test in which they decried the color and taste of soy pastrami as "vile," likened barbecue-flavored tofu to "overcooked scrambled eggs," and played with a soy hot dog after someone discovered that the rubbery concoction could bounce.[1] Humorist Dave Barry aptly describes a fake burger sold under the name Harvest Burger as "a well-constructed extremely cylindrical frozen unit of brown foodlike substance. The package states that it contains '83 percent less fat than ground beef': I believe this, because it also tastes exactly 83 percent less good than ground beef. Nevertheless, I highly recommend it for anybody who needs more 'soy' or a backup hockey puck."[2] Hard as it is to believe, the soy industry boasts that the taste, smell and appearance of such products *have* improved dramatically over the past few years.

That's primarily due to food technology specialists and their lavish use of sugar and other sweeteners, salt, artificial flavorings, colorings, preservatives and MSG. It also hasn't hurt that newer refining techniques yield blander and purer soy proteins than the "beany," hard-to-cover-up flavors of the past. Cargill even bills its new soy protein isolate as "inconspicuously good."[3] Now that processors have succeeded in eliminating more and more of the troublesome soy fats and carbohydrates, the new soy products are less likely to drive consumers away from the table because of their "off fla-

---

VINTAGE HARVEST BURGER INGREDIENTS: FOODLIKE SUBSTANCE OR HOCKEY PUCK?

Water, SPC (soy protein concentrate), partially hydrogenated vegetable oils, SPI (soy protein isolate), methylcellulose, natural flavors, onion powder, salt, maltodextrin, modified food startch, corn syrup solids, dehydrated Worcestershire sauce, malt extract, beet powder, zinc oxide, niacinamide, ferrous sulfate, copper gluconate, vitamin A palmitate, calcium pantothenate, thiamine mononitrate (vitamin B1), pyridoxine hydrocholoride (vitamin B6), riboflavin (vitamin B2) cyanocobalamin (vitamin B12).

vors" or out the back door after the production of offensive gas.

What food processors call "functionality" has also greatly improved. Soy protein products such as textured soy protein (TSP), soy protein isolate (SPI) and soy protein concentrates (SPC) survive use under heavy processing conditions such as sterilization, freezing, thawing, recooking and microwaving.

INVISIBLE SOY

Soy proteins have been hiding in chopped meat mixes such as preformed hamburger patties, readymade meat loaves, spaghetti sauces and even some brands of fresh ground beef for years. Food companies make money by "extending" ground beef with the addition of cheaper soy protein products such as defatted soy flour, texturized soy protein, soy protein concentrate and/or soy protein isolate. In theory, cost savings are passed on to the consumer. Soy-meat mixes also make economic sense because the soy protein granules soak up water and fats, resulting in less shrinkage during cooking.[4-6]

For years, government regulations protected the public by limiting the amount of soy protein that could be included in meat products. In the 1970s and earlier, the law required that soy protein carry a "tag" of 0.1 percent titanium in the form of titanium dioxide. This was done to ensure that companies couldn't get away with sneaking soy protein isolate into a meat product. More recently antibody assays have been used. This would appear to be fail-proof technology, but researchers report frustration because so many chemical changes occur during the processing of soy protein that the final products cannot always be identified in the laboratory as "soy."[7-9]

Actually, enforcement was not completely necessary because shoppers unilaterally rejected the off taste and gas production of textured soy proteins, toasted flours and grits. Consequently, excessive amounts of soy rarely appeared in products other than those earmarked for institutional use, giveaway programs or disaster relief. Indeed, the old soy-ground beef products gave soy such a bad name that marketing efforts today center on helping consumers forget the horrible-tasting, gas-producing, soy-sodden abuses of the past. While taste *has* improved, the key has been combining better taste with a health claim—and never, ever referring to these "natural" products in public using industry terminology such as "comminuted-cured meat food mixes with texturized soy proteins and plasticizers."

Writers for The Illinois Center for Soy Foods found that in blind taste tests, "Consumers who ate products which mentioned soy on the package described the taste as more grainy, less flavorful, and as having a strong aftertaste compared to those who ate the product but saw no soy label." Combined with a health claim, however, consumers' attitudes improved, although their descriptions of taste often did not.[10]

Today's more popular products are "extended" with the blander, more refined soy protein concentrates (SPC) and soy protein isolate (SPI). These also appear in dairy analogues such as nonfat dry milk replacers, whipped toppings, coffee whiteners, non-dairy ice creams and infant formulas.[11] As a result, more and more Americans are unknowingly eating soy protein hidden in their fast-food burgers, spaghetti sauces, breads, cookies and other processed foods sold in restaurants, supermarkets and other outlets. They appear even more heavily in cheap food served in school lunch programs, nursing homes, hospitals and other institutional settings, as well as in food giveaway programs here and abroad. This has created a nightmare for people allergic to soy who must avoid it completely, and a challenge for those who seek to minimize their intake of soy because of health concerns.

Soy protein is rarely the only additive in these partial meat products. To help hold patties, meat balls and frankfurters together, "plasticizers" such as egg albumen, wheat gluten or—increasingly—functional forms of SPC are added. Taste, appearance and shelf life are enhanced with artificial flavorings, colorings, MSG and preservatives.[12]

Not all products are "analogues" made to imitate meat. Products known as "meat alternatives" are targeted at vegetarians who would prefer not to eat something that looks and tastes like meat, and to vegetarian sympathizers who take pride in the occasional meatless meal.[13]

THE SOY REFORMATION

"Progress" continues with what is known in the industry as "reformed meat technology" or "pumped meats." To create simulated "whole cuts" of meat, poultry or fish, food processors start with pieces of real meat or poultry then mix in—or inject—some form of soy protein along with soy or another vegetable oil, food colorings, salt, phosphates, flavorings and other additives. These are then massaged, shaped and bound into familiar meat-like shapes—such as chicken nuggets. After fabrication, these products may be sliced, ground or dried.[14,15]

Such products sell poorly in supermarkets, but briskly at fast food establishments where customers don't ask nosy questions about what's really in those meaty nuggets and nobody is required to tell them. Clyde Boismenue, a longtime distributor for Archer Daniels Midland said in a 1990 interview that the main problem in the United States was "the obnoxious meat labeling requirement. For example, if isolates are injected into ham, it must be sold as 'smoked pork ham with soy protein isolate product.'" Boismenue blamed this requirement on the USDA being "staffed largely by veterinarians."[16] The November 1969 issue of *Soybean Digest* reviewed the regulatory problems faced by the industry and expressed concern that "new product concepts" would be canceled because of "standard of identity" problems as well as failure to secure prompt government approvals.[17]

TEXTURED SOY PROTEIN: THE EX-TRUDER FILES

TSP is the generic term for textured vegetable protein or TVP, a product patented by Archer Daniels Midland (ADM) and sold as granules, particles and chunks and used by fast-food companies and food processors as a meat substitute or extender. Vegetarians often buy it in the bulk bin section of health food stores and use it in place of ground beef in chili, spaghetti sauce, tacos, sloppy joes and other strongly spiced recipes.

In 1973, *Business Week* indicated that "TVP got its first big boost when the USDA approved its use in the national school lunch program in 1971. By the end of 1972 total demand had grown to about 55 million pounds a year with ground beef as the largest single market."[18]

TSP is produced by forcing defatted soy flour through a machine with a spiral, tapered screw called an extruder. This occurs under conditions of such extreme heat and pressure that the very structure of the soy protein is changed. What comes out is a dried out, fibrous and textured alien protein product that can survive just about anything that a home cook or food processor might later do to it. Red or brown colors and flavorings may be added to the soy protein before texturization, drying and packaging.[19-21]

Soy protein extrusion differs little from extrusion technology used to produce starch-based packing materials, fiber-based industrial products or plastic toy parts, bowls and plates. The difference is that extruded "foods" such as TSP are designed to be reconstituted with water, at which point they resemble ground beef or stew meat. By the time the TSP products appear steaming hot at your dinner table, they've been heated at least three times.

Textured soy protein usually refers to products made from defatted soy flour, though the term may be applied to textured soy protein concentrates and spun soy fiber. Compared to soy flour, TSP has a very long shelf life, provided it is tightly sealed to keep out moisture. The intense heat and pressure of the extrusion process deactivates many of the antinutrients present in soy flour, but alters amino acids and may create other processing toxins (see Chapters 11 and 13). TSP is often flavored to taste like ham, beef or chicken using natural and artificial flavorings and MSG.

eight: second generation soy products

SOY PROTEIN CONCENTRATES: FORM AND FUNCTION

Soy protein concentrate (SPC) comes from defatted soy flakes, consists of 70 percent protein, and retains most of the soybean's fiber. The first 70 percent SPC was manufactured by Mead Johnson Company in the mid-1930s but was discontinued due to lack of markets for the product.[22] Producers don't sell it directly to consumers

---

FOWL PLAY

The Insta-Pro extruder—developed to turn defatted soybean meal into textured vegetable protein and other modern food products—is being used to extrude "secondary resources."

Nabil Said, Ph.D., Director of Research and Development at Insta-Pro, discovered that poultry poop can be cooked, dehydrated and sterilized into a valuable source of protein. Mixed with soy protein, it is then formulated into pet kibble, livestock feed and fish-farm rations. "We're not just an equipment company," said Said. "We're a nutrition company first."

Said was hired to assist Hy-line, an Iowa-based poultry genetics company, when they learned that waste from their hatchery would no longer be welcome at the local landfill. Transformed into tasty animal feed, however, Iowa chicken doody is now welcomed by herds of hungry, local cows. Pig poop, too, tested well, with no cows on record complaining that it was a "bitter swill to swallow." Though the soy industry is most enthusiastic about this inexpensive way to "add value" to soy, mass production has not yet begun, nor have product names and slogans been developed. Truth in advertising suggests "Caca Crispies," with the jingle "Snap, Crapple and Poop."

SOURCES:
Insta-Pro Extruder Provides a Money-Saving Solution, Soya Bluebook Update, April-June 1996.

Phone interview with Dr. Nabil Said, November 5, 2002.

---

in stores, but to food processors churning out meat and dairy analogues. The concentrate is made by precipitating the solids with aqueous acid, aqueous alcohol, moist heat and/or organic solvents. These "immobilize" the protein, which is then removed along with some of the soy carbohydrates and salt residue. Different processing methods favored by different manufacturers affect the quality of the protein, the levels of the antinutrients and toxic residues, solubility, emulsifying ability and texture.[23,24]

Two types of SPC are in general use. Textured soy concentrate—a subtype of textured soy protein (TSP)—is put through an extruder and turned into the familiar flakes, chunks and granules of ersatz meat. "Functional" soy concentrate is used by food processors in the binding phase of production to guarantee firmness, cohesion and juiciness. By combining both of these two very different forms of SPC, food processors have concocted many moist "meaty" products. Though best known for its use as a fake meat, SPC can replace almond paste in marzipan recipes, cream filling in chocolates, and numerous other ingredients.[25]

SOY PROTEIN ISOLATE: NEVER IN ISOLATION

Soy protein isolate (SPI) is mixed with nearly every food prod-

---

REAR GUARD

Back in 1979 the U.S. military dictated precise specifications for purchase of 60 million pounds of ground beef extended with soy protein concentrate at a level of 20 percent. The military approved SPC—even though it is considerably more expensive than soy flour—for two reasons: better taste and lower flatulence potential.

SOURCE: Report of the Working Group. Joint FAO/WHO Food Standards Programme Codex Committee on Vegetable Proteins, Fifth Session, Ottawa, Canada, 6-10 February 1989.

---

uct sold in today's stores—energy bars, muscle-man powders, breakfast shakes, burgers and hot dogs. SPI is also the major ingredient in most of today's soy infant formulas. Consisting of 90 to 92 percent protein, SPI is a highly refined product processed to remove "off flavors," "beany" tastes and flatulence producers and to improve digestibility. Vitamin, mineral and protein quality, however, are sacrificed. Indeed soy isolates increase the requirements for vitamins E, K, D and B_{12}. Among the minerals, phosphorous is poorly utilized, and calcium, magnesium, manganese, molybdenum, copper, iron and especially zinc deficiencies appear in animals fed SPI as the primary source of protein in their diets. Soy protein isolates are also more deficient in sulfur-containing amino acids than other soy protein products.[26-28] What's increased during the production of SPI are levels of toxins and carcinogens such as lysinoalanines and nitrosamines.[29-32] (See Chapter 11.)

The manufacture of SPI has always been a complicated, high-tech procedure. There's nothing natural about it—it takes place in chemical factories, not kitchens. Although the manufacturing process varies and some companies hold patents on key elements of the process, the basic procedure begins with defatted soybean meal, which is mixed with a caustic alkaline solution to remove the fiber, then washed in an acid solution to precipitate out the protein. The protein curds are then dipped into yet another alkaline solution and spray dried at extremely high temperatures.[33-36]

GAG ME WITHOUT A SPOON!

In an episode of *The Simpsons*, Lisa, the vegetarian, goes to a vending machine for a snack and buys a "Soy Joy" energy bar. The wrapper does more than make inflated health claims. It boasts, "Now with gag suppressor!"

SPINNING DOPE

SPI is often spun into protein fibers using technology borrowed from the textile industry. The only difference is that fat, flavor, color and fiber-binding agents are incorporated into the fibers during processing. This process—introduced in 1957—involves preparing a protein solution with a soy protein content of 10 to 50 percent at a very alkaline pH that is above 10. The solution is aged at about 121 degrees F until it becomes as viscous as honey at which point it is called "spinning dope." The dope is next forced through the holes of an extrusion device, coagulated with an acid bath, stretched long

SEAL OF APPROVAL

Soy protein isolate (SPI) appears in so many food products today that consumers would never guess that it was not originally developed for food. In the late 1970s, the Federation of American Society for Experimental Biology (FASEB) concluded that the only safe use for soy protein isolates was as a binder and sealer for cardboard boxes.

Although investigators were concerned about the leaching of the carcinogen nitrosamine and the toxin lysinoalanine from the SPI of the cardboard into the food contents, they decided the amounts would be too low to pose a health hazard. The committee, however, expressed concern about infants exposed to SPI, which the industry was beginning to use in soy infant formulas. The idea that manufacturers would one day purposely put soy protein isolate *into* boxes—and sell it with a health claim no less—would have been inconceivable to the original investigators.

SOURCE: Evaluation of the health aspects of soy protein isolates as food ingredients, 1979. SCOGS-101. Prepared for Bureau of Foods, Food and Drug Administration by the Life Sciences Research Office, FASEB.

and thin, bound with edible binders such as starch, dextrins, gums, albumen and cellulose, and coated with fat, flavor, color and other substances. The idea is to attain the fibrous "bite" of animal muscle meats.[37,38] Spun soy protein fibers are not much different from plastic fibers; both are difficult to digest, have a "scouring effect" on the GI tract and cause marked amounts of flatulence.[39]

For chunkier, less well-defined fibers, processors prefer the textured soy protein (TSP) extrusion process discussed earlier. The synthetic meat business has cooked up many variations on these basic processes and can turn out soy protein in sheets, strings, chunks, granules, and gels. SPI products work well functionally, and so are used heavily by food processors to improve texture, retain moist-

EAT HERE, GET GAS!

Many health experts believe that soy burgers, soy hot dogs, TVP chili and other modern soy products provide high octane fuel. Figures released by the American Oil Chemists' Association prove them right!

SPI (soy protein isolate)—the ingredient that provides the familiar ground meat-like texture in soy lasagna, soy chili and hundreds of other products—contains some 38 petroleum compounds including, but not limited to: butyl, methyl and ethyl esters of fatty acids; phenols, diphenyls and phenyl esters; abietic acid derivatives, diehydroabietinal, hexanal and 2-butyl-2-octenal aldehydes; dehydroabietic acid methyl ester; dehydroabietene and abietatriene.

The American Oil Chemists' Association did not provide data on what kind of mileage soy eaters can expect.

SOURCE: Boatright WL, Crum AD. Nonpolar-volatile lipids from soy protein isolates and hexane defatted flakes. *J Am Oil Chem Soc*, 1997, 74, 461-467.

ness, bind with fat, increase protein levels and reduce shrinkage during cooking. Food processors can also use SPI as a replacement for flour, eggs or milk.[40-42]

HVP/HSP: NO VIP

Hydrolyzed vegetable protein—usually a synonym for hydrolyzed soy protein—is a brown powdery substance used widely by the food industry as a flavoring additive. Consisting of a mixture of amino acids and peptides obtained from soy flour, isolate or concentrate using acid and alkaline solutions and a fast hydrolysis process, HVP is most commonly found in quantity in cheap commercial soy sauce. The food industry also likes to use HVP as a substitute for egg whites for confections.[42] The chemical process that breaks down the soybean's protein structure into free amino acids also releases the excitotoxins glutamate and aspartate (see Chapter 11). Yet HVP or HSP are often included in products labeled with words like "all natural." Because of recent lawsuits, fewer companies dare use the words "No MSG."

AGENT ORANGE

Soy protein shows up in many food products, but who would suspect that manufacturers might add it to orange juice? A document filed with the Patents and Trademarks Office reveals that beverages such as orange juice can be "stably clouded by the suspension of soy protein particles therein. A new procedure is provided to cause such suspension, in which pectin prevents suspended protein particles from aggregating to the point of settling out."

SOURCE: Patent #5286511, Docket #303191, Serial #7965308, Date patented 2/15/94. www.ars.usda.gov/research/patents/patents.htm?serialnum=07965308.

9
FAT OF THE LAND
soy oil and margarine

Most of the vegetable oils sold in supermarkets are either 100 percent soy oil or a blend of soy oil with corn, cottonseed and other cheap oils. There's nothing natural about them.

Soybeans don't willingly or easily give up their oil. The only economical way to obtain it is to use a complicated high-tech process that includes grinding, crushing and extracting, using high temperature, intense pressure and chemical solvents such as hexane. During these processes, the oil is exposed to light, heat and oxygen, all of which damage the oil by creating free radicals. The resulting rancidity affects taste and smell, giving rise to off flavors, variously described as "green," "grassy," "beany," "fishy," "painty" or just plain "bitter."[1-5]

Because consumers turn their noses up at rancid oils, processing companies have learned to remove or cover up the "off" tastes and odors with very high-temperature refining, deodorizing and light hydrogenation. Heavily treated in this way, soy oil becomes bland

enough to appeal to the American public. By 1962, soy oil had captured more than 50 percent of the U.S. cooking and salad oil market.[6]

Even so, most of the world's soy oil never gets poured into a
vegetable oil bottle. Instead, it undergoes a process known as hydrogenation, which turns polyunsaturated oils that are liquid at room
temperature into fats that are solid at room temperature. The soy oil
is thus made over into a bland, odor-free solid fat that is dyed pale
yellow if it is to be sold as margarine or bleached virginal white if it
is intended as shortening. Neither refined soy oil nor hydrogenated
soy oil products were ever eaten as part of traditional diets in China,
Japan or other countries in Asia. They are modern, western, indus-
trial-era food products.

SOY OIL IN CHINA: A BURNING PROPOSITION

Soy oil production began hundreds of years ago in China when
people extracted a crude, dark-colored, unpleasant smelling oil from
the soybean using a crush stone mill or wedge press. Unlike today's
gigantic soybean crushing operations, oil pressing was a small cottage industry run by peasants in the village or supervised by eu-
nuchs in the palaces. In the old days, soy oil was burned like kero-
sene in lamps with wicks, and also used to make soap, caulk boats,
grease axles and otherwise lubricate machinery.[7,8] The nitrogen-rich
soy meal left over from the extraction process was used as a fertilizer, never as a feed for people and rarely for animals.[9]

In the 1860s, large scale soybean-crushing operations began in
the northern province of Manchuria. After the Sino-Japanese War of
1894-1895, the Manchurians began shipping crude soy oil and meal
to Japan, the United States, Europe and other parts of the world.
This business collapsed in the late 1920s when importers realized it
would be more economical to grow or import the soybeans and to
process them locally using the more efficient, modern solvent extraction systems.[10]

The Chinese have never preferred soy oil for cooking. The traditional favorite is lard (pig fat), followed by sesame oil produced by street vendors using stone grinders. Today, peanut and rapeseed oil are favorites. Soy oil is almost never chosen for cooking in southern China but is sometimes used in the northeast provinces, although some reports indicate that even turnip-seed oil is preferred. European visitors in the 19th and early 20th centuries reported the use of soy oil, but mention of it is conspicuously missing from earlier encyclopedias and historical accounts.[11,12]

In 1911 a Customs official named Shaw wrote: "The oil is used, as a substitute for lard, in cooking. Although it is inferior to rapeseed and sesamum oils for this purpose, these oils cannot compete with it in point of price. . . in spite of its unpleasant characteristic odour and unpalatability, the poorer classes in China consume it in its crude state, but among the rich it is boiled and allowed to stand until it has become clarified."[13]

Traditionally, soy oil seems to have been utilized for its pharmaceutical rather than its nutritional properties. Ancient Chinese medical texts referred to soy oil, variously, as "acrid, sweet, heating, mildly toxic and slightly deleterious" and recommended it for poultices on ulcers, wounds, skin irritations and bald heads.[14]

Up until the post-World War II period, all soy oil in China was a crude soy oil extracted by mechanical pressing. Today refined soy oil is gaining popularity in China, Japan, Korea and other countries along with other highly processed western foods. Ironically, western companies are marketing a refined form of soy oil there that was never used traditionally in Asia while promoting a crude "natural" soy oil similar to that burned in oil lamps back home to the health-conscious American consumer.

NATURAL SOY OIL: OUT IN THE COLD

"Natural" soy oil is a light brown or yellow-brown, marked by a strong odor and flavor and some laxative properties. In the U.S., this product is generally labeled "cold pressed," a term that Hain, a manufacturer of foods for health food stores, introduced into health food store labeling in the early 1950s and which was appropriated by other major sellers of "natural" oils.[15] The term "cold pressed" is deceptive because oil easily reaches a heat of 160 degrees F even during mechanical pressing. This is less than the heat of solvent extraction, but if the "cold pressed" oil is deodorized during refining, it may reach temperatures as high as 440 degrees F. On a positive note, the product does not contain petroleum residues, chemical additives or the *trans* fatty acids found in refined soy oils (because "light" hydrogenation improves stability under high temperature cooking). However, unrefined "natural" soy oil smokes at low temperatures and goes rancid quickly, making its bad taste and odor even worse. Not surprisingly, consumers have given natural soy oil the cold shoulder, and it enjoys only a minuscule share of the vegetable oil market.

MARKET SATURATION: MARGARINE AND SHORTENING

Many people don't realize that they consume soy oil. In 1978, the American Soybean Association learned that while soy oil accounted for nearly 84 percent of all edible vegetable oils and 58.3 percent of all oils and fats in the U.S., most customers were ignorant of the fact that they were buying and eating soy.[16] In most cases, refined soy oils are still identified either as "vegetable oil" or by brand names such as "Wesson Oil." Although calling an oil "vegetable oil" gives the manufacturer freedom to throw in whatever vegetable oil happens to be cheap and available, companies also know that older Americans have long memories of gagging on the beany, smelly and greasy soy oils of the past.

Soy oils also go incognito because most are processed by hydrogenation into products known as margarine or shortening. Many people consume some soy oil in the form of margarine at the dinner table, but far more in the form of the shortening used by fast-food outlets and food manufacturers who make French fries, baked goods and other processed and packaged, readymade foods. Soy oil margarines and shortenings have been widely consumed since the 1950s and have dominated the market since the 1960s in countries such as the United States and Northern Europe that traditionally used solid fats. Most of these people would prefer butter but buy the substitutes because of the cheaper price. In India, a shortening known as *vanaspati* is sold as a substitute for the clarified butter known as *ghee*. *Vanaspati* is often made with soy oil.

MARGARINE

The first margarines came out in the 1860s. In the early days, they were butter substitutes made from animal fats (such as lard or tallow) or saturated vegetable oils (such as coconut or palm oil). Today 90 percent of margarines are made from soy oil. Today's "regular" stick margarines are usually 80 percent hydrogenated soy, corn or cottonseed oils, with most of the remainder comprised of milk solids. Other likely ingredients are soy protein, colorings, flavorings and preservatives.

Kraft came out with the first commercially successful soft margarine in 1952. Soft or tub margarines contain greater amounts of unhydrogenated or "lightly hydrogenated" liquid vegetable oils. Whipped versions are "whipped up" with nitrogen gas so that the product contains more air. These contain *trans* fats, but fewer than the stick margarines. The remainder of the margarine market is taken up by various "spreads," liquid margarines in squeezable bottles and diet "imitation" margarines, which are "low calorie" imitations of a product that is itself an imitation. Premium brands may contain some butter and in Europe there is a popular product called Half Butter.[17-19]

SHORTENING

Shortenings are solid fats used for baking, frying and creaming. The word "shortening" derives from the old-fashioned definition of "shorten," which means to add fat to pastry dough to make it tender and flaky. Until the 1930s, shortening referred to butter or lard when used by bakers. Now it refers to vegetable shortenings made with partially hydrogenated vegetable oils such as soy, cotton-seed or canola oil. Unlike margarine, shortenings are all fat. The best known brand is Crisco, a product named after its main ingredient, crystallized cotton seed oil. Procter and Gamble introduced Crisco with a great fanfare in 1911 as an innovative new product and not just another poor lard substitute. Most of its competitors today are a blend of a saturated vegetable fat such as palm oil (50 percent saturated fat) or cottonseed oil (25 percent saturated fat) with a hydrogenated soy oil base. In most cases manufacturers aim for a flavor that is as bland as possible and that will remain stable.[20-22]

VANASPATI: GHEE WHIZ

Vanaspati is made from hydrogenated vegetable oils and artificially colored and flavored to resemble clarified butter, known in India as *ghee*. Soft in cool weather and liquid in hot, it is kept slightly grainy as part of the effort to simulate *ghee*. The *vanaspati* business first developed in the 1930s with a product that consisted of 85 percent peanut oil, 10 percent cottonseed oil and 5 percent sesame oil, fortified with vitamins A and D. The formula changed in the early 1960s after the Soybean Council of America gave *vanaspati* manufacturers 3,021 tons of soybeans, provided technical consultants and showed them the money to be saved using hydrogenated soy oil.[23,24]

According to Dr. K.T. Achaya, Emeritus Scientist with the National Aeronautical Laboratory in Bangalore, the soy industry's start-up gifts did not instill long-term loyalty. "The oils manufacturers can use in making *vanaspati* are constantly under review, and many unfamiliar oils which would otherwise have been difficult to market came into the food stream as a component of *vanaspati*. These include imported soya, rape, sunflower and palm oils, and indigenous cottonseed and rice bran oils. Eventually the lowest-price imported edible oils were allotted by the government for *vanaspati* manufacture. This seems anomalous considering the fact that *vanaspati* is a processed and packaged product purchased mostly by the affluent sections of Indian society."[25]

nine: soy oil and margarine

HOW SOY OIL TOOK OVER IN INDIA

In India, mustard or rapeseed oil is a traditional cooking oil. It was extracted as needed with small oil presses and sold directly to housewives. This small-scale oil processing provided employment for thousands of artisans and ensured that the households had a fresh product.

Within a few months of the advent of "free trade" allowing soybean oil into India, thousands of Indians fell ill with "dropsy" due to a mysterious adulteration of mustard oil. The government banned the sale of all unpackaged edible oils, thus ensuring that all household and community-level processing of edible oils came to a halt. Edible oil production became fully industrialized, and local processing became a criminal act. Thousands of workers were dispossessed of their livelihood and millions of Indians were denied traditionally processed cooking oil. Cheap, highly processed soy oil immediately replaced mustard oil in the markets. During the crisis, the U.S. Soybean Association pushed for soybean imports as the "solution." "U.S. farmers need big new export markets..." reported one business publication. "India is a perfect match."

In the wake of the soy oil takeover, other products soon appeared in the form of "analog dals—soybean extrusions shaped into pellets that look like black gram, green gram, pigeon pea, lentil and kidney bean."

SOURCE: Shiva, Vandana. *Stolen Harvest* (South End Press, 1999).

THE HYDROGENATION STORY

Historian William Shurtleff of the Soyfoods Center in Lafayette, CA, calls hydrogenation "the single most important technical advance leading to the increased consumption of soy oil."[26] Chemists began dreaming of converting liquid oils into solid fats during the second half of the 19th century when butter became scarce and expensive in Europe. The first patent for a hydrogenation process went to Paul Sabatier in 1897 who received the Nobel Prize in chemistry in 1912 for his work with the catalysts used in the process. During that period, numerous other hydrogenation patents were issued in Germany and England, soon making the process commercially practical and profitable.[27,28]

No one seems to know when soy oil was first hydrogenated. More than 321 tons of soybean oil went into margarine in 1912 but this oil was not hydrogenated; it was included for its yellow coloring. In 1914, American travelers to Europe reported the use of hydrogenated soybean oil used to make soap and candles.[29] In 1921, William J. Morse of the USDA's National Center for Agricultural Utilization Research in Peoria, Illinois, wrote that soybean oil was "employed very extensively in the manufacture of lard and butter substitutes and quite largely in the manufacture of soap and paints. That the demand for soy bean oil in this country is very large is borne out by the large importation of the oil from Oriental countries."[30] At the 1928 Berlin Exhibition, soy oil was promoted as one of the "preferred materials" for the manufacture of margarine, although the "preferred formula" was only 8 to 25 percent soy oil with 63 to 80 percent coconut or palm oil.[31]

HEIL SOJA!

During the 1930s, Germany used more soy oil than other European countries thanks to vegetarian Adolf Hitler's favorable opinion of the soybean. His support of the soybean, however, did not extend to its use in margarine. Der Führer considered the product to be "unnatural."[32] The German people apparently considered soy oil in margarine to be in poor taste. Although Germany was the world's largest consumer of margarine until 1951 (when the U.S. moved into first place), the principal ingredients were palm kernel and coconut oils. After World War II, British Intelligence agents reporting on technical developments in the margarine industry noted that the Germans accepted no soy oil in its Grade A margarines, only 4 percent soy oil in Grade B and no more than 16.5 percent in the bottom-of-the-line Grade C.[33]

In the United States, all-vegetable oil margarines hit the marketplace in the 1930s, first made from cottonseed oil alone, then from a blend of cottonseed and soy. By 1939, soy oil accounted for 29.2 percent of all oils and fats used in margarine.[34] A product known as Soy Butter, introduced in 1942, consisted of liquid and hydrogenated soy oils, soy milk, soy lecithin, salt, carotene, vitamin A and

---

APPROPRIATE USES OF SOY: LUBE JOBS

Afraid to eat up that soy oil in your cupboard? You needn't throw it out even though it's sure to be rancid. Joseph Mazzela, an eighth grader at Maris Academy who exhibited at the 2002 California State Science Fair, proved that old vegetable oils can shine as lubricants for skateboards, bikes, boats, cars or door hinges. Before the Industrial Revolution, what we now consider cooking oils were routinely used as lubricants. Although the mechanically pressed crude vegetable oils of the past broke down under conditions of immense heat and pressure, today's highly refined oils survive nicely, thank you. Unlike their low-tech predecessors they've come to the marketplace after having been subjected to repeated assaults by heat and pressure. Indeed all that's needed to make today's vegetable oils perform as well or even better than the commercial standard 10W-30SG is a "proprietary additive" developed by doctoral student Svajus Asadauskas at Penn State.

SOURCE: Harris, Doug. Vegetable Oils as Lubricants? Student Research says 'yes' — with some modifications. ScoutNews, 9/17/2002 www.healthscout.com

butter flavor.[35] Although lard and cottonseed oil-based products dominated the industry during the 1940s, soy oil passed cottonseed to become the number one ingredient in margarine in 1951. Today soy oil dominates the market and is used in nearly 80 percent of all hydrogenated oils.[36,37]

A COLORFUL HISTORY

Dairy farmers as well as consumer advocates opposed to fraud and fake food lobbied repeatedly and often successfully for special tariffs, taxes and restrictions designed to slow the margarine juggernaut. For years, manufacturers were either forbidden to dye their product yellow to look like butter or taxed excessively if they did so. Sometimes companies sidestepped that regulation by giving customers little dye packets to color their own or used unbleached peanut or soy oil as ingredients during manufacture to provide a natural-looking buttery yellow. In 1967, North Dakota legislators made a last ditch attempt to single margarine out for opprobrium by pressing for a law that would have forced manufacturers to dye it pink or green.[38]

No margarines ended up pink and green, but all sorts of phony ingredients began to appear in the products of the 1950s to 1970s. These included artificial colors and flavors, mono- and diglycerides, dispersing agents, anti-foaming agents, emulsifiers, stabilizers, fillers, anti-spattering agents, metal scavengers, crystallization inhibitors, and the preservatives BHA (butylated hydroxyanisole), BHT (butylated hydroxytoluene), PG (propyl gallate) and TBHQ (tertiary butylhydroquinone)[39,40]

Some of these technical developments were the result of food preservation efforts during World War II. Although they improved shelf life, taste, color and texture, it took creative advertising by the American Soybean Association and margarine manufacturers to convince the public that margarine was a tasty and healthy alternative to butter and not just a cheap, second-class imitation. To maintain the illusion of healthfulness, the vegetable oil industry has kept people in the dark about the sordid secrets of margarine manufacture, particularly the crucial process of hydrogenation.

PROCESSING MATTERS

Hydrogenation begins with a cheap oil derived from corn or soybeans, one that is already probably rancid from the process of extraction. It is mixed with a catalyst—usually nickel oxide—then blasted with hydrogen gas in a reactor under conditions of intense pressure and temperatures as high as 400 degrees F. Although this changes the oil into the desired solid or partially solid state, the lumpy consistency, foul smell and dirty-gray appearance require further processing. Accordingly, soap-like emulsifiers and starch are mixed in, followed by a high temperature steam cleaning, bleaching, dyeing and flavoring. The spanking fresh product is then compressed into the sticks, bars or tubs that will be sold at the market.[41-44] Although the words "hydrogenated" and "partially hydrogenated" tend to be used interchangeably, partially hydrogenated is the correct term. Fully hydrogenated soybean oil would be as hard as wax.

From the food industry's point of view, hydrogenation serves several useful purposes. Shelf life is extended indefinitely in that margarines and shortenings almost never go bad. (More accurately, they never *seem* to go bad, as they've been mostly rancid from the start.) Secondly, soy oil is lousy for baking or frying unless it is first changed from liquid oil to a solid.

Mary G. Enig, Ph.D, author of *Know Your Fats*, explains that cookie dough made by creaming a cup of fat into a cup of sugar and two cups of flour will bake up into a well-shaped, nicely textured, non-greasy cookie. Replace the fat with oil, though, and the dough runs all over the baking sheet to produce flat, greasy cookies that burn at the edges. Likewise, French fries cooked in liquid vegetable oil come out exceptionally greasy, even by the loose standards of "greasy spoon" restaurants.[45] In contrast, the partially hydrogenated shortenings made from soy oil perform very well in the kitchen, and cost less than saturated animal fats (such as butter, lard and tallow) or saturated tropical oils (such as coconut and palm) that have traditionally excelled as baking fats. Accordingly, soy margarines and shortenings are used in nearly all readymade foods, from baked goods to frozen dinners to fast-food fries and non-dairy whipped toppings.

Commercially, they work very well. Healthwise, they wreak havoc throughout the body. The culprit is *trans* fat, an artificial form of fat formed during the hydrogenation process that has been implicated in heart disease, cancer, learning disabilities, autism, obesity, and other ills (see Chapter 10). Because of the *trans*-fat threat, food companies in Europe have already lowered the *trans*-fatty acid con-

---

CONSUMER ALERT:
FAT *TRANS*-ACTIONS

The Food and Drug Administration (FDA) does not yet require the listing of *trans* fats on food labels. This makes it difficult but not impossible for consumers to gauge how much *trans* they are eating.

Until the recently passed disclosure rule goes into effect in 2006, consumers need to read ingredient lists carefully and fill in the blanks. If "partially hydrogenated" oils or fats are included on the label, the food contains *trans* fat. Knowing how much is the challenge. If the label claims a total of six grams of total fat and only three grams are accounted for in the saturated, polyunsaturated and monosaturated fat counts, that leaves three grams of fat unaccounted for. Most of that will be *trans* fat. However, food labels are notoriously inaccurate, often misreporting the amount and kinds of fats in the product.

SOURCE: For up-to-date and accurate information on *trans* fats, visit Dr. Mary G. Enig's website www.enig.com

tents of foods. Americans are lagging behind, although some companies are already advertising their products as low in *trans*-fatty acids or even *trans*-free.

LOW-*TRANS* TUB SPREADS

To lower the levels of *trans* fats, some companies dilute hydrogenated oil with liquid oil while others avoid hydrogenation altogether. Although the latest "low-*trans*" tub spreads are promoted as health foods and positioned to appeal to upscale consumers, they are also highly processed products, usually consisting of rancid vegetable oils plus a host of additives, including soy protein isolate. As Joseph Mercola, D.O., warns, "Don't let these companies fool you with their expensive alternatives to the real thing: butter. This new non-*trans* fat margarine is still liquid plastic."[46]

The safest way to make margarines without partially hydrogenating the oil is to do it the way it was done in the good old days—that is formulate them with palm oil, palm kernel oil or coconut oil—oils with enough naturally occurring saturated fats to crystallize satisfactorily. A newer process called interesterification also produces a *trans* fat-free product, but consumers have been put off by the poorer quality and higher price.[47,48]

Meanwhile, researchers are developing new and "safer" hydrogenation techniques. One of these involves the use of a solvent known as supercritical carbon dioxide in conjunction with higher pressures and lower temperatures. The firm margarine or shortening that results contains less than 10 per cent *trans* fats, compared with the 10 to 30 percent typically found in hydrogenated oil. Compared to the usual hexane solvent processes, this is non-toxic, nonexplosive and relatively inexpensive.[49,50]

Whether this new manufacturing process will ultimately prove safer or create another whole set of problems remains to be seen. What's certain is that until the new technique becomes fast, easy and cheap, the vegetable oil cartel will continue business as usual. On the defensive, it continues to repeat claims that *trans* fats aren't really so bad after all and that there are aren't so many of them in the food supply anyway. Until Food and Drug Administration (FDA) rules requiring the listing of *trans* fats on food labels go into effect in 2006, it is difficult for consumers to gauge how much they are eating. This has led to the nickname of "phantom fat" for *trans*-fatty acids.[51,52]

PUMPED UP ON STEROLS

The latest development in soy margarine is a super-priced superspread doctored with added sterols, an estrogenic component found naturally in small quantities in soy oil. Sterols are produced as byproducts in the manufacture of vegetables oils. In the past they

---

APPROPRIATE USES OF SOY: BUG OFF

U.S. researchers have discovered a new use for soybean oil—as a mosquito repellent. "In a pan of 100 larvae we will get 100 percent mortality," says Robert Novak, a medical entomologist at the University of Illinois. The larvae suffocate from the soy oil, just as they do when immersed in the petroleum-based products widely used to control mosquito larvae in wetland habitats. Novak's team is "also looking at using secondary compounds found in soybeans that can kill insects, primarily mosquitoes." Preliminary research indicates that the pests die from being sprayed from these compounds. Whether the soy saves the mosquitoes from cancer, heart disease, hot flashes and osteoporosis is not known.

SOURCE: NSRL Bulletin, 2, 295. National Soybean Research Laboratory, University of Illinois at Urbana-Champaign. www.nsrl.uiuc.edu

were incinerated as industrial waste because it was difficult to separate them from other byproducts.[53]

Two of the best known of these so-called "functional foods" are Benecol, which contains a hydrogenated phytosterol ester derived either from soy or crude tall oil (a wood pulping byproduct), and Lipton's Take Control, which contains sterol esters derived from soy oil. When Take Control entered the marketplace, news stories indicated that it had been "proven to lower cholesterol in 31 clinical studies." No mention was made of the fact that 30 of the 31 studies were supported by Unilever Bestfoods, the world's leading manufacturer of margarines and spreads.[54]

CLASS ISSUES

The fact that soy protein enjoys an excellent reputation but soy oil has been disgraced has led to a marketing split along class lines. Upscale consumers pay dearly for the supposedly beneficial soy protein products in health food and gourmet stores. The masses, meanwhile, get the soy oil in the form of the deadly hydrogenated oils lurking in nearly every fast food or packaged product—from crackers, cookies and other baked goods to canned foods, frozen French fries and TV dinners.

Upscale soy products are trickling down as the word "soy" becomes associated in the popular mind with "healthy." Although average Americans still won't accept soy protein in the form of a "Fake Steak," "Sham Ham" or "Foney Baloney" they don't seem to mind the fact that the industry has slipped "invisible" soys into every supermarket food imaginable, from Chef Boyardee ravioli to Bumblebee canned tuna. Provided that the prices are low, and flavor and textures remain familiar, soy is now perceived as a "healthful" additive—a "plus value." Meanwhile, over in the upper-crust neighborhoods, soy oil has begun feeding off soy protein's healthy reputation and is starting to pop up in high-priced baked goods sold to the health food crowd, and not all of it is in the unrefined, cold-pressed "healthy" form.

GREASING THE WAY

The United Soybean Board (USB) has decided to help soy oil overcome its unhealthy image. In December 2004, the USB announced that its 2005 Soy Health Research Program will fund the preparation of at least two proposals designed to establish a positive connection between soybean oil and health. A total of 10 proposals will be funded at $10,000 each, with most expected to link the consumption of soy protein and isoflavones to healthy heart, bones, cognitive function, weight, "natural" hormone replacement therapy and the prevention of breast and prostate cancer. The incentive grants help researchers prepare elaborate applications to be submitted the National Institutes of Health (NIH). Proposed research must be "new and innovative and lead to greater understanding of how soy can affect human health," be "deemed acceptable" by the USB and require an annual budget to be funded primarily by the NIH (i.e. the American taxpayer) of between $150,000 and $500,000 in direct costs annually for at least three years. This is the sixth year of the Soy Health Research Program and NIH grants won have returned the USB's investment many times over.

SOURCE: Yancey, Sarah. Letter to researchers about incentive grants available through the Soy Health Research Program, December 7, 2004.

10

SOY LECITHIN
sludge to profit

Lecithin is an emulsifying substance found in the cells of all living organisms. The French scientist Maurice Gobley discovered lecithin in 1805 and named it "lekithos" after the Greek word for "egg yolk." Until it was recovered from the waste products of soybean processing in the 1930s, eggs were the primary source of commercial lecithin. Today lecithin is the generic name given to a whole class of fat- and water-soluble compounds called phospholipids. Levels of phospholipids in soybean oil range from 1.48 to 3.08 percent, which is considerably higher than the 0.5 percent typically found in vegetable oils but far less than the 30 percent found in egg yolks.[1-6]

OUT OF THE DUMPS

Soybean lecithin comes from the sludge left after crude soy oil goes through a "degumming" process. It is a waste product containing residues of solvents and pesticides and has a consistency ranging from a gummy fluid to a plastic solid. The color of lecithin ranges from a dirty tan to reddish brown. Manufacturers therefore subject lecithin to a bleaching process to turn it into a more appealing light yellow hue. The hexane extraction process commonly used in soybean oil manufacture today yields less lecithin than the older ethanol-benzol process, but produces a more marketable lecithin with better color, reduced odor and less bitter flavor.[7]

Historian William Shurtleff reports that the expansion of the soybean-crushing and soy oil refining industries in Europe after 1908 led to a problem—getting rid of the increasing amounts of fermenting, foul-smelling sludge. German companies then decided to vacuum dry the sludge, patent the process and sell it as "soybean lecithin." Scientists hired to find some application for the substance cooked up more than a thousand new uses by 1939.[8]

Today lecithin is ubiquitous in the processed food supply. It is most commonly used as an emulsifier to keep water and fats from separating in foods such as margarine, peanut butter, chocolate candies, ice cream, coffee creamers and infant formulas. Lecithin also helps prevent product spoilage, extending shelf life in the marketplace. In industry kitchens, it serves to improve mixing, speed crystallization, prevent "weeping," and stop spattering, lumping and sticking. Used in cosmetics, lecithin softens the skin and helps other ingredients penetrate the skin barrier. A more water-loving version known as "deoiled lecithin" reduces the time required to shut down and clean the extruders used in the manufacture of textured vegetable protein and other soy products.[9,10]

In theory, lecithin manufacture eliminates all soy proteins, making it hypoallergenic. In reality, minute amounts of soy protein always remain in lecithin as well as in soy oil. Three components of soy protein have been identified in soy lecithin, including the Kunitz trypsin inhibitor, which has a track record of triggering severe allergic reactions even in the most minuscule quantities. The presence of lecithin in so many food and cosmetic products poses a special danger for people with soy allergies.[11-13] (See Chapters 24 and 25.)

ten: soy lecithin: sludge to profit

LEC IS IN—THE MAKING OF A WONDER FOOD

Since the 1920s, health writers have touted lecithin as a wonder food capable of combating atherosclerosis, multiple sclerosis, liver cirrhosis, gall stones, psoriasis, eczema, scleroderma, anxiety, tremors and brain aging. These claims are based on the fact that the human body uses phospholipids to build strong, flexible cell membranes and to facilitate nerve transmission. A. A. Horvath, Ph.D., an early purveyor of soybean health claims, recommended lecithin as a component in "nerve tonics" or to help alcoholics reduce the effects of intoxication and withdrawal. In 1934, Chinese researchers published an article entitled "A Comfortable and Spontaneous Cure for the Opium Habit by Means of Lecithin" in an English-language medical journal.[14]

Lecithin captured the popular imagination during the 1960s and 1970s when the bestselling health authors Adelle Davis, Linda Clark and Mary Ann Crenshaw hyped lecithin in their many books, including *Let's Get Well; Secrets of Health and Beauty;* and *The Natural Way to Super Beauty: Featuring the Amazing Lecithin, Apple Cider Vinegar, B-6 and Kelp Diet.*[15-17]

Lecithin did not become a star of the health food circuit by accident. Research took off during the early 1930s, just as lecithin production became commercially viable. In 1939, the American Lecithin Company began sponsoring research studies and published the most promising in 1944 in a 23-page booklet entitled *Soybean Lecithin.* The company, not coincidentally, introduced a health food cookie with a lecithin filling known as the "Lexo Wafer" and a lecithin-wheat germ supplement called "Granulestin." In the mid-1970s, Natterman, a lecithin marketing company based in Germany, hired scientists at various health clinics to experiment with lecithin and to write scientific articles about the product. These "check book" scientists coined the term "essential phospholipids," an inaccurate term since a healthy body can produce its own phospholipids from phosphorous and lipids.[18]

In September 2001, lecithin got a boost when the U.S. Food

and Drug Administration (FDA) authorized products containing more than traces of lecithin to bear labels such as "A good source of choline." Producers of soy lecithin hope the new health claim will raise demand for lecithin and increase prices in what has been a soft market. Eggs, milk and soy products are the leading dietary sources of choline, according to recent research conducted at the University of North Carolina at Chapel Hill and at Duke University.[19-21]

LEC THAT'S MORE—PHOSPHATIDYL CHOLINE (PC)

Because many lecithin products sold in health food stores contain less than 30 percent choline, many health professionals prefer to use the more potent phosphatidylcholine (PC) or its even more powerful derivative drug glycerylphosphorylcholine (GPC). Clinicians are recommending both products to prevent and reverse dementia, improve cognitive function, increase human growth hormone (hGH) release, and to treat brain disorders such as damage

SOY, SOY EVERYWHERE, DROPS OF SLUDGE TO EAT

Try to find a chocolate bar, ice cream or other readymade food at the supermarket or health food store that doesn't contain small amounts of soy lecithin. That's the challenge for people who are allergic to soy. Lecithin isn't supposed to contain any of the soybean's allergenic protein, but there's always the chance that a bit might remain. For the allergy sufferer, that little bit could cause anything from gastrointestinal upset to life-threatening anaphylactic shock (see Chapters 24 and 25). For everyone else, a little lecithin sold from the sludge left over from soy oil manufacture isn't really a big deal. There are many worse additives in processed foods, namely soy protein, soy oil, soy isoflavones and soy sterols.

from stroke. PC and GPC may help build nerve cell membranes, facilitate electrical transmission in the brain, hold membrane proteins in place, and produce the neurotransmitter acetylcholine.[22-24] However, studies on soy lecithin, PC, and brain aging have been inconsistent and contradictory ever since the 1920s. Generally, lecithin is regarded as safe except for people who are highly allergic to soy. The late Robert Atkins, M.D., advised patients not to take large doses of supplemental lecithin without extra vitamin C to protect them from the nitrosamines formed from choline metabolism.[25] Trimethylamine and dimethylamine, which are metabolized by bacteria in the intestines from choline, are important precursors to N-nitrosodimethylamine, a potent carcinogen in a variety of animal species.[26,27]

PHOSPHATIDYL SERINE (PS)

Phosphatidyl serine (PS)—another popular phospholipid that

MY SOY STORY:
EVEN ALLERGIC TO SOY LECITHIN

My mom switched me to formula when she found out she was pregnant with my sister, less than a year after I was born. She thought I was colicky and gassy but never imagined an allergy at the root. In high school I became a vegetarian. My gas was horrible and I went to a dietitian who said I was "swallowing air." After I acknowledged my soy allergy and stopped swallowing soy products I learned that even soybean oil or soy lecithin would give me bad gas. Chocolate with soy lecithin will even give me diarrhea, soy-free chocolate will not. You can seriously taste the difference—traditionally made chocolate bars don't have that greasy feeling. They are more expensive, but it's worth it to get to eat chocolate.

S.L., Easton, MD

improves brain function and mental acuity—nearly always comes from soy oil. Most of the scientific studies proving its efficacy, however, come from bovine sources, which also contain DHA as part of the structure.[28-31] Plant oils never contain readymade DHA. Indeed, the entire fatty acid structure of soy-derived PS is different from that of bovine-derived PS. The latter is rich in stearic and oleic acids, while soy PS is rich in linoleic and palmitic acids.[32] Complicating matters further, the PS naturally formed in the human body consists of 37.5 percent stearic acid and 24.2 percent arachidonic acid.[33] Yet soy-derived PS seems to help many people[34-36] and because of the Mad Cow scare, bovine-derived PS isn't likely show up in the marketplace anytime soon.

Russell Blaylock, M.D., author of *Excitotoxins, the Taste that Kills*, believes that PS may protect us from glutamate toxicity.[37] Ironically, many people are taking the expensive soy-derived supplement PS in order to undo the damage that may be caused in part by the cheap soy protein in processed foods.

LYSOPHOSPHATIDYLETHANOLAMINE (LPE)

The Environmental Protection Agency (EPA) has approved lysophosphatidylethanolamine (LPE), another phosphatidyl substance commercially extracted from soybeans, for use as a fruit ripener and shelf-life extender. The produce industry now uses LPE—once called cephalin—to treat grapes, cranberries, strawberries, blueberries, apples, tomatoes and cut flowers.

When applied to fruits that are nearly ripe—going into puberty, so to speak—LPE promotes ripening. When applied to picked fruit or cut flowers that are already ripe or blooming, however, it will "reduce senescence by inhibiting some of the enzymes involved in membrane breakdown." This can dramatically extend shelf life.[38] Whether the substance could also keep human bodies fresh for funeral home viewings is a topic that has not yet been investigated.

MY SOY STORY:
LECITHIN AND GOITER

Approximately 16 months ago I felt a large almond-shaped mass on my thyroid. It was quite noticeable to me when I looked in the mirror and also when swallowing. For several years I have taken supplements, but only in the past year did I add soy lecithin. The ultrasound recommended by the endocrinologist revealed a multinodular goiter, with a few larger nodules. These were biopsied and diagnosed as follicular neoplasms. Since follicular cells on aspiration cannot be ruled out as benign or malignant, it was recommended I have the thyroid lobe surgically removed.

After talking with a friend who owns a health food store, I decided to stop taking the soy lecithin as this was the only supplement I had added in the past year and the evidence seemed questionable as to the safety of soy. Now 16 months later, my nodule is significantly smaller, which the oncology surgeon said would not happen.

R.E., Holstein, IA

11
NOT TRUSTING
THE PROCESS

Second generation soy foods are manufactured using high-heat and pressure, chemical solvents, acids and alkalis, extruders and other harsh tools that are very likely to contain or produce toxic or carcinogenic residues. This is also true of highly processed products using fractions of milk, eggs, meat, grains, oils or vegetables.

The difference is that second generation soy foods are billed as "health foods" whereas other processed foods are widely acknowledged to be what they are—junk foods that do not support health. The soy industry typically puts a positive spin on their products by claiming all the health benefits found in soy while insisting that levels of toxins are too low to pose any hazard to the consumer.

But risk is always a product of dose and duration of exposure. Vegans who favor soy protein, wheat gluten and other heavily processed plant protein products as their primary sources of protein are regularly exposed to relatively high levels of toxins. Indeed, warnings have begun appearing on websites advising vegans and other visitors not to fall prey to industry propaganda touting health benefits of soy-based junk foods.[1]

The usual suspects are nitrosamines, lysinoalanines, heterocyclic amines, excitotoxins, chloropropanols, furanones, hexane and other solvents.

NITROSAMINES

Nitrates occur naturally in vegetables, water and just about everything else we eat or drink. Nitrate is harmless until reduced to nitrite either in the body as part of the digestive process or through spray drying and other harsh processing methods that occur during the manufacture of soy protein isolate (SPI), casein and other highly

---

SMOKING GRAS

Soy protein, added to thousands of grocery items, has *never* received GRAS (Generally Recognized as Safe) status as an additive to food. In 1958 and 1960, an amendment to the U.S. Food Drug and Cosmetic Act permitted food additives already in use that were "Generally Recognized as Safe." Thousands of items that have been in the food supply for many years (such as salt and sugar) or additives approved by FDA before 1958 went on the GRAS list. The margin of safety for most additives was established as a daily intake no more than 1/100 of the amount thought to be hazardous, provided the substance was not carcinogenic. The Delaney Clause specified that *no* substance be added to the food supply if it has been shown to cause cancer in people or animals. Although soy protein isolate (SPI) was certainly in use prior to 1958, it was only as an industrial product to bind and seal paper products, not as a food. It does not qualify as a product having a long history of safe use in the food supply and it is also known to include toxins and carcinogens.

---

eleven: not trusting the process

In 1979, the Select Committee of GRAS Substances (SCOGS) took a look at safety issues in the manufacture of soy protein isolate. It advised establishing acceptable levels of the carcinogens nitrite and nitrosamines and the toxic amino acid lysinoalanine "to avoid future problems" and urged a close monitoring of the levels of these substances in edible food products. To date, these safety levels have not been established, soy protein as a food has not been given GRAS status, and no monitoring is being carried out by people outside the industry itself. As SPI does not have GRAS status, manufacturers must by law attain "Pre-Market Approval" before adding SPI to any food item, yet SPI is now routinely added to food products, including baby formula, without safety checks or prior approval.

In October 1999, the FDA approved a health claim for soy protein at the amount of 25 grams, an action the SCOGS committee would have found inconceivable. The committee considered a mere 150 mg per day of soy protein to be the maximum safe dose. In its Final Ruling on the 1999 soy protein health claim, the FDA dismissed the matter of dangers from nitrites, nitrosamines and lysinoalanines with the recommendation that "good manufacturing practices are and should be employed." In other words, the FDA has stepped aside to let the fox guard the hen house.

SOURCES:
Evaluation of the health aspects of soy protein isolates as food ingredients. Prepared by Life Sciences Research Office, Federation of American Societies for Experimental Biology for the Bureau of Foods, Food and Drug Administration, 1979. Contract # FDA 223-75-2004.

Food and Drug Administration, Final Rule. Food Labeling: Health Claims; Soy Protein and Coronary Heart Disease, Federal Register 64FR 57699, October 26, 1999.

FDA Backgrounder: Milestones in U.S. Food and Drug Law History http://vm.cfsan.fda.gov

processed, fractionated food products. Nitrites are also added directly to foods, as in the curing of meat and fish. Nitrites are very reactive chemically and are precursors of nitrosamines. We have known since 1937 that nitrosamines damage the liver; and since 1956 that nitrosamines are mutagens and carcinogens.[2,3]

In 1979, an independent committee known as the Select Committee of GRAS Substances (SCOGS) reported to the FDA that the nitrites found in soy protein—either directly in soy food or indirectly from migration from the soy protein isolate used in packaging—was likely to be so small (50 parts per million) that it would not pose a health hazard. After all, people at the time rarely consumed more than 150 mg (about one-fourth teaspoon) per day of soy protein. The committee, however, recommended the establishment of safe levels as well as routine monitoring of nitrites and nitrosamines in soy protein isolate.[4] Today, more than 30 years later, these studies have yet to be carried out.

Today Americans eat ten times more soy protein isolate (SPI)—and other highly processed forms of soy included in readymade foods—than they did in 1979. Vegetarians who rely on second generation meat substitutes, analogues, energy bars, shakes and other products made with soy protein isolate could easily consume 100 times more than the 150 mg SCOGS determined as safe.

Even at today's higher levels of soy consumption, soy apologists dismiss concerns about nitrites, pointing out that the microbes in our saliva and intestines manufacture far more nitrites from the nitrates in food and drink. Although this is correct, those extra nitrites *do* matter. The rate of nitrosamine formation in the body proceeds exponentially—slowly at low nitrite concentrations, but more and more rapidly as nitrites enter the body from the diet or water supply. People with low hydrochloric acid (HCL) levels in the stomach are especially likely to be nitrite producers because adequate HCL prevents microbial overgrowth.[5] HCL levels tend to decrease with age and most people over the age of 40 are at least mildly deficient.[6]

eleven: not trusting the process

Although high levels of nitrites in processed foods lead to nitrosamine formation, the most serious problem comes from the pre-formed nitrosamines. These occur in soy protein isolates and other products that have undergone acid washes, flame drying or high temperature spray-drying processes. In USDA studies undertaken in the 1980s, researchers found that soy protein isolate contained about twice the nitrite content found in other soy protein products, including overly toasted soy flour. They also found levels of 1.5 parts per billion of a potent nitrosamine known as N-nitrosodimethylamine (NDMA) in soy protein.[7] More recently, scientists have found this highly volatile nitrosamine in significant quantities in SPI, malt and malt beverages, non-fat dry milk and dried cheeses.[8] Soy sauce also contains high levels of tyramine, a derivative of the amino acid tyrosine and a potent precursor of mutagens produced by nitrites.[9-14]

The California Environmental Protection Agency Office of Environmental Health Hazard Assessment has established safe levels for nitrosamines ranging from 40 ng (billionths of a gram) per day for NDMA to 80 ug (millionths of a gram) per day for the relatively weak nitrosamine N-nitrosodiphenylamine. Environmental Scientist Mike Fitzpatrick, Ph.D., points out that a person who eats 100 grams of soy protein would exceed safe levels if NDMA is present in excess of 0.20 parts per billion in steam-treated soy flour or 0.36 parts per billion in soy protein isolate. The safe level of N-nitrosdiphenylamine would be exceeded if present at levels in excess of 0.42 parts per million in steam-treated soy flour or 0.72 parts per million in soy protein isolate. Though there seems to be very little information on the levels of nitrosamines in soy products—and levels vary from batch to batch—this level of toxicity is not only possible but likely. Taking the USDA finding of 1.4 parts per billion, people eating 100 grams per day of soy protein—a goal promoted as healthful by Protein Technologies International (PTI) in a 1999 petition to the FDA—could be exposed daily to 35 times the safe limit of NDMA. Finally, Fitzpatrick notes that the safe levels are defined for a 70 kg adult male and that lower levels should be established for adult women, teenagers, children and infants.[15]

LYSINOALANINES

Lysinoalanine is a cross-linked amino acid that is produced when the essential amino acid lysine is subjected to strong alkaline treatments. The soy industry uses alkali to turn soybeans into soymilk, tofu, TSP, SPI, SPC and other products quickly and profitably. Only the old-fashioned, fermented "good old soys," or tofus and soymilks made at home or by cottage-type industries, can bill themselves as "lysinoalanine-free."[16,17]

The highest levels of lysinoalanines occur in soy protein isolates manufactured for use as sizing and coating adhesives for paper and paperboard products. Such products are produced at high alkaline pH levels. Rats fed soy proteins processed using similar high-alkali baths have suffered kidney damage, specifically increased organ weights, lesions and kidney stones. The soy industry assures us that soy proteins intended for human consumption are safer because they are extracted at a pH level below 9.[18-21]

A look at new processes receiving patents today, however, reveals that keeping alkaline levels low is not a high priority for much of the food-processing industry. For example, Kraft recently developed a process to "deflavor" soy milk, flour, concentrates and isolates by adjusting the pH to levels ranging from 9 to 12. This makes it possible to dissolve the soy proteins and release the "beany" flavors through a special ultrafiltrated membranous exhaust system.[22]

Lysinoalanine toxicity can be hard to pin down. It varies depending upon the species of test animal, the total diet and the form of lysinoalanine consumed. Some studies show that the type of lysinoalanine found in hydrolyzed vegetable proteins (HVP) will display toxicity while those in other forms of soy protein exhibit low levels or none at all. Confusing matters further, heavily heated proteins that have not been subjected to alkaline baths have nonetheless tested positive for lysinoalanines.[23,24] There is no confusion, however, about the fact that most commercial soy products are produced using alkaline baths and high temperatures, both of which create by-products that are best avoided.

Other cross-linked amino acids, whose toxic effects are suspected, but not yet thoroughly researched, may also occur. Arginine, an important amino acid for proper growth, may be kicked up a notch into the amino acid ornithine and from there into the problematic ornithinoalanine. Threonine produces methyl-dehydroalanine, which can undergo further reactions to form methyl-lysinoalanine and methyl-lanthionine. Cysteine can produce dehydroalanine and methyl-dehydroalanine.[25-27]

Toxic byproducts are not the only problem with modern soy products. Ghulam Sarwar, Ph.D., of the Nutrition Research Division, Health Canada, Ottawa, has found that as lysinoalanines are formed, 19 to 20 percent of the essential amino acid lysine is lost. At the same time, heat and alkaline treatments destroy 73 to 77 percent of cystine, 35-45 percent threonine, and 18-30 percent serine. Furthermore, the natural forms of amino acid-isomers may be converted to the less usable or unusable analogues, resulting in a dramatic loss in protein digestibility and protein quality.[28] (See Chapter 13.)

Alkaline processing also compromises mineral status. Iron levels in male and female rats fed SPI dropped to half those of controls while copper levels increased threefold.[29] Practitioners are increasingly concerned about copper toxicity—generally seen in conjunction with a zinc deficiency and skewed zinc-copper ratio—as it has been linked to mental health problems such as depression, mood swings, anxiety, panic attacks, as well as a host of diseases ranging from anorexia to diabetes to rheumatoid arthritis.[30]

According to Sarwar, "The data suggested that LAL (lysinoalanine), an unnatural amino acid derivative formed during processing of foods, may produce adverse effects on growth, protein digestibility, protein quality and mineral bioavailability and utilization. The antinutritional effects of LAL may be more pronounced in sole-source foods such as infant formulas and formulated liquid diets which have been reported to contain significant amounts (up to

2400 ppm of LAL in the protein) of LAL."[31]

EXCITOTOXINS

Excitotoxins are amino acids such as glutamate and aspartate that wreak havoc on neuroreceptors in the brain. Glutamate and aspartate are created when food processors hydrolyze soy protein to make hydrolyzed vegetable protein (HVP), commercial soy sauces and other products. MSG is the sodium salt of glutamate, and aspartate is a component of aspartame, the artificial sweetener used in many "lite" products.

Excitotoxins exist naturally in the body and are normally used by the brain in small, carefully controlled concentrations. Problems arise, however, when people eat excessive amounts of processed foods. Soyfoods deliver a double whammy. Glutamate is formed as a byproduct of processing, and MSG and other "natural flavorings" are often added to improve taste and smell. The makers of health food-store soy products boast "all natural" on their labels yet sometimes list hydrolyzed vegetable protein, vegetable protein, hydrolyzed plant protein and "natural" flavorings likely to contain glutamate. This is why the FDA ordered the company that makes Bragg's Amino Acids to cease and desist from using the "No MSG" claim on its label. (See Sidebar, Chapter 5.) Dangers from excitotoxins increase when two or more are present in the same food or when nitrosamines or other toxins are also present.[32-34]

HETEROCYCLIC AMINES (HCAs)

Ordinary cooking procedures such as broiling, frying and barbecuing, and industrial processes such as heat processing extrusion and pyrolysis can form potent mutagenic and carcinogenic compounds known as heterocyclic amines (HCAs). In rats, mice and monkeys, the organ most vulnerable to HCAs is the liver, but lung and stomach tumors, lymphomas and leukemias also occur, as well as myocardial lesions in monkeys. The higher the heat and pressure, the longer the duration, the more HCAs are formed.[35-39] Thus, industrially processed foods are likely to contain much higher levels of HCAs than foods prepared at home. Because modern soy products such as TVP, SPI, SPC, and HVP may undergo three or more heat treatments before they reach the supermarket, they can carry high levels of HCAs.

Although people generally expect to find HCAs in fried or grilled beef and fish, similar HCAs are formed in any pyrolyzed, protein-rich food. Soy globulin protein plus sugar under heat and pressure combine to form potent mutagens such as 2-amino-9H-pyrido (2,3-b) indole and 2-amino-3-methyl-9H-pyrido (2,3- b) indole. Commercial soy sauce is rich in an HCA known as 1-methyl-1,2,3,4-tetrahydro-beta-carboline-3-carboxylic acid (MTCCA).[40] Nitrites increase the mutagenicity of HCAs in foods—and vice versa. As discussed above, mutagen precursors isolated from nitrite-containing soy sauce have been identified as either tyramine or beta-carboline derivatives.[41,42]

Soy sauce plus sugar—a combination found in many marinades and barbeque sauces—also form heterocyclic amines. The more soy sauce in the marinade, the more HCAs. Soy sauces, ketchups and fish sauces containing beta carbolines are also commonly used in recipes used by food processors, spurring the formation of even more HCAs.[43-45]

The more types of HCAs found in a given product or meal, the greater the risk. As T. Sugimura of the National Cancer Center Research Institute in Tokyo puts it, "Heterocyclic amines are probably involved in the development of human cancer in the presence of other carcinogens, tumor promoters and factors stimulating cancer progression."[46]

HCAs appear naturally in the body, but never in the quantities provided by today's overly—and repeatedly—heated food products. In animal studies, mutagenic HCAs have been shown to be more likely to turn carcinogenic when eaten regularly than sporadically. HCAs are also most likely to trigger human cancer in the presence of other carcinogens. Thus the consistent presence of nitrites, glutamate and HCAs in heavily processed soy foods poses a triple threat. Soy sauces, bouillons, flavor enhancers and other ingredients used to flavor meat analogues and other ersatz soy products contain HCAs, nitrites or nitrosamines and MSG or glutamate—HCA reactions involving glutamate are highly mutagenic. Sometimes nitrites initially turn mutagens into nonmutagens—a fact that will surely lead to soy industry claims that the nitrites in soy prevent cancer. The reality is that these nonmutagens are a just a step in an ongoing process that creates new mutagens.[47-49]

To date, much of the research on HCAs has centered on grilled and barbecued meats, fish and poultry. Grilled tempeh, tofu and other soyfoods could probably gain HCAs this way as well. However, most HCAs in soy foods are formed at the processing plant, not in the home kitchen or on the patio.

FURANONES

A byproduct of processing known as furanones intensify flavor. They appear in foods cooked at high temperatures when Maillard —known as "browning"—reactions occur between sugars and amino acids. Furanones that are mutagenic to bacteria and cause DNA damage in lab tests have been identified in soy sauces and hydrolyzed vegetable protein (HVP). However, furanones have also proved anticarcinogenic in animals treated with known cancer-inducing compounds.[50-54] One furanone is identical to a male pheromone produced by the cockroach, so it might be best not to spill much furanone-rich soy sauce in the kitchen.[55]

CHLOROPROPANOLS

Hydrolyzed vegetable protein (HVP) and commercial soy sauces may also contain dangerous levels of chemicals known as 3-MCPD (3-chloro-1,2-propanediol) and 1,3-DCP (1,3-dichloro-2-propanol), both of which have been linked to liver cancer. The two belong to a group of chemicals known as chloropropanols, which are produced when soy sauce production is speeded up using acid hydrolyzation methods. Most modern companies use some form of this method

SOY MYSTERY:
THE CASE OF THE SQUIRT ATTACKS

A Brisbane, Australia, man was arrested for repeatedly squirting soy sauce at another man in a shopping mall. The victim was riding up an elevator to return to work after his lunch break when he was squirted on the back of his trousers. He reported feeling slight pressure and wetness on the back of his legs before turning around to find his assailant aiming a plastic packet of sauce at him. When he called police, he revealed that he had been the victim of similar soy sauce attacks from the same man in the past. He told police that he did not know the man or agree to—or in any way encourage—a soy sauce squirting game.

The soy sauce assailant refused to talk to police or explain his behavior in court. He was ordered to pay $300 to replace the man's trousers and a fine of $150. No damages were awarded for exposing the man to the health dangers of the excitotoxins glutamate and aspartate or to the mutagens and carcinogens, chloropropanols, furanones, salsolinols or ethyl carbamates. He hadn't been forced to eat them, after all.

SOURCE: Financial Times Information Limited – Asia Africa Intelligence Wire, AAP News via NewsEdge Corporation, October 23, 2002. Posted 10/24/02 on www.soyatech.com

and exercise less-than-perfect quality control. Product recalls have occurred in Great Britain and New Zealand, and the safety of all modern commercial soy sauces is in doubt.[56-61]

HEXANE

Organic solvents—such as acetone, benzene, chloroform, cyclohexane and ether—are used by the vegetable oil industry to extract oil from beans and seeds. Years ago, chlorinated solvents were popular because they are nonflammable and efficient. However, the dark side appeared in 1916 when 54 cows in Scotland died from trichloroethylene, the solvent used to extract the soybean meal used for their feed. Similar problems appeared in Germany in the 1920s and the United States in the 1950s. The cows died from severe aplastic anemia—a rare blood disease caused by destruction of the bone marrow—and soy feed suffered a blow to its "healthy" image.[62-64]

In the United States, the dangers of hexane solvents were well publicized in the 1930s because of explosions triggered by volatile hexane vapors in the Glidden Plant and other processing facilities. Even so, hexane became the most widely used solvent by 1941.[65] Today, the primary concern is hexane's toxicity. It irritates the lungs and depresses the central nervous system. Ingestion has been linked to Parkinson's disease, and workers exposed to hexane may develop polyneuropathy. Although the industry insists that "desolventizing" processes remove hexane residues from soy oil or meal, some traces always remain.[66]

12
FORMULA FOR DISASTER

Soy infant formula was never used traditionally in Asia. Babies who could not be breastfed by their birth mothers received homemade dairy formulas made with mare, water buffalo, cow or goat's milk, were breastfed by a wet nurse. . . or died. The inventors of the first soy formulas were westerners with very good intentions—to save babies that would not otherwise have survived.

Yet the myth persists that soy formula has been around for centuries and so must be safe. Mark Messina, Ph.D., a spokesperson for the soy industry, defended soy formula at the Fifth International Symposium on the Role of Soy in Preventing and Treating Chronic Disease, in Orlando with the words "Asian babies have been raised on soy products for centuries with no apparent ill effects."[1] This is not true, and the first soy formula was not even invented in Asia.

Historian William Shurtleff of the Soyfoods Center in Lafayette, California, confirms that the earliest known document on use of soybean in infant feeding is an article by John Ruhrah, M.D., published in the *Archives of Pediatrics* in 1909.[2] Dr. Ruhrah, a pediatrician from Baltimore, presented a paper at the 21st annual meeting of the American Pediatric Society entitled "The Soy Bean in Infant Feeding: A Preliminary Report" and argued that his soybean gruel formula made from boiled beans was "useful as a substitute for milk in diarrhea and in intestinal and stomach disorders and in diabetes mellitus." By 1915, he had also experimented with soy flour formulas and mixtures of soy gruel with barley flour, salt and condensed milk.[3-5] In 1916, the *Journal of the American Medical Association* reported that a soy flour-based formula was tried on 74 cases of infants with diarrhea with a success rate of 59.4 percent.[6]

SOY FORMULA IN THE EAST

In China, Ernest Tso announced the invention of the first soy formula in Asia that could sustain an infant for the first eight months of age in 1928. Writing in the *Chinese Journal of Physiology*, Tso informs us that "soybean milk" is a native food used in certain parts of the country as a morning beverage but it is little used as part of the diet for children. He states that its nutritive properties as a food for young infants are practically unknown. Tso's formula consisted of wet-ground soybean flour supplemented with salt, sugar and other substances. After carrying out metabolic studies, he concluded that the calcium was inadequate. By 1931, he had not only added calcium lactate but also more sugar and sodium chloride plus cod liver oil (for vitamins A and D) and cabbage water for vitamin C.[7-9]

In 1936, R.A. Guy of the Department of Public Health of Peiping Union Medical College provided additional background information in three articles for the *Chinese Medical Journal:*[10-12] "It seems pertinent here to note that we have never found soybean 'milk' naturally used by Peiping women to feed their children. This beverage is not made in the home in Peiping, but is sold by street vendors, as a hot, very weak solution of soybean protein and is usually drunk by old people in place of tea. The 'milk', as reinforced for the feeding of young infants, is rather tedious and difficult to prepare. As dispensed recently by the various health stations, it is in demand, but is just as artificial in this community as cow's milk. One must bear in mind that the successful feeding of very young infants with milk other than human, has only been done in the past twenty years or so. Such feeding is highly artificial, since it depends for its success not only on the equipment and care in preparation in the home, the measured administration of the food and conscious attention to the inclusion of vitamins, but also on the whole machinery of modern government for the production and distribution of good milk. That artificial feeding has become necessary in some countries is no argument against giving the human infant the milk of his own species. Aside from the disputed physiological and psychological benefits of maternal nursing, it is more economical, cleaner, safer and less trouble for the mother to prepare the milk '*in vivo*' than '*in vitro*' as it may be so put."[13]

Likewise, an investigation by C.Y. Chou in the 1980s found no evidence to indicate that soy infant formula was developed in China prior to the late 1920s.[14]

The first manufacturer of soy formula in China was Harry W. Miller, M.D., a Seventh Day Adventist medical missionary from Ohio who developed a soy milk that "could be built up into a satisfactory formula for babies." Dr. Miller's goal was to nourish babies, children and adults where animal milk "is not available, and which for economic reasons can never be a dependable source of food supplies for the masses." He noted that the people had "built up a number of soy protein dishes, called 'meat without bones'" for adults but had not "taken into consideration the nutritional needs of infants and growing children, and malnutrition is seen everywhere in these developing countries." Dr. Miller helped set up plants in China, the Philippines, Taiwan, Japan, Singapore, Thailand and Hong Kong by providing "American knowhow."[15]

Despite Dr. Miller's efforts, soy formula was not widely accepted in Asia and is still not the preferred formula today. Most babies in Asia are breastfed for a few months, then switched to a dairy-based infant formula. Orphans and other babies that cannot be breast fed by a wet nurse receive milk-based formulas.[16]

SOY FORMULA IN THE WEST

Dr. Ruhrah's 1909 soy formula was designed for sick infants who experienced severe diarrhea on the early cow's milk formulas and was intended as a "temporary therapeutic procedure." The formula consisted of a tan or caramel-colored thin gruel with a nutty odor made from boiled soybeans. No sugars or starch were added in order not to exacerbate the infant diarrhea. Those who responded favorably began producing brown "malt" stools.[17]

Bowel health of the infants is a running theme of the pre-1960 soy formula literature, with recurring reports of the soy flour-based formulas causing diarrhea, foul smells and flatulence.[18] Researchers often expressed astonishment at the sheer bulk. "The residue is at least twice that of human or cow's milk," wrote two Cleveland pediatricians in 1932. Testing soy formula on 205 infants, they reported that the healthy babies had three or four very large, soft, green stools per day and that infants whose green stools totaled six or seven per day "failed to thrive." Although the most obvious cause was indigestible cellulose roughage, the number of bowel movements decreased and stool size shrank if the mixture was well boiled before serving. The researchers thus concluded that home cooking rendered the formula more digestible.[19,20] In all probability, the manufacturing process had inadequately deactivated the soybean's trypsin inhibitors and other antinutrients, making it very hard to digest the soy protein (see Chapter 16).

Manufacturers faced other problems as well. According to A. A. Horvath, Ph.D.,—an employee of several U.S. government agencies and world traveler who "went soybean one hundred percent" after a trip to China[21]—the biggest problem was the tendency of soy flour to go rancid.[22] However, new processing methods were coming on the market and producing soy flours that could be kept for longer periods without turning rancid.[23] (See Chapter 7.)

The more difficult task was to pump up soy formula's soggy

TESTING FORMULA

Infants who participated in the early soy formula studies not only failed to receive the emotional and nutritional benefits of breast milk, but were sometimes taken away from their parents or guardians for days at a time. To determine nitrogen retention and compare the protein quality of several new soy formulas, a research team in Cleveland tested a total of 205 infants over a three-and-one-half year period in small groups as follows:

"The infants, seven in number, were selected from those coming regularly to the dispensary and had been fed exclusively on one of the soy bean preparations for some time prior to admission to the hospital. They were placed on a canvas bed strapped at the four corners to the upright supports of the crib and strapped to the canvas, the buttocks resting on a padded rim of an aperture cut in the canvas support. A stool pan was held in place beneath the buttocks and a special tube was attached to the infant for the collection of the urine.

"A sample of food sufficient for the entire experiment was thoroughly mixed and daily portions weighed from this sample. In this way it was possible to determine accurately how much nitrogen, calcium and phosphorus were provided in the quantity given to the baby. Any portion of the food refused was measured and proper allowance made.

"The infants were kept on the metabolism bed for a total of four days, during which twenty-four hour collections of the urine and feces were made. The samples were thoroughly mixed and portions for analysis taken. . . . All the infants were offered liberal feedings, depending on appetite and tolerance and were fed at four-hour intervals. . ."

SOURCE: Rittinger F, Dembo LH, Torrey G. Soy bean (vegetable) milk in infant feeding: Results of three and one-half years' study on the growth and development of 205 infants. *J Ped*, 1934, 6, 517-532.

nutritional profile. A common tactic—tried early on by Dr. Ruhrah—was to combine soy flour with milk powders or condensed milk "with the object of rendering them suitable for infant feeding." Many recipes were tested over the years, and they varied widely in terms of protein power, fatty acid profile, vitamin and mineral content, digestibility, oligosaccharide levels and "keeping properties."[24] Not surprisingly, many of the test-case infants failed to thrive.

In the early days of soy formula, many infants suffered from vitamin A deficiency. One of the worst cases reported was a soy formula-fed baby diagnosed with keratomalacia, an eye disease in which the cornea is dry and ulcerated as a result of severe vitamin A deficiency.[25] Although the Chinese solved the problem with the addition of cod liver oil, the Americans labored under the still commonly held misconception that beta-carotene and vitamin A are identical. A typical statement made by researchers at the time was that "the soybean is a legume that is noted for its vitamin A content."[26-29] True vitamin A is never found in soybeans (or any other plant food) and infants cannot easily convert its precursor beta-carotene into the true vitamin A it needs for metabolism and growth.

Calcium presented another difficulty. Soybeans do not naturally contain much calcium, but do contain phytates, a type of antinutrient that interferes with calcium absorption. (See Chapter 17.) Early researchers struggled mightily to find the best form of supplemental calcium and the right ratio of calcium and phosphorous.[30]

These and other problems were widely acknowledged in medical journals of the time, yet a 1938 *Readers Digest* article stated that Madison Foods (a company affiliated with the Seventh Day Adventist Madison College in Tennessee) had been busy developing a soy milk that "is now not only cheaper than cow's milk but, on the authority of the American Medical Association, better for babies."[31]

A more truthful picture emerged in the *Archives of Diseases of Children*. Helen MacKay, M.D., of the Medical Research Council and Queens Hospital for Children in London, reviewed the entirety of the soy formula literature through 1938 and concluded: "Babies on soya flours without any admixture of cow's milk do not, on the whole, make as good progress as babies having milk as the basis of their diet." She noted that researchers of the 1930s had put great effort into finding ways to mix soybean milk (because it was cheap) with dairy formulas (to prop up the nutritional value) in order to create a formula that would serve in parts of the world "where a sufficiency of milk alone is beyond the means of the people."[32]

From the 1940s to 1960s, reports surfaced of deficiencies of vitamins A, K and B_{12} and of the minerals zinc, iron and calcium from soy formula. As manufacturers got the message, they solved the deficiencies in the cheapest and most expedient way possible—by fortifying with the vitamins and minerals or the adding an enhancer (such as vitamin C to enhance the uptake of iron).[33-35]

In 1939, the specter of thyroid damage emerged when soy feed was found to be goitrogenic to poultry. Over the next two decades, researchers learned that soy formula damaged the thyroids of human infants. By 1961 formula manufacturers routinely added iodine to soy formula. But although iodine prevents overt damage, long-term risks to the thyroid remain. (See Chapter 27.)

The issues for consumers were the same as back in 1909—taste, odor and "undesirable gastrointestinal side effects and stool patterns." These problems were not solved until a second generation soybean formula was developed based on soy protein isolate. Unlike the soy-flour formulas, these are largely free of the gas-producing oligosaccharides and have eliminated the irritating fiber and roughage.[36-38]

SECOND GENERATION SOY FORMULAS

Soy formulas made with soy protein isolate (SPI) came on the market in the early 1960s despite the fact that this substance did not have a long history of safe use in the food supply. This fact greatly concerned scientists at the Federation of American Society for Experimental Biology (FASEB), who determined in 1979 that the only safe use for soy protein isolates was to strengthen the sealers of card-

HIGH FIVE—THE DIONNE QUINTUPLETS

In the 1930s, reports linked soy formula to the miraculous survival of the Dionne quintuplets. Actually, "the miracle bean" didn't deserve much credit. The quints did receive soy acidophilus milk from Dr. John Harvey Kellogg, but what saved their lives was breast milk donated by women in the United States and Canada.

Shortly before the quints' birth in 1934, Dr. Kellogg discovered that soymilk was a good medium in which to grow the healing acidophilus bacteria that he liked to plant into his patients' intestinal tracts. When Dr. Kellogg heard that Marie, the smallest of the Dionne quintuplets, was suffering from bowel trouble, he wired the quints' physician Dr. Allan Roy Dafoe, sent a supply of soy acidophulus milk and learned that it had helped her problem. Dr. Kellogg wrote: "It cured the quintuplets of serious trouble and keeps them in good health. They have been using it regularly in their daily food for more than a year and a half. Dr. Dafoe writes me that he cannot get along without it. When he stops the use of it the bowels get bad and he has to resume its use at once."

What the immodest Dr. Kellogg didn't mention was that the quintuplets owed their very survival to another physician, Herman Bundeson, M.D., of Chicago. An expert on premature infants, Dr. Bundeson telephoned Dr. Dafoe and provided him an incubator and donated breast milk two days after their birth. In Toronto, members of the Junior League responded by collecting breast milk daily and shipping it by overnight train to northern Ontario. Breast milk was eventually shipped in from Montreal as well. Five months later, the quints were weaned on a dairy formula.

Dr. Kellogg was not the only person to take credit for

the health of the quints. Carnation ads boasted that the quintuplets had consumed 2,500 tins of their milk. The truth was
that the quintuplets refused to drink it.

SOURCES:
Schwarz, Richard W. *John Harvey Kellogg, MD* (Nashville, TN, Southern Publishing, 1970) 123.

INFACT Canada. The Milk of Human Kindness: The History of Milk Banking in
Canada. www.infactcanada.ca.

Berton, Pierre. *The Dionne Years: A Thirties Melodrama* (NY Norton, 1977). 50,
62, 147.

board packages. The evaluators determined that the leaching of carcinogens produced during soy processing from cardboard boxes into
the food stored in those boxes would be too low to pose a health
hazard to adults, but warned that infants on soy formula consumed
up to 27 grams SPI per day—80 times the adult average.[39] (See Chapter 11.)

Top pediatricians were also troubled. Edmund J. Eastham, M.D.,
Consultant Pediatric Gastroenterologist at Royal Victoria Infirmary,
Newcastle-upon-Tyne, England, wrote in a 1989 textbook: "Their
current use has, in my opinion, tended to be indiscriminate and led
to conflicting evidence and confusion among the medical and health-
care professionals. There are strong advocates for their use, backed
by their high-powered sell of the manufacturers, but there are those
who feel that they should not be freely available without prescription and should only occasionally be prescribed."[40]

GROWTH

As soy formulas became standardized, the soy formula-fed babies began to match growth rates of those who were breast and dairy
formula fed. Before the 1970s, this wasn't always the case, and the
cause was identified as a shortage of the essential amino acid methionine.[41-44] (See Chapter 13.) Supplementation of soy infant for-

mula with methionine was eventually required by law. Before this became routine, infants with undiagnosed, untreated cystic fibrosis were at special risk for hypoalbuminemia and edema when fed soy proteins.[45]

Today's soy formulas also include added carnitine, required for the optimal mitochondrial oxidation of long-chain fatty acids, and taurine, a "conditionally essential" amino acid which functions as an antioxidant and conjugate of bile acids during infancy.[46] (See Chapter 13.)

Growth problems have also been traced to the presence of protease inhibitors in soy formula. These antinutrients block the action of trypsin and other enzymes needed for normal infants to properly digest their meals. Although most protease inhibitors are deactivated during the heating of soy formula, processing methods are imperfect and leave many inhibitors intact.[47] Manufacturers are not required to state trypsin inhibitor content on labels or even to meet minimal standards. Nor are they required to warn consumers that trypsin inhibitors have been shown to stress the pancreas (see Chapter 16).

BIOAVAILABILITY OF MINERALS

The American Academy of Pediatrics reports that prior to the 1980s "mineral absorption from soy formulas was erratic because of poor stability of the suspensions and the presence of excessive soy phytates in the formula." Although manufacturers have learned how to better mix ingredients and stabilize their products, phytates remain a problem.[48]

Phytates are antinutrients that bind minerals such as calcium, zinc, iron and copper, causing them to be excreted from the body unused (see Chapter 17). Because soy protein isolate formulas contain 1.5 percent phytates and up to 30 percent of the total phosphorous in the soybean is bound up in phytic acid, manufacturers of soy formula must provide a total phosphorous and calcium content that is 20 percent higher than cow's milk-based formula and in the proper ratio.[49] Even so, problems with inadequate or slower bone mineralization remain.[50-55]

As early as 1967, researchers found that phytates caused zinc deficiency unless the formula contained high levels of supplemental zinc.[56] Even with additional zinc added, high phytate levels in soy formula caused the worsening of symptoms in a child with acrodermatitis enteropathica, a rare disease caused by zinc malabsorption and marked by skin inflammation, hair loss, diarrhea and failure to thrive.[57] Phytates also negatively affect iron. To avoid serious iron deficiencies, soy formulas are now heavily fortified with iron.[58]

In 1980, investigators discovered two other mineral problems connected with soy infant formula: chloride deficiencies and manganese toxicity.

In 1980, 13 infants between two and ten months of age who had been fed Neo-Mull-Soy formula developed hypochloremic alkalosis. The symptoms included lethargy, anorexia, spitting up, diarrhea, hematuria (blood in the urine) and growth failure. All responded promptly to supplemental salt. One infant redeveloped alkalosis when the supplemental salt was discontinued. Two of nine apparently normal infants on this formula were also diagnosed with hypochloremia. Three of four infants on a different formula known as Prosobe had low urine concentrations. The researchers concluded that the chloride content of some infant formulas was insufficient to offset salt losses following mild stress."[59]

The manganese problem does not stem from manufacturing error but from the soybeans themselves. Levels of manganese in soy formula are far higher than those found in either breast or cow's milk. Per liter, breast milk contains 3 to 10 ug manganese, cow's milk formula 30 to 50 ug, and soy formula 200 to 300 ug. Newborns exposed to such high levels of manganese are vulnerable to brain damage associated with learning disabilities, attention deficit and other behavioral disorders, and violent tendencies. Although healthy toddlers, children and adults who ingest excess manganese can usually eliminate most of it, infants cannot because of their immature livers. Because the manganese problem comes from the soybean it-self, the only way to solve the problem is to take soy formula off the market (see Chapter 21).

SUGAR BLUES

Human breast milk is naturally sweet because it contains lac-tose or human milk sugar. Lactose is broken down by the enzyme lactase, produced by virtually all infants, into galactose, a primary constituent of the myelin in the nerve cells. Lactose is therefore critical to the optimal development of the nervous system.

Manufacturers use lactose in the more expensive, milk-based powdered infant formulas but sucrose and corn syrup in the less expensive formulas, including soy formula. Manufacturers play on concerns about "lactose intolerance" to transform cheap ingredi-ents into a marketing asset. In reality, very few infants are lactose intolerant, although many are allergic to the processed proteins and other ingredients in milk-based formula. Adverse effects of sucrose consumption include alterations in insulin secretion and stimula-tion of sympathetic nervous system activity.[60,61]

FAT AND CHOLESTEROL

Soy infant formula manufacturers have also failed to match the fatty acid profile of breast milk. Although the quantity of spe-cific fats varies by manufacturer and is usually similar to those in each company's corresponding cow's milk-based formula, commer-cial formulas almost always exclude EPA and DHA, long chain, poly-unsaturated fatty acids that are crucial to proper brain development. Soy formulas also lack cholesterol, a vital substance needed by the growing baby's brain and nervous system. (Mother's milk is very rich in cholesterol and contains a special enzyme to ensure that the baby absorbs all the cholesterol available.)[62-64]

IMMUNOLOGY

From the outset, soy formulas were billed as "hypoallergenic"—

the failproof solution for babies allergic to cow's milk formula. Dr. John Harvey Kellogg and Dr. Harry W. Miller both claimed that their formulas "solved the allergy problem."[65,66] Advertisers plugged the same message. Loma Linda Food's Soyalac Infant Powder—introduced in 1951—was intended "for infants allergic to dairy milk."[67] A 1960 textbook edited by Herman Frederic Meyer, M.D., of Northwestern University in Illinois even listed several soy milk products under the category "hypoallergenic."[68]

In fact, research showing that soy is indeed allergenic dates back at least to the 1930s. Babies who are allergic to cow's milk are highly likely to be allergic to soy formulas as well. Symptoms run the gamut from rashes to diarrhea, asthma and anaphylactic shock. (See Chapter 24.) In its most recent policy statement, the Australian College of Paediatrics (ACP) stated: "The indiscriminate use of soy formulae for vague symptoms and signs not proven to be due to cow's milk protein intolerance is to be avoided. Casual treatment in this manner is undesirable because it leads to over-diagnosis of food intolerance with potential long-term effects on child health and behavior. Soy formulae should not be used routinely as prophylaxis in infants thought to be at risk for the development of allergy. Soy protein is a potential allergen in its own right. . ."[69]

Soy formula also adversely affects the immune system, causing lower immunoglobulin levels and more infections than breast milk or cow's milk formulas.[70]

Finally, pediatricians have seen lowered antibody responses to vaccinations as early as the 1980s. As Dr. Eastham explained in his 1989 textbook: "They have also recently published data looking at antibody responses to polio virus, diphtheria, pertussis and tetanus vaccine in a group of infants fed exclusively for 5 months on the breast or on one of four types of artificial feed varying in quality and quantity of protein. Antibody levels measured at 5 and 8 months showed a much lower response to all vaccines in those infants fed on the soy formula and the authors concluded that vegetable protein should not be given in infant feeds during the first months of life. Although this has been thought by some to be too dogmatic, the figures are nevertheless impressive and worrying."[71]

QUALITY CONTROL

Quality control problems have caused vitamin deficiencies since the early days of soy formula. In 1990, Loma Linda Foods considered ditching its infant formula division because of "legal liability" problems, watchdogging by the FDA and the fear that there could be future expensive recalls of improperly supplemented cans of soy formula, based on one incident involving a "small shortage of vitamin A."[72]

Another fat-soluble vitamin—vitamin K—has also come up short. In 1968, a seven-week old infant developed a bleeding disorder known as hypothrombinemia while being fed a new soy formula (Isomil). The bleeding ceased and clotting time quickly improved with the administration of intramuscular vitamin K.[73]

Shortages of vitamin B_{12}—another vitamin that is rarely if ever found in plant foods—were documented in the 1950s and 1960s[74] and a case of B_1 deficiency came up in 1958.[75]

In the autumn of 2003, B_1 deficiency made the six o'clock news. Three babies in Israel who had been fed the Remedia brand of soy formula died from beriberi, an extreme deficiency of vitamin B_1 (thiamine). Another eight babies were hospitalized, of which four may have suffered permanent brain damage. The babies were admitted to the hospital suffering from disquiet, followed by apathy, vomiting and then coma and breathing difficulties. The problem was identified after doctors at Schneider Medical Centre for Israel in Petah Tikva (the largest children's hospital in the Middle East) noted that three infants had been admitted with encephalopathy within a week. Epidemiologists examined more than a dozen recent infant encephalopathy cases and found a common denominator: all had been exclusively or mainly fed Remedia-brand soy infant formula. At least 17 babies may have been hospitalized prior to the discovery of the soy formula connection.[76,77]

twelve: formula for disaster

The Remedia formula, manufactured by Humana in Berlin, contained only one tenth of the B_1 that it was supposed to have. A lawyer representing Remedia claimed that Humana removed the vitamin from the formula on the assumption that the soybean itself contained plenty of vitamin B_1. The Israeli Health Ministry urged parents who had fed their infants this formula to immediately go to their doctors to receive booster shots of B_1.[76,77]

PROCESSING MATTERS

Soy protein isolate (SPI), the key ingredient in today's soy infant formula is the product of high-tech industrial processing involving high temperatures, high pressures, solvent extraction and alkaline baths. These processes compromise protein, vitamin and mineral quality and create toxins such as lysinoalanine and carcinogens such as nitrosamine. (See Chapters 11 and 13.)

Soy formula also contains levels of aluminum 10 times greater than milk-based formula and 100 times greater than breast milk, a fact that can negatively affect bone and nervous system development.[78] (See Chapter 23.)

The ingredient lists of most brands of soy formula reveal many additives of questionable safety such as carrageenan, guar gum, sodium hydroxide (caustic soda), potassium citrate monohydrate, tricalcium phosphate, dibasic magnesium, phosphate trihydrate, BHA and BHT.

ESTROGENS

Worst of all, soy formulas contain high levels of the phytoestrogens (plant estrogens) known as isoflavones. These put the infant's developing endocrine, nervous and immune systems at risk (see Chapters 26-28). Although it is possible to remove the isoflavones from soy formula using an expensive solvent extraction process, manufacturers have chosen not to.[79]

Dave Woodhams, Ph.D., of the SoyOnline Network in New Zealand, concludes that the many problems of soy formula lead to

JUST SAY "NO" TO SOY FORMULA

Parents turn to soy-based formula for infants who are allergic to dairy-based formulas because of the lack of other commerical options. Some babies do better on hydrolyzed (predigested) casein formulas, but these present their own dangers, including high levels of neuro-toxic free glutamic acid or MSG. Gerber's used to make a meat-based formula for allergic infants, but cheap soy formula has pushed this alternative off the market.

Homemade formulas are another option, but parents must make sure that the recipes are based on solid science. *Nourishing Traditions* by Sally Fallon and Mary Enig, Ph.D., (Washington, DC, New Trends, revised second edition, 2000) not only offers three whole food-based formulas but ways to improve the best of the commercially available formulas. Fallon's and Enig's milk-based and meat-based formulas are based on recipes given in textbooks on infant feeding published during the 1940s with the addition of recent information on fatty acids and other crucial nutrients. They contain only whole foods and are designed to provide a nutrient profile as close as possible to human breast milk. The recipes are also posted under Children's Health at www.westonaprice.org.

"Soya-based infant feeding should be used *only* where there is a clear medical indication," warns Bernard Zimmerli, Ph.D., of the Swiss Federal Office of Health. "It should *never* be used for ecological or ideological reasons such as strict vegetarianism."

Zimmerli warns that the isoflavones in soy formula have a history of playing havoc with hormones and jeopardizing the infant's reproductive growth and development. Furthermore, he reports increased levels of hypothyroidism and autoimmune thyroid diseases among infants fed soy formula.

twelve: formula for disaster

Finally, he condemns soy formula for the nutritional deficiencies and poor digestibility of all soyfoods, which pose special risks to infants because of their immature gastrointestinal tracts and small stomachs.

Don't feed your infant soy formula. The risks *can* be avoided.

an appreciation of "the immense and apparently inexhaustible subtlety and complexity of nature in the evolution, over long ages, of these foods for the young.

"A recent symposium 'New Perspectives in Infant Nutrition' (Renner and Sawatzki 1993) provides ample evidence of the importance of the minor constituents of human milk. According to the authors of the report, at least with cow's milk, the basic components (proteins, fats, carbohydrates, vitamins and minerals) are very similar to those in human milk and have evolved to perform similar functions (the building of bone, muscle and other tissues and the provision of metabolic energy). If there are any minor constituents in human milk which, in the formulation of a dairy-based formula, are overlooked in ignorance, they may well be partly compensated for by similar or identical factors from the cow's milk.

"The problem of emulating human milk with plant proteins, and other components that are taken out of the role for which they developed naturally, is of an entirely different order, particularly when the subtlety and complexity of the biochemistry of the plant world, evolved for plant functions, is taken into account. In this situation, factors which are essential for the complete nutrition of the infant must be known before they can be provided for. If they are unknown, obviously they cannot be included. Any toxins or anti-nutritive components in the raw materials which adversely affect the infant must first be identified and then removed. If they are unknown or unidentified, of course, their removal will be a matter of chance.

"These problems are inherent in the manufacture of infant formula based on soybeans. The soybean has evolved for the survival of the soybean species, not for benefit of human infants. The process of evolution has bequeathed us human milk for our newly born and young children; the further we stray from that natural standard, the greater is the risk that we will seriously compromise the nutritional needs of the infant child."[80]

Despite such clear and present dangers, sales of soy infant formula have been rising and now represent a 25 percent market share in the United States.

GROWING PAINS

Soy formula should not replace breast milk. And soy-oil implants should not be used to increase the size of a woman's breasts.

That's the word from the United Kingdom's Medical Devices Agency and the Belgian National Ministry of Health. The two agencies have urged plastic surgeons to contact any patients who have had soy-oil implants and to have them removed. The advice contrasts sharply with the message sent out in the mid-1990s that "trilucent breast implants filled with soy oil were the ultimate prostheses for breast augmentation." But ruptures have occurred in so many patients that the only safe course is to "explant" them. Problems have included inflammation, bleeding and the circulation of toxic, oxidated soy-oil byproducts.

In the future women might take their cue from the ancient Chinese. Archaeologists recently dug up a thousand-year-old silk push-up bra with cotton padding.

SOURCES:
Monstrey S et al. What exactly was wrong with the Trilucent breast implants? A unifying hypothesis. *Plast Reconst Surg*, 2004, 113, 3, 847-856.

1000–year old push up bra discovered in Mongolia, *New Zealand Herald*, June 11, 2004., www.livingontheplanet.com.

part three
MACRONUTRIENTS
IN SOY

13
SOY PROTEIN
the inside scoop

Coined from the Greek word "protos," protein means "first" or "of primary importance." We need high-quality protein in our diets for growth, repair, immune function, hormone formation and all metabolic processes. We cannot live without protein.

Our bodies contain more than 50,000 types of proteins, all built from the building blocks known as amino acids. Nine of these amino acids are considered "essential" for humans because we cannot manufacture them on our own and must obtain them from the diet. If the "essential" amino acids are present in sufficient quantities, we can build the "non-essential" amino acids. But if one or more are missing, the body will fail to synthesize many of the enzymes, antibodies and other proteins it needs.

For most of us, protein synthesis breaks down not only when the essential amino acids are missing but also when supplies are low. We also lose the ability to produce sufficient amounts during periods of infection, chronic poor health, physical or mental duress, and rapid growth (infants and children). Consequently, many respected scientists believe we need to obtain many more amino acids than the ones considered essential from our food, and that as many as eight other amino acids should be considered "conditionally essential." These include arginine, glycine, proline, glutamine, tyrosine, serine, cysteine and taurine.[1-4]

Traditionally animal products such as eggs, milk, fish, poultry and meat have been valued as sources of the best proteins. They contain a "complete" set of the essential amino acids in desirable proportions. In contrast, plant proteins are "incomplete" because they are low in some of the essential amino acids. The amino acids that are in short supply in these foods are known as the "limiting amino acids." It only takes a shortage of one of these to slow down or even shut down the body's protein-manufacturing process. In soybeans and other legumes, the limiting amino acid is methionine. In grains, it is lysine. Accordingly, beans and grains are traditionally eaten together to maximize protein quality. In Mexico that might mean corn tortillas with beans, in the Middle East chick peas and pita bread, and in Asia, soybeans with rice. In all cultures, animal foods, at least in small amounts, are added to the grain-legume combinations to ensure a complete supply of amino acids. In Japan that means that the little cubes of tofu are almost always served in a broth along with fish and rice.[5]

BEAN SUPREME?

Compared to other plant foods, soybeans earn a high rating in terms of both quantity and quality of protein. Between 35 and 38 percent of the soybean is protein compared to 20 to 30 percent in other beans.[6] The percentage of protein goes up to 70 percent or more in processed soy protein products such as soy protein concentrate and isolate in which much of the fat and carbohydrate have been removed.

Soy also enjoys status as the highest quality plant protein because it contains all of the essential amino acids. Although "contains all" is not the same as "contains a complete and balanced ratio" of essential amino acids, the World Health Organization (WHO), the U.S. Food and Drug Administration (FDA) and many governments now accept a rating system that puts soy on a par with casein and egg white as a high quality protein.[7]

How this recognition came about is a tribute to the power of profits and politics over the rigor of science.

RATINGS WARS

In 1919, scientists came up with a method of evaluating protein quality known as the Protein Efficiency Ratio (PER). The PER is based on how well rats grow on a specific protein, and the findings are then extrapolated to humans. The problem is that rats grow up faster and furrier than people. These differences dictate different amino acid requirements. Humans have a lower need for methionine—the amino acid that is "limiting" in soy and other legumes, and this shortage causes rats to grow poorly on soy. Accordingly, PER gives soy protein a rating of 70, compared to 100 for casein and 82 for beef. [8]

Soy protein scores only slightly better using a system called Biological Value (BV), which measures the amount of protein deposited compared to the amount of protein absorbed. The highest BV protein is whey (104), followed by whole egg (100), egg white (88), casein (77) and soy protein (74).[9] Other systems in use such as Relative PER (RPER), Net Protein Ratio (NPR) and Relative NPR (RNPR) rank protein products in much the same order, with soy consistently turning in a mediocre performance.[10]

These poor test scores have not pleased the soy industry.

AFFIRMATIVE ACTION

To make soy look smarter, researchers in the late 1970s came up with a system known as the Protein Digestibility Corrected Amino Acid Score (PDCAAS). Scientists have praised PDCAAS not because of its impressively long string of initials but because it calculates human (not rat) amino acid requirements, corrects for digestibility and bases scores on the protein needs of two- to five-year-old children, the human group with the greatest need for protein (other than infants). This system gives soy protein a high rating of 100, right up there with casein (a milk protein) and egg white protein and a bit ahead of meat.[11] With this new A+ rating the soybean seems to live up to its Chinese nickname of "the meat without a bone."

The catch is that PDCAAS was set up so that no protein can score higher than 100, the score of the reference protein. Egg white and casein match soy because they cannot score higher.[12] In other words, C students get the same high honors as the more deserving A students—a clear case of industry-sponsored affirmative action.

In the past, soy always fell short in protein quality analyses because of its limited amount of methionine. Less well known are its other problems. Ghulam Sarwar, Ph.D., of the Nutrition Research Division of the Banting Research Centre in Ottawa, warns us that PDCAAS scores "clearly overestimate the protein quality of sources that contain anti-nutritional factors."[13]

As we will see in Part Four, soy contains many antinutrients. They include trypsin inhibitors, lectins, saponins, phytates, all naturally occurring growth-depressing factors. Soy's protein quality is also compromised by toxins formed during processing. Soybeans today are routinely treated with heat, oxidizing agents (such as hydrogen peroxide), organic solvents (such as hexane), alkalis and acids, or combinations of such treatments, to improve flavor, texture and other functional properties, to deactivate the natural anti-nutritional factors, and to prepare concentrated protein products. These treatments result in lower amino acid bioavailability and poorer protein quality. For example, the PDCAAS for the alkaline-treated soy protein isolate (SPI) is 49 percent of the value for untreated soy protein, though charts seen by the public provide the more favorable latter figure.[14]

It gets worse. Amino acid testing methods used to determine PDCAAS scores do not distinguish between the Dr. Jekyll and Mr. Hyde forms of amino acids. High heat, pressure and chemicals can transform usable and needed L-form amino acids into the potentially toxic D-forms. Testing techniques that could make the crucial distinction are available, but not in use.[15,16]

Such a flawed system could only have been rigged by the food industry.

Soy Protein in Human Nutrition, a collection of papers read at a May 22-25, 1978 conference in Keystone, CO,[17] tells a revealing soy story. The event was sponsored, in part, by Ralston-Purina, a major manufacturer of soy protein isolate, and brought together researchers who had been testing new methods of analyzing protein quality in humans. These methods measure nitrogen consumption and excretion because nitrogen is the element that exists in proteins but not in fats and carbohydrates. As we use up protein in our bodies, we excrete nitrogen in our urine and feces. Researchers measure the amount of nitrogen lost to determine how much protein is used and how much is needed to replace it.

Throughout the conference, researchers expressed reservations about the new test designs, the accuracy of the methods, and the motivation that drove their development. Many seemed to be struggling mightily to find some way, somehow, to make soy protein look better, to make it look very good indeed. One participant came right out and said, "We are mainly trying to help the food industry."[18] The end result—the PDCAAS system—shows that the food industry doesn't care how good the protein really is so long as it just looks good.

Before PDCAAS could be accepted, however, soy had to prove its mettle as the primary protein in the human diet. This required human, not animal, subjects. Ralston Purina jumped in to sponsor a short-term study in Central America entitled "Nutritional Quality of Soy Bean Protein Isolates: Studies in Children of Preschool Age."[19] Although it lasted only two weeks, the study is routinely cited to justify the nutritional adequacy of soy protein. It is accurately summed up as follows:

"A group of Central American children suffering from malnutrition was first stabilized and brought into better health by feeding them native foods, including meat and dairy products. Then these traditional foods were replaced by a drink made of soy protein isolate and sugar for a two-week period. All nitrogen taken in and all nitrogen excreted were measured in truly Orwellian fashion (children weighed naked every morning, all excrement and vomit gathered up for analysis, etc.) The researchers found that the children retained nitrogen and that their growth was 'adequate,' and declared the experiment a success.

"Whether the children were actually healthy on such a diet, or could remain so over a long period, is another matter. The researchers noted that the children vomited 'occasionally,' usually after finishing a meal; that over half suffered from periods of moderate diarrhea; that some had upper respiratory infections; and that others suffered from rash and fever. It should be noted that the researchers did not *dare* to use soy products to help children to first recover from malnutrition and were obliged to supplement the soy-sugar mixture with nutrients largely absent in soy products, notably vitamins A, D, B_{12}, iron, iodine and zinc."[20]

Scientists pinpoint many problems with such studies. Children retain nitrogen at higher rates than normal when they have been malnourished and need to catch up on their growth. Soy or other protein sources used on such children will always achieve higher scores than would be expected from normal children. And protein usage always varies depending upon our physiological state, activity level and other factors.[21] In addition, protein quality differences rarely show up unless intake levels are inadequate because quantity can, to a large extent, compensate for quality. Foods such as soy that supply all the amino acids (although with less-than-ideal ratios) will achieve maximum positive nitrogen balance provided they are swallowed in sufficient quantity. The fact that proteins such as beef prove satisfactory at a much lower level is not plugged into the equations.[22]

Ethical guidelines on experiments using human subjects require only studies of short-term duration, making them essentially worthless. The Central American study lasted two weeks—although the children tested were propped up before the study began with meat and dairy foods for a month or more! [23] (Note that the researchers did not risk the health of U.S. children for this study.)

The short duration of this study was not unusual. In the mid-1960s, a series of nitrogen balance studies to evaluate vegetable proteins lasted only 16 days.[24] And a PDCAAS study on adults was referred to as "long term" even though it lasted only 11 weeks.[25] Short-term or long-term, such studies provide no sound, scientific evidence that people can safely adopt soy as their main protein source for life. Vegetarians and others who choose soy year after year as their principal source of protein are unwittingly volunteering themselves and their children to serve as guinea pigs in a truly long-term, unmonitored epidemiological study.

The results are already coming in, at least anecdotally. Doctors and nutritionists are hearing more and more complaints of dry skin, lusterless hair, balding, poor muscle tone, weight gain, fatigue, brain fog, digestive distress, allergies, immune breakdown, thyroid dysfunction, reproductive disorders and so on.

These complaints are entirely predictable, when one considers the amino acids that are poorly represented in soy protein.

AMINO CHALLENGED: METHIONINE

Methionine, a sulfur-based amino acid, always comes up short in soybeans. Although present, it is so underrepresented that it must be added to soy infant formula and to animal feeds based on soy. Without methionine, babies don't grow big enough fast enough. Soy formula only matches cow's milk formula in terms of growth rates if extra methionine is added.[26]

Studies on adults are less clear. Most establish that extra methionine need not be added to soy protein unless people's total protein intake is so low that they suffer from protein malnutrition. Minimum sulfur amino acid needs seem to be met at a daily protein intake of 38 g and higher (about the amount of protein in 119 g of beef chuck pot roast, 158 g of cheddar cheese or almost 5 cups of whole milk), although some researchers have found that many people benefit from considerably more.[27,28]

This is hardly surprising, given methionine's role as one of the body's most important methyl donors. This means it excels at donating a single carbon atom with three tightly connected hydrogen atoms, the very molecule needed for many biochemical conversions in the body. Liver disease, brain disorders, osteoarthritis, fibromyalgia, chronic fatigue and depression are just a few of the disorders that have responded to supplements of methionine.

Methionine is also the precursor of SAM (s-adenosyl methionine) made by our liver *if* it is healthy enough and *if* it has enough methionine at its disposal. Kilmer McCully, M.D., author of *The Heart Revolution: The Extraordinary Discovery that Finally Laid the Cholesterol Myth to Rest*[29] and *The Homocysteine Revolution,*[30] and winner of the 1998 Linus Pauling Award, notes that diets high in soy protein can lead to reduced SAM synthesis because of methionine deficiencies.[31] That, in turn, leads to increased levels of homocysteine, an atherogenic amino acid which, if elevated in the blood, indicates greater risk of heart disease and stroke. Back in the 1950s, studies with Cebus monkeys showed that diets containing soy protein isolates were atherogenic, but feeding of methionine to the monkeys prevented atherogenesis, probably because of reduced plasma levels of homocysteine resulting from increased SAM synthesis.[32,33] Recently, a study of retired school teachers in Baltimore found that increased dietary protein led to decreased plasma homocysteine and decreased dietary protein led to increased plasma homocysteine.[34] This suggests that a diet rich in soy protein is highly unlikely to be good for preventing heart disease.

Finally, methionine is critical because it is the precursor for two "conditionally essential" amino acids, cysteine and taurine.

CYSTEINE

Cysteine is the instable form of the amino acid cystine, and the body converts one to the other as needed. Healthy blood sugar levels depend on cysteine for the production of glucose tolerance factor (GTF) and insulin. Cysteine is considered to be a "conditionally essential" amino acid because premature and full term newborn infants need it for proper nitrogen balance and growth. The inability of the premie to manufacture cysteine from methionine and serine is due to the fact that the activity of the enzyme cystathionase is low during fetal development.[35]

Clinical nutritionists who test their clients' amino acid status with assay tests see many methionine and cysteine/cystine deficiencies, particularly among people on soy-rich diets. One of the hottest supplements on the market right now is MSM (methylsulfonylmethane), a usable form of sulfur that helps methionine-deficient people heal their skin, intestinal tract and joints. All this suggests that a whole lot of people need more methionine and other sulfur-containing amino acids—much like our smaller furry friend the rat. Humans who boast beautiful, moist skin and thick, shiny hair invariably live on sulfur-rich diets. Sulfur has been nicknamed the "beauty mineral" for it provides the cross links that make the elastin and collagen of our skin strong, flexible and youthful.

The beauty provided by methionine and cysteine/cystine is more than skin deep. These sulfur aminos optimize immune system function and the body's ability to produce glutathione. Cysteine is also one of the three amino acids comprising glutathione, one of the most important anti-oxidants found in the body. Glutathione (gamma-glutamyl cysteinyl-glycine) protects cells by detoxifying harmful compounds such as hydrogen peroxide, free radicals and carcinogens, including the nitrosamines in modern soy products (see Chapter 11).

Glutathione is partly responsible for keeping LDL-cholesterol from oxidizing and clogging arteries. Though soy has a reputation for reducing cholesterol, rats fed soy protein that was *not* fortified with methionine showed an increased total cholesterol and an increased susceptibility of LDL-cholesterol to peroxidation. These rats were found to have low levels of glutathione and also did not grow as well as the control group fed casein.[36]

TAURINE

Taurine is the other sulfur-containing amino acid underrepresented in soyfoods. As is the case with cysteine, the formation of taurine requires active enzymes and working pathways, not yet developed in newborns. Taurine is the second most plentiful amino acid in human milk, a "conditionally essential" amino acid that is routinely added to infant formula.[37,38]

Taurine depletion affects adults as well. Edema, high blood pressure, seizures, macular degeneration, diabetes, poor fat digestion, heart disease and asthma are all linked to taurine deficiencies.[39] Taurine also plays a role in normalizing the balance of other amino acids. For example, GABA levels in the brain are raised by taurine. GABA (short for gamma-amino-butyric acid) is both an amino acid and a neurotransmitter. The gift of GABA is its ability to quell anxiety. Over-the-counter GABA supplements are often prescribed as natural tranquilizers.[40]

The late Robert Atkins, M.D., found that estrogen replacement therapy (ERT) blocked the manufacture of taurine,[41] a fact that brings into question the wisdom of taking any artificial estrogens, including soy phytoestrogens.

LYSINE

Lysine levels naturally occurring in soybeans are adequate. Unfortunately, modern high-tech processing can degrade lysine so severely that it becomes largely unusable. Lysinoalanine, an unnatural amino acid derivative produced during processing, causes the loss of bioavailable lysine as well as cystine and phosphoserine. This dramatically reduces the nutritional quality of the entire protein[42] and in sufficiently large doses, lysinoalanine can induce renal toxicity.[43,44] Infertility from loss of sperm motility, cold sores, herpes and heart disease have all been linked to lysine deficiencies.[45,46]

Lysine also degrades whenever proteins are cooked with sugar. The Maillard reaction—the "browning reaction"—commonly occurs during the production of cereals and grains. Maillard reactions can occur during soybean manufacture when sweeteners in the form of barley malt, rice malt or other sugars are added to mask the beany taste of soy. Because the body finds it difficult to hydrolyze the protein chain that contains the carmelized lysine molecule, lysine deficiencies may occur. And should this undigested protein enter the bloodstream, allergies and immune responses may result.[47]

CARNITINE

Lack of sufficient methionine and high-quality lysine can lead to yet another likely deficiency—carnitine. We need carnitine for high energy, healthy heart function and fat metabolism. It's so necessary for infants, that witty researchers have suggested the nickname "vitamin Bb."[48] Babies get plenty of carnitine through breast milk, and some formulas are fortified with carnitine. However, since we can only get carnitine from meats and animal products, vegetarian moms who breastfeed almost always need carnitine supplements to adequately nourish their babies. Vegans—strict vegetarians who consume no eggs or dairy products—tend to be deficient not only in carnitine itself but in its precursors methionine and lysine. People with low thyroid function, a common health problem among soy-eating vegetarians, also need extra.[49]

NO CLASS PDCAAS

The PDCAAS method does not take into account individual amino acids. Individually, these may be less bioavailable than the various protein scores might suggest.[50] As Sarwar puts it, "The PDCAAS method may give misleading results about the quality of proteins co-limiting in more than one essential amino acid."[51] Although methionine is generally the first limiting amino acid in soy products, lysine, threonine and tryptophan also affect soy's true protein quality. In studies using chicks, soybean meal was found to be

SOY CONFUSING:
SOY FOODS VERSUS SOY PROTEIN

Many people use the words "soy" and "soy protein" interchangeably, perhaps because soy foods are the chief source of protein in their diets. Foods made from the whole soybean such as tofu, however, contain only 8 to 15 percent protein along with fat and carbohydrates. In contrast, fat and carbohydrate are mostly removed from products such as soy protein isolate (SPI), textured vegetable protein (TVP) and soy protein concentrate (SPC). About 90 percent of the soy consumed in the United States comes in the form of such fractionalized soy protein added to shakes, bars, canned and frozen spaghetti sauces, fast food burgers, and other products. To know how much protein you are getting in a given soy dish, see below:

SOY FOOD (per 100g)	PROTEIN
Miso	11.8 g
Natto	17.7 g
Soy flour (defatted)	47.0 g
Soy flour (full-fat, raw)	34.5 g
Soy flour (full-fat, roasted)	34.8 g
Soy flour (low fat)	46.5 g
Soy milk	2.8 g
Soy protein concentrate	58.1 g
Soy protein isolate (SPI)	80.7 g
Soy sauce (tamari)	10.5 g
Soybeans (cooked, boiled)	16.6 g
Soybeans (dry, roasted)	39.6 g
Soybeans (raw)	36.5 g
Soymeal (defatted)	45.0 g
Tempeh	19.0 g
Tofu (raw, firm)	15.8 g
Tofu (raw, regular)	8.1 g

SOURCE: Composition of Foods: Legumes & Legume Products, USDA, Human Nutrition Information Service Agriculture Handbook, no 8-16.

limiting, as expected, in methionine and cysteine. But soybean protein concentrate and soy protein isolate (SPI) were limiting in methionine, cysteine and also threonine.[52]

Specific amino acid deficiencies lead to deficiencies of the amino acids that the body is ordinarily able to make. For example, creatine, an amino acid manufactured from methionine, glycine and arginine, may well be in short supply among soy eaters. It is needed for muscle tone, heart rhythm and cancer prevention. Threonine supplies serine, which is not considered essential, but is easily used up in methionine metabolism and synthesis of acetylcholine and glycine.

In most cases soy would provide adequate quantities of threonine, arginine and other essential amino acids needed for bodily growth and repair. However, all of these are altered by the high-temperature, high-pressure modern processing methods. The damage may not be as extensive as that done to lysine, but it is real nonetheless. These methods—used to eliminate anti-nutrient proteins (such as protease inhibitors)—have the unhappy effect of wasting necessary proteins as well. One protein cannot be dismantled without affecting the others.[53-57]

The bottom line is that the only way to preserve lysine and the other amino acids while deactivating antinutrient proteins is to practice the time-consuming, old-fashioned soaking and fermenting techniques traditionally used in Asia. Even then, soyfoods come up short in methionine.

TWINKIES VS SNICKERS

Farmers and veterinarians know that the way to pump up the performance of soy feeds is to add methionine. Rats fed soy protein fortified with methionine grow on a par with those fed casein according to Protein Digestibility Corrected Amino Acid Score (PDCAAS) standards. However, both soy feed and casein feed fall short of the PER or BV of whole egg or a good quality whey protein because both soy and casein lack adequate amounts of the sulfur-containing amino acids.[58] Both are fractionated products, with soy protein taken from the whole soybean and casein taken from whole milk. Neither serves the human body well. Yet soy and casein are routinely compared in studies touting soy's ability to prevent and reverse disease. Discovering that soy protein is better than casein as a cancer preventer doesn't mean much. It's like designing a study that pits Snickers against Twinkies. Neither offers a healthy option, but Snickers would likely come out on top because it contains a few nuts.

Soy does not. At least not yet. In a recent attempt to improve the quality of soy protein, scientists spliced a methionine-rich nut protein into soybean DNA. The new bean boasts better methionine levels, but the nut protein adds another potent allergen to a food that is already full of them.[59] (See Chapters 24 and 25.)

EGG ON ITS FACE

The genetically engineered, methionine-fortified bean has received sufficient bad press for the soy industry to begin promoting the idea that "soy protein is best just the way it is."[60] The industry now claims soy's inherent methionine shortage as an asset, based on a theory that the sulfur found in eggs, meat and animal products can cause calcium loss and osteoporosis.

The study most often cited to justify this claim involved 15 healthy young people, divided into three groups. All three groups ate foods that contained identical amounts of sodium, potassium, calcium, phosphorous, magnesium and protein, but differing amounts of sulfur. The first group (least sulfur) consumed soy products; the second (moderate sulfur) consumed soymilk, TSP, cheese and eggs; and the third (most sulfur) animal protein from meat and cheese. Those who got their protein from the animal products lost 50 percent more calcium from their bodies than did those who had only soy protein. The soy, egg and dairy people were in the middle. The researchers concluded, "The inability to compensate for the animal protein-induced calciuric response [meaning calcium in the urine] may be a risk factor for the development of osteoporosis."[61]

What is never mentioned when this study comes up—as it does in Mark Messina's *The Simple Soybean and Your Health*[62] and *Earl Mindell's Soy Miracle*,[63] among other books promoting soy—is that the 15 subjects spent a grand total of 12 days testing each type of food. That was just enough time for their bodies to react to unexpectedly high levels of sulfur proteins, but not enough time for the body to normalize and handle the sulfur load. Calcium homeostasis is normally well regulated so that increased calcium loss through the urine results in increased calcium absorption from the gut. This adaptive process may fail to occur during short-term studies but the human body is more than capable of adjusting to the sulfur load of real food, given a proper time frame.

Sulfur is not a problem provided our levels of vitamin B_6 are adequate. Pyridoxal-5-phosphate (the most active form of vitamin B_6) is the coenzyme for cystathionine synthetase, the enzyme needed for proper conversion of sulfur-containing amino acids. It's in short supply in most American diets. The obvious solution is to optimize vitamin B_6 levels, not to cut back on foods containing sulfur.

The fallacy of most other studies linking sulfur-rich animal foods to high calcium excretion is equally easy to find. The majority of the experiments feature overdoses of the isolated amino acids methionine, cysteine and cystine without providing adequate levels of vitamin B_6 and the extra hydrochloric acid needed to process this high amino acid load. Notably, people and animals fed real food have not experienced the same problems so cutting back on sulfur-rich foods is not the solution to osteoporosis.[64,65]

One more thing about soy sulfur. Deficiencies occur not only because soy is short in methionine but because the protease inhibitors create a greater need for this amino acid. The pancreas must use sulfur-containing amino acids when it produces extra digestive enzymes to compensate for losses caused when the enzyme trypsin is bound by trypsin inhibitors and excreted in the feces. This leads to a deficiency of amino acids, particularly the sulfur-containing amino acids that would ordinarily be used for growth and repair processes. Protease inhibitors also affect other amino acids needed for health and growth, notably threonine and valine, which are routinely added to rat and other animal chows to achieve proper growth.[66] (See Chapter 16.)

If consumers are ever to achieve anything close to peak performance on soy protein, people chow will need the same bulking up.

BOON TO THE INDUSTRY: THE FDA'S SOY PROTEIN HEALTH CLAIM

In November 1999, the FDA approved a health claim that permits food processors to label many soy products with the phrase "Diets low in saturated fat and cholesterol that include 25 grams of soy protein a day may reduce the risk of heart disease."[67] The soy industry has taken this claim straight to the bank. Sales of soy products have achieved double-digit growth rates since the FDA allowed the industry to claim that soy products are not only safe to eat but also "health foods."[68]

The FDA bills itself as "The Nation's Foremost Consumer Protection Agency,"[69] and its mission statement ends with the phrase "helping the public get the accurate, science-based information they need to use medicines and foods to improve their health." Yet the agency's handling of this dubious claim suggests nothing so much as an unholy alliance with big business.

The original petition—submitted by Protein Technologies International—requested the health claim not for soy protein but for soy isoflavones, the plant estrogens found abundantly in soybeans.[70] Provided with only weak and conflicting proofs that isoflavones lower cholesterol and besieged by strong evidence of toxicity and endocrine disruption, the FDA had a duty to throw out the PTI petition. Instead, the agency took the unprecedented step of rewriting PTI's petition and substituting a claim for soy protein for the original one of isoflavone-rich soy protein.[71] Because the FDA is authorized to make rulings only on substances presented by petition, this initiative violated the agency's own regulations.[72]

Worse, the FDA hastened the decision-making process by reducing the time in which members of the public could protest to only 30 days.[73] In addition, they disregarded the testimony of top scientists at the FDA's own National Center of Toxicological Research, British government researchers, and other qualified experts providing evidence of possible danger from allergens, protease inhibitors, phytates and goitrogens, as well as the hormonally active isoflavones.[74-78] In the end, meticulously evidenced concerns were dismissed in favor of weak evidence that soy protein *might* lower cholesterol and in support of the widely held—but still unproven—theory that cholesterol-lowering is the key to preventing heart disease.

Although Congress mandated that the FDA obtain "sufficient scientific evidence" of cholesterol-lowering properties before approving any health claim to that effect, it relied almost entirely on just one study—a 1995 meta-analysis by James W. Anderson, Ph.D.[79] Meta-analyses are popular with researchers—and their industry sponsors—who wish to draw general conclusions. Many in the scientific community have criticized the authors of meta-analyses for making faulty assumptions, indulging in creative accounting and for leaving out studies that contradict or dilute the conclusions desired.

Meta-analysts are especially tempted to leave out studies that skew the conclusions desired by the study's sponsor, which in this case was none other than Protein Technologies

International. Indeed, Anderson chose to discard eight such studies. As for the 29 studies that better met his and PTI's needs, they offered *some* proof that substituting soy protein for animal protein would bring about a 7 to 20 percent lowering of cholesterol among hypercholesterolemic individuals with levels over 260 mg/dl but that soy would do *little* or *nothing* for individuals whose cholesterol was lower than 250 mg/dl. In plain English, soy protein is *not* likely to lower the cholesterol of the average person and might even raise it. Meanwhile, 25 grams of soy protein a day has been shown capable of disrupting the endocrine system, with the most immediate effects felt on the thyroid.[80,81] (See Chapters 26-30.)

The health claim that now appears in big, bold letters on packages of soy foods fails to warn the hapless consumer that the benefits are spurious, that the risks are grave and that the public's "number one consumer protector" is not only asleep on the job but in bed with big business.

14
SOY FAT
shortening life

Fats profoundly affect every cell, tissue and organ in our bodies. We need them for optimum energy, endurance, immunity, brain power and health. Fats stave off food cravings, carry the fat-soluble vitamins A, D, E and K, facilitate mineral absorption, cushion vital organs, build hormones, contribute to moist, young-looking skin, and construct strong, flexible, fully functioning cell membranes. It's smart to appreciate fat—and no accident that fats make up more than 60 percent of the brain.[1-3]

Yet Americans demonize fat. Health-conscious consumers scarf down "low-fat" and "no-fat" products in the sure, though mistaken, belief that "less is more." Indeed fat has been blamed for nearly every ill that can befall the human body. Obesity, heart disease, cancer, diabetes, multiple sclerosis, and other scourges have all been blamed on fat.

The problem is that fats both heal and harm. Fats destroy health when they are either bad fats to begin with or good fats gone bad due to improper processing, storage or cooking. Contrary to popular belief, the worst of these are not animal fats or tropical oils, but the refined and processed polyunsaturates that come from plants.[4,5]

Some of the most dangerous of these come from the soybean.

THE SOY-LING OF AMERICA

Between 77 and 79 percent of the vegetable oils consumed in America come from the soybean. This figure includes the bottled oil plus margarines, shortenings and other butter substitutes commonly made of soy oil.[6-8] Soybean oil is the oil chosen for 90 percent of salad dressings, 72 percent of baking and frying fats, 88 percent of margarines and 76 percent of salad and cooking oils.[9] Its bland flavor and cheap price make it the oil of choice in supermarket brands of mayonnaise, salad dressings, frozen foods, imitation dairy and meat products, and every imaginable baked good, including cookies, crackers, cakes, chips and other snacks. Nearly all the soy oil used in such products has been partially hydrogenated—a process that turns unstable liquid oil that is likely to go rancid into a stable, solid fat that is good for a long shelf life.[10]

The chief problem with soy oil is the processing. But because it is virtually impossible to buy a high-quality, non-rancid or non-hydrogenated soy oil product, even health experts hawking soy protein as a "miracle food" steer consumers away from the oil. "Before you look for ways to increase your intake of soy oil, we have to interject a note of caution," warns Mark Messina, Ph.D., in *The Simple Soybean and Your Health*.[11] "It is unfortunate that much of the soybean oil used in the North American diet is the unhealthy hydrogenated type," adds Stephen Holt, M.D., in *The Soy Revolution*.[12] "Soybean oil, if hydrogenated, is *not* recommended for everyday use," agrees Neil Solomon, M.D., in *Soy Smart Health*. [13] Even industry spokesperson Peter Golbitz of Soyatech urges caution: "Preliminary evidence suggests that hydrogenated soybean oil is not a healthful fat, so you might want to limit your intake until more information is available."[14] In fact, the information already available would fill a small library, and the news is not good.

fourteen: soy fat, shortening life

Ironically, the soy protein Messina and his followers revere is the waste product of margarine manufacture—a leftover that was once thrown away after the soy oil was removed from the bean.

UNITED IT STANDS, DIVIDED IT FALLS

Soybean oil is healthiest when left intact in the whole bean, as found in fermented whole soy products such as miso, tempeh and *natto*. The soy fat found in tofu and soymilk is also safe, although phytates, isoflavones and other antinutrients and hormones make these products less than ideal. Organically grown soybeans are definitely preferable in that many pesticide and fertilizer chemicals accumulate in the fat portion.

Few people, however, eat many whole soy products. Average Americans shun them, and health-conscious consumers find that they don't fit the low-fat profile they expect from "health foods." Indeed, soybeans—with 17 to 27 percent oil—are higher in fats than most other plant foods.[15] Accordingly, the soy industry has taken advantage of the public's fat phobia to come up with low-fat versions of tofu and soymilk. As is usually the case when food processors decide to improve upon nature, nutritional value goes down as the profits—from the sale of both the protein *and* the oil—go up.

There's nothing "natural" about separating the soybean's protein and fat fractions. As we described in Chapter 9, it is a complicated high-tech process accomplished by grinding, crushing and extracting, using high temperatures, intense pressures and chemical solvents. During these processes, the oil is exposed to damaging light, heat and oxygen. Rancidity is inevitable so companies remove or cover up the "off" tastes and odors with refining, deodorizing and "light" hydrogenation. Virtually none of the soy oil sold to the public escapes this fate.

Consumers who buy soy protein—an ingredient in numerous products from energy bars to veggie burgers—are correct in assuming that the products contain very little soy oil, but might be surprised to learn that what little remains is damaged during the extraction process. It is not hydrogenated, but it is almost certain to be rancid and tainted with petroleum-solvent residues.[16-18]

THE NATURAL SOY-LUTION

Natural soy oils are a bit better than their commercial counterparts. Small companies are more likely to choose organic soybeans, which contain lower residues of agricultural chemicals. The beans are then extracted mechanically, under lower temperatures, with minimal exposure to light and oxygen, and without the use of petroleum solvents. These low-tech methods result in an oil with greater food value, lower toxic residue and virtually no *trans* fatty acids. The downside is that the oil is far more prone to rancidity.[19,20]

Compared to the volume of liquid and hydrogenated soy oil sold to the supermarkets and fast food franchises, natural soy oils constitute a tiny segment of the market. More accurately, it is almost nonexistent, given the health food industry's love affair with canola oil. The irony is that many health-conscious consumers avoiding the *trans* fats of partially hydrogenated soy oil choose canola, a product also likely to contains *trans* fats even in its liquid form.[21, 22] Unrefined soy oil would be a better—though far from optimal—choice.

RANCID AND RANDY

Whether natural or commercial, soy oils go bad easily because they contain the agent of their own destruction—the enzyme lipoxygenase, also known as lipoxydase—which catalyzes the oxidation and forms free radicals.[31] Soybean seeds contain the richest known source of lipoxygenase, and it is such a problem for the soy industry that whole books have been written about the technologies needed to handle it.[32] The spots in polyunsaturated fatty acids that are most vulnerable to oxidation are the unpaired electrons of the molecule's double bonds. These easily attract attacks from oxygen—and other chemicals called "free radicals"—and break down in a process similar to rusting. Free radicals are solo molecules that are perpetually on the prowl, compelled to mate and break up molecular marriages, leaving hoards of newly single, highly reactive molecules in their wake. Free radicals not only turn oils rancid, but turn *us* rancid. Eating rancid oils sets off chain reactions in our bodies that destroy cells, damage DNA, promote disease and accelerate aging.[33]

GOING, GOING, GONE: THE FATE OF OMEGA-3s

Omega-3 fatty acids are the latest darling of the health industry. Soy oil contains relatively large amounts of omega-3s compared to other commercial vegetable oils, but if the steam and pressure of the refining process doesn't kill them, the deodorizing intended to cover the telltale rancid smells and tastes will. More than half of the omega-3s and some of the omega-6s are destroyed during processing, leaving the oil with a lowered essential fatty acid (EFA) value.[34]

In the late 1950s and early 1960s, the USDA Northern Regional Research Center in Peoria, Illinois, discovered that the omega-3 component in soy oil was responsible for the undesirable odors generated during frying and that it could be removed by "selective hydrogenation." This process uses copper catalysts to hydrogenate the omega-3 fatty acids 15 to 20 times faster than the omega-6 fatty acids, reducing the former from about 8 percent to 3 percent or less. This was the key to the mass marketing of soy oil.[35] It is the reason *trans* fatty acids are in liquid oils, at amounts known back in the 1970s to be between 2.7 and 5.4 percent.[36]

Even though most of the omega-3s are gone, the soy industry considers the remaining ones a big problem. Kraft recently applied for a patent for a process to inhibit the oxidation of soy oil's polyunsaturated omega-3 component in order to extend shelf life. The process calls for mixing the lipids with polyamines, compounds that contain two or more amine groups such as spermidine, spermine and putrescine.[37] Polyamines function as antioxidants, but also as growth factors for microorganisms and cell proliferation, facts that certainly suggest caution.

SOY OIL FATS AND FIGURES

Like all fats and oils, soy oil consists of a mixture of polyunsaturated, monounsaturated and saturated fatty acids. The percentages vary because of plant breeding.

POLYUNSATURATED FAT: Unrefined, unhydrogenated soy oil contains 61 percent polyunsaturated fatty acids, of which 53 percent are linoleic acid (omega-6s) and about 8 percent alpha-linolenic acid (omega-3s), found in a 6.5 to 1 ratio.[23] These constitute both of the Essential Fatty Acids (EFAs) that we must get from our diet in order to maintain good health. The ideal ratio of omega-6s to omega-3s is 2:1.[24] Given that the ratio in American diets goes as high as 20:1 or higher, it is clear that most Americans have far too many omega-6s in their diets, and that omega-3s almost always go missing.[25]

The richest plant source of omega-3s is flax oil—used by many health-conscious consumers to provide omega-3 fatty acids. Flax oil provides 60 grams of omega-3 per 100 grams. Walnut, canola and soy oils offer 12, 10 and 6.8 grams respectively, compared to the one percent or less commonly found in corn, sunflower, safflower, and sesame.[26] The fact that soy oil contains more than trace amounts of omega-3s gives promoters something to brag about. However, most are lost or damaged during processing and soy oil's ratio of omega-6 to omega-3 is still greater than the ratio that scientists consider optimal.

MONOUNSATURATED FAT: Soy oil has been touted for its 23 percent monounsaturated fat, the type of fatty acids found mainly in olive oil and considered to be "heart healthy." This content is actually low compared to 78 percent for olive, 56 percent for canola (if unhydrogenated), 81 for high-oleic sunflower, and 74 for the high oleic form of safflower. Even animal fats have higher levels of monounsaturates, with tallow at 48, lard at 44, and butter at 29 percent.[27]

SATURATED FAT: Soy oil contains 15 percent saturated fat, of which 11 percent is palmitic acid and 4 percent stearic acid. Stearic acid happens to be the chief fatty acid in beef fat. These saturates are not what people expect in soy oil, and soy proponents almost never mention them. Whether the erroneously low figure of 10 percent used in the data banks of the National Health and Nutrition Examination Survey (NHANES) II of the Public Health Service is the result of wishful thinking, a careless error, or industry coddling is not known. However, laboratory analyses provided by Durkee, a fats and oil company, show 15 percent; the USDA reports 14.1 percent; and lipids researchers at the University of Maryland check in at 14.8 percent.[28] The respected five-volume textbook *Bailey's Industrial Oil and Fat Products* also places the average saturated fat content in soy oil at 15 percent.[29]

In fact, the natural saturated fat in soy oil is nothing to be ashamed of. Along with the monounsaturated fraction, its chemical stability helps keep the oil from going bad. Even so, soy oil has such a high polyunsaturated content that it is highly prone to rancidity. This, of course, is a problem with all polyunsaturated vegetable oils, not just soy.

Finally, the polyunsaturated fractions in soy and other vegetable oils may not be as healthful as most people assume. Strong evidence links polyunsaturated oils to cancer, heart disease, inflammation and premature aging *if* they are consumed in anything more than very small amounts. Caution is advised until we know whether the problem comes exclusively from processing and/or rancidity or from the vegetable oils themselves. They don't seem to be a problem consumed in whole food rather that extracted oil.[30]

DuPont took the different tack of hiring plant engineers to breed out the omega-3s and came up with a genetically modified soybean with higher levels of the monounsaturated oleic and saturated stearic acids (both very stable and resistant to rancidity) and an omega-3 content that has been lowered from 8 to 3 percent.[38] Interesting indeed that in public, the soy industry has been boasting about its new genetically engineered low stearic-acid bean—a leguminous wonder offering super-low levels of "dangerous" saturated fat. But in private, it is taking advantage of a genetically-engineered model that is higher in saturated fat and lower in the rancidity-prone superpolyunsaturated omega-3s. The new oil is particularly useful in baked goods and confections.[39]

Another new soybean called "Satelite" (pronounced "Sat–e-light") has a lower saturated fat content and low polyunsaturated omega-3 levels but 40 percent more monounsaturated fat. This variety was designed to cut out most of the unstable omega-3s and help manufacturers reduce the levels of *trans* fat needed in their final products.[40]

The fact that most of the omega-3s in soy oil have either been killed off or never existed to begin with hasn't prevented soy proponents from spreading the good word about soy's omega-3s.

SOMETHING FISHY

Soybeans are not fish. This would appear obvious, yet the presence of omega-3s in unrefined cold-pressed soy oil has led vegetarian spokespersons to claim that it provides all the health benefits—from cardiovascular protection to brain power enhancement—attributed to fish consumption.[41] This claim is both irrelevant and inaccurate. Irrelevant because the only soy oils most people ever eat are the refined and hydrogenated types proven to cause heart disease, cancer and other health problems; inaccurate because the fatty acids in soy oil are not interchangeable with those in fish oil.

Confusion arises because our bodies can convert ALA (alpha-linolenic acid, the omega 3s found in small quantities in soy oil) into the EPAs (eicosapentaenoic acid) and DHAs (docosahexaenoic acid) found readymade in fish oil. Yet most of us are unable to make the conversion efficiently—if at all. The reasons are many, and include widespread deficiencies of enzymes, zinc, vitamin B_6 and other key nutrients; the presence of *trans*-fatty acids from partially hydrogenated soy oils—used to improve the stability of vegetable oils— and a lack of sufficient saturated fat in the diet. Illness and genetic propensities also inhibit the pathways. Vegans and others who decline to eat fish—as well as the breastfed infants of such mothers— consistently suffer deficiencies, as shown in laboratory testing. This holds true no matter how much omega 3-rich flax, walnut, canola or soy oil they squeeze into their diets.[42-46] Only animal sources can provide the elongated forms of DHA and EPA so vital to neurological function, primarily cod liver oil, oily fish, shellfish and also organ meats and egg yolks from grass-fed animals.

TRANS STATES

Most soy oils are never sold in bottles, but as partially hydrogenated fat. Commercially, hydrogenation works. Healthwise, it does not. The culprit is *trans* fatty acids.

Chemical changes that occur during the hydrogenation process create what are known as "*trans* fats." Hydrogen atoms—subjected to high temperatures, catalysts and intense pressure—switch positions on the fatty acid chain. Thus hydrogen atom pairs that once lived amicably side by side in what is technically known as a *cis* formation are separated. One hydrogen atom is moved to the other side of the molecule into the *trans* configuration. Whereas *cis* molecules bend and sway, *trans*-formations go stiff and straight. Because this change does not occur to every double bond in every molecule, the term "partially hydrogenated" is correct, though "hydrogenated" and "partially hydrogenated" tend to be used interchangeably. Fully hydrogenated soy oil is as hard as wax.[47]

Superficially, *trans* fats don't look or behave much different from saturated fats, so our bodies are easily fooled into incorporating them into the cell membranes. Here is where problems begin because, once there, *trans* fats operate about as well as a key that slips into a lock but won't turn. *Cis* fats provide needed structure, yet bend as required to allow cellular respiration, nutritional transport, elimination of toxins, hormone messaging, immune system functioning, and other vital functions. *Trans* fats stiffen the membrane, inhibit enzyme activity, block transport of nutrients and inhibit elimination of wastes. Optimally functioning cell membranes are constructed of a combination of saturated fats and *cis* unsaturated ones. By bollixing up the machinery, *trans* fats negatively affect health at every level.[48]

FAT LIES AND HALF TRUTHS

Soy proponents try to defuse the *trans* fat issue by stating that *trans* fats are present in variable amounts in a wide range of natural foods, including meats and dairy products. True, but not all *trans* fats are alike. Natural *trans* fats do exist in butterfat and meat fat in small quantities, however these don't foul up the working of our cell membranes. Ruminant animals such as cows and sheep convert these naturally occurring *trans* fatty acids into conjugated linoleic acid, a useful fat that enhances immunity and fights cancer.[49] Known as CLA, it is now a popular supplement, often promoted to fight the very damage sustained from eating the unnatural *trans* fats found in soy margarine and shortenings.

The soy industry also likes to spiff up the image of *trans* fats by repeating what "everyone knows" about saturated animal fats— namely that they are "dangerous" and to be "avoided at all costs." "*Trans* fats aren't perfect," concede the editors of the industry newsletter *The Soy Connection*, but they are "the best, and in many cases, the only available alternative" to saturated fats.[50] The Land of Lincoln Soybean Association explains: "Even when hydrogenated, soybean oil retains a 2:1 ratio of unsaturated to saturated fats."[51]

Honest Abe would be less than impressed with the accuracy of that statement. The proportion of unsaturated to saturated varies widely from product to product, with a few going as high as 9:1—a ratio that the industry would surely like to brag about—but with many as low as 1:1.[52]

MEDIA SATURATION

Mounting evidence suggests that *trans* fatty acids—not saturated fats—are what contribute to and even cause heart disease and cancer. Early researchers lumped butter and margarine together—as though they had equivalent effects. This error confounded innumerable test results, and has confused health experts to this day.[53]

Epidemiological, clinical and laboratory studies in which natural saturated fats are carefully separated from artificial *trans* fats yield very different results—ones that the vegetable oil industry has discounted and not seen fit to publicize. Such studies exonerate saturated fats and build a tight case against soy margarine as well as other products full of *trans* fatty acids.

Hundreds of medical and scientific journal articles link hydrogenated oils to heart disease, cancer, obesity, diabetes, immune disorders, birth defects, infertility, vision problems, allergies, attention deficit and hyperactivity disorders and senility.[54-68] *Trans* fatty acids consumed by pregnant women cross the placenta to reach the fetus and after birth will alter the lipid profile of breast milk.[69-72] Because soy oil is not the only culprit, just the dominant vegetable oil in today's market, we will not review these studies here. Corn, cottonseed, canola and other heavily refined and partially hydrogenated vegetable oils all contain high levels of *trans* fats and cause similar health problems.

Trans fats pose such a danger that the National Academy of Science's Institute of Medicine concluded recently that the only safe level of *trans* fat is zero and that people should consume as little *trans* fat as possible."[73] The panel's report has led the Food and Drug Administration (FDA) to move ahead with plans—stalled since 1999—to require food processors to disclose the *trans* fatty acid content of foods on packaging. The initial proposal—widely criticized by such diverse groups as the American Dietetic Association (ADA) to the Weston A. Price Foundation—was to combine *trans* and saturated fats into one category, which would have deceptively implied that *trans* fats and saturated fats have the same effect.[74,75] Until foods are properly labeled, *trans* fat enjoys the nickname "phantom fat" or "stealth fat" because it is rarely listed on food labels and many consumers don't even know that it exists.[76]

Impending *trans* fat labeling is not good news to margarine manufacturers. Accordingly the industry has been talking rapidly out of two sides of its mouth—first saying that *trans* fatty acids are not so bad for us, then adding that we don't consume that many anyway.

FAT-FINDING MISSION

So how much *trans* fat *do* Americans eat? Pioneer researcher Mary G. Enig, Ph.D., set out to answer that question in 1978, and has published two editions of her *Trans Fatty Acid Report,* which currently contains reports on more than 500 commonly eaten foods. In addition, she has released her findings on her website, her book *Know Your Fats* and in several journal articles.[77-80]

In 1990, Enig estimated an average of 13.3 grams per person per day, but with a typical range of anywhere from 1.6 to 38.7 grams of *trans* fats per day. Junk food eaters, such as teenagers who subsist on deep-fried nuggets, fast-food fries, doughnuts, chips and cookies, eat far more. With as much as 19 grams of *trans* fats in a single McDonald's meal and 22 grams in typical snacks, a fast-food junkie can easily take in 60 grams (4 tablespoons) of *trans* fats every day.

Enig's estimates are considerably higher than the American Dietetic Association estimate of 5.3 grams of *trans* fatty acids per day.[81] Over the years, the ADA has been a cheerleader for the processed food industry, and earns money for its journal by running advertisements for processed food. Lower figures also come from J. Edward Hunter and Thomas H. Applewhite, defenders of the safety of *trans* fatty acids in the *American Journal of Clinical Nutrition,* whose sponsors include General Foods, General Mills, Nabisco and Quaker Oats. Hunter and Applewhite offered low estimates of 7.6 grams per day per person until 1984, and 8.1 grams for 1989, with a note that *trans* fatty acids would likely increase by about 0.3 gram per person per day because fast food establishments were switching from tallow to partially hydrogenated vegetable (usually soy) oils for frying.[82,83]

Hunter and Applewhite were not disinterested researchers but paid affiliates of the Institute of Shortening and Edible Oils, an industry special interest group that has provided flawed figures for the *trans* fat content of various brands of margarine and shortening over the years. Applewhite has also served on the payroll of Kraft, and as chairman of the National Association of Margarine Manufacturers' Technical Committee.[84,85]

Estimates of *trans*-fat consumption have also varied considerably over the years because of inaccurate national food data bases, industry misrepresentations, reformulations of products, variability among products of the same type and other factors. Higher figures tend to come from food availability data and lower from food frequency data.[86] This is not surprising in that most people tend to underestimate the quantities they eat.

The Institute of Shortening and Edible Oils, for example, claims that margarines and shortenings contain no more than 35 percent and 25 percent *trans* fat, respectively, and that most contain considerably less. Tests by Enig and her colleagues, however, have revealed that most margarines contain at least 31 percent and that many shortenings contained more than 35 percent. Parkay margarine leads the pack with 45 percent *trans* fats. Enig also discovered that many baked goods and processed foods contained considerably more fat from partially hydrogenated vegetable oils than is listed on the product label.[87] Although the vegetable oil and soy industries have been harshly critical of Enig, she was vindicated in 1993 when researchers from the Health Protection Branch of the Canadian Health and Welfare department in Ottawa measured the fatty acid composition of 100 common food items and found similar levels of *trans* fats.[88]

The last word goes to Enig, who asks, "If the trade association truly believes 'that *trans* fatty acids do not pose any harm to humans and animals,' why are they so concerned about any levels of consumption and why do they so vehemently and so frequently attack researchers whose findings suggest that the consumption of *trans* fatty acids is greater than the values the industry reports?"[89]

15
SOY CARBOHYDRATE
the flatulence factor

Soy is an incomparable gas producer—the King of Musical Fruits. Vegetarians and other heavy soyfood eaters experience so much abdominal bloating, rumbling and flatus that soy is the butt of a great deal of bathroom humor. Unfortunately it is no laughing matter for the many people struggling with health problems who have been advised to eat more soy but cannot abide the consequences to their marriages, relationships, jobs and self image. Such people often ask Andrew Weil, M.D., and other soy proponents to help them choose the types and brands of soy that will give them the supposed health benefits of soy minus the killer gas.[1]

THE BOTTOM LINE

In fact, neither Dr. Weil nor anyone else has completely solved this problem. The obvious solution is to steer clear of soy. Since the average American prefers to do just that, the soy industry has acknowledged that the "flatulence factor" must be overcome if soyfoods are ever to become a major part of the American diet."[2,3]

Accordingly, research dollars have poured into studies with titles such as "Flavor and flatulence factors in soybean protein products," "Effects of various soybean products on flatulence in the adult man," "Development of a technique for the *in vivo* assessment of flatulence in dogs" and so forth. Studies comparing types of soyfoods (tempeh, tofu, soy protein isolate, etc.) and/or different strains of soybeans (hybrid or genetically engineered) in terms of their flatulence potential are commonplace. Test subjects have included rats, college students and other animals. "Containment devices" have included gas-tight pantaloons sealed to the skin at the waist and thighs using duct tape and equipped with two ports. Among the objective measurements have been the numbers of incidences per hour and day; the quantities of gas ejected per incident; the proportions of hydrogen, methane, carbon dioxide, hydrogen sulfide, methanethiol and other gases; even propulsion force and noise levels. In addition, subjective measurements of odor have been made by professional "odor judges."

Despite these fine efforts, researchers have not completely identified the "flatulence factor" in soybeans and have been unable to come up with definitive solutions to the problem.

THE TWO STOOGES: RAF AND STACH

The chief culprit, as with all beans, is the oligosaccharides in the carbohydrate portion. The word oligosaccharides comes from oligo (few) and saccharides (sugars). The best known oligosaccharides in beans are raffinose and stachyose. They require the enzyme alpha-galactosidase to be digested properly. Unfortunately, humans and other mammals do not come so equipped.

The result is that the pair—whom we'll call Raf and Stach—pass through the small intestine unscathed to arrive in the large intestine, where they are attacked by armies of hungry bacteria. The digestive fermentation that takes place always results in gas and sometimes in odor. The precise amount and specific smell varies widely from person to person and also depends upon gender, age and the

fifteen: soy carbohydrate, the flatulence factor

demographics of each individual's gut population.[4] Several reports indicate that the increased availability of flatulent foods cause anaerobic bacteria to reproduce. Eating more such foods results in a "rapid rate of gas production," with the possibility of faster, more explosive results every time additional foods of this ilk appear in the intestine.[5-7]

Although a few people seem able to eat soy without gassing up, "excessive volume" and "noxious odor" are commonly noted in studies on soybean digestion. Infants fed soy formula produce greater

---

SOY BOMBS

ABC News reports that the U.S. Department of Defense is working on a "stink bomb" designed to disperse crowds and to drive terrorists from networks. Developed as part of the Nonlethal Weapons Program, it causes shortness of breath, nausea and panic.

What smells have such an effect? Researchers at the Monell Chemical Senses Center in Philadelphia analyzed a variety of horrid smells ranging from burning hair and rotting flesh to human waste. The two rankest by far were rotting garbage and human waste full of sulfur-containing gases — the very stuff generated in the human gut from soy oligosaccharides.

The Defense Department plans to recreate the two foul smells chemically, but a more natural solution to the human waste smell would be to create it by feeding recruits surplus soy. As yet, stink bomb weaponry has not gone into development. Seems the chief problem to be solved is that of "friendly fire." Whether released by a spray or bomb, it often backfires, so to speak.

SOURCE: Stink Bomb Science: A Weapon of the Future that Assaults the Senses. ABC News, January 7, 2002. http://abcnews.go.com/sections/scitech/DailyNews/stinkbomb020107.html

amounts of malodorous methane (CH_4) and hydrogen sulfide (H_2S) gases.[8] The highly volatile and toxic H_2S has been linked to many intestinal disorders, particularly ulcerative colitis.[9]

Over the years, scientists have done their darndest to find a way to either reduce the presence of Raf and Stach in soybean products or to cut out the entire carbohydrate load. Carbohydrates in soy generally constitute 30 percent of the bean and break down into soluble sugars of sucrose (5 percent), stachyose (4 percent), raffinose (1 percent) and insoluble fiber (20 percent). The insoluble fiber consists of cellulose and pectins, which are not digested by the enzymes of the GI tract, and which absorb water and swell considerably. Unlike other beans, soybean carbohydrate contains very little starch— less than 1 percent.[10,11]

Neither home cooking nor high temperature industrial heating processes dispatch Raf and Stach. They are stubbornly heat stable. However, germination, which occurs during the fermentation process, will dramatically reduce the amount of these sugars, with a complete disappearance of the oligosaccharides on the third day. Incubation with microrganisms or enzymes derived from microorganisms also has this good effect.[12] Thus, old-fashioned soy products such as miso, tempeh and *natto* rarely cause gas but modern, heat-processed products that still contain the carbohydrate portion of the bean (soy flour, for example) create copious amounts. Among the modern processed products, soy protein concentrate is said to produce the least gas because its carbohydrates have been extracted by alcohol. Soy protein isolate (SPI) being almost pure protein is also considered to be practically free of "flatulence factors."[13-17]

In theory, tofu should be a low gas producer because oligosaccharides concentrate in the whey (the soaking liquid) and not the curds (the part sold as tofu).[18] Some Raf and Stach remain, however, and tofu is a gas producer for many consumers, probably because westerners tend to eat such large quantities that even the small proportion of Raf and Stach remaining in the curd are enough to set off a feeding frenzy among the colon's bacteria.

fifteen: soy carbohydrate, the flatulence factor

In fact, science confirms the anecdotes of many soy consumers—that eating a little soy produces minimal gas, but eating just a bit more can result in discomfort or embarrassment. A study published in the *American Journal of Clinical Nutrition* showed no significant increase in flatus frequency after ingestion of 34 grams (about two tablespoons) of soymilk, but a major increase after 80 grams (about one-third cup). The researchers found that as the rate of gas production in the colon increased, smaller proportions were absorbed by the body and more expelled through the rectum.[19] Thus, it is no wonder that soy consumption can so easily become a social problem. At least part of the cause may be inhibition of a zinc-containing enzyme known as carbonic anhydrase, which helps transport gases across the intestinal wall. If carbonic anhydrase is neutralized, gas builds up in the colon. Hydrogen sulfide in the cecum has been reduced fivefold by supplementing with zinc, a mineral blocked by the phytates in soy and in short supply anyway in many soy-eaters' diets.[20]

The question remains of why certain individuals experience stupendous amounts of gas even when eating soyfoods that are virtually devoid of Raf and Stach. Imbalances in gut flora caused by trypsin inhibitors—which inhibit protein digestion (see Chapter 16)—may be part of the problem, although undigested protein itself is not. Circulating levels of insulin, gastrin, gastric inhibitory polypeptide, pancreatic polypeptide and neurotensin are affected by trypsin inhibitors, but do not seem involved in flatulent dyspepsia.[21]

The likeliest explanation is that soy-food eaters who suffer from truly excessive amounts of gas may be victims of undiagnosed soy allergies or sensitivities and/or celiac disease. Obvious allergies to soy include sneezing, runny nose, hives, diarrhea, facial swelling, a swollen tongue, shortness of breath and anaphylactic shock. Delayed allergic responses are less dramatic but even more common, and may manifest as gastrointestinal disturbances, including excess gas. Diarrhea, bloating and flatulence in celiac sufferers result not only from the consumption of wheat gluten and dairy products, but from even tiny amounts of soy in the diet.[22] Soy saponins and lectins, which damage the mucosal lining of the intestine, may also be contributing to gas and bloating problems (see Chapters 18 and 19).

One solution proposed by the soy industry is genetically modified strains of soybeans that are low in the two stooges Raf and Stach. Scientists have already developed a strain known as "High Sucrose Soybeans" which contains more sucrose and less indigestible carbohydrates than ordinary beans. It also lacks the lipoxygenase-2 enzyme that results in soy's famous "beany" taste. With taste improved and flatulence eliminated, it is expected to be popular with makers of soy milk and tofu.[23,24]

Another possibility—not proposed for humans but for animals—is antibiotics. Animal studies have shown that antibiotics destroy the anaerobic bacteria in the intestinal tract that eat Raf and Stach and cause gas, thus improving the smell of chicken coops and barnyards.[25]

FULL OF BEANO

Until such "low gas" beans come on the market, soy proponents recommend that afflicted parties take Beano™ with their soy. This was suggested by soy industry spokesperson Clare Hasler, Ph.D., to a consumer who said he enjoyed eating tofu and drinking soymilk but wondered what to do about levels of gas that were "almost too embarrassing to discuss" and which made him unable to "stand the smell of myself."[26] Beano™ is an over-the-counter supplement containing alpha-galactosidase, the enzyme required to breakdown the raffish oligosaccharides into simple digestible sugars. Sometimes this works, many times it doesn't. Beano™ will not affect gas caused by soy allergies or intolerances, or by celiac disease.

The best all-around solution for people who wish to eat soy is to choose old-fashioned fermented soy products such as miso, tempeh and *natto*. With soaking and fermenting, the content of the oligosaccharides decreases while the levels of alpha-galactosidase increase.[27] The process neutralizes trypsin inhibitors, saponins and other contributors to indigestion along with the gas-producing duo Raf and Stach.

For gas-afflicted folks who are addicted to the taste of tofu or to modern soy products, there is one other solution—a seat cushion packed with a charcoal filter. The medical journal *Gut* recently reviewed this product favorably, concluding that it "effectively limits the escape of these sulfur-containing gases into the environment."[28] *Current Treatment Options in Gastroenterology* further recommended the cushion as a viable solution for "the noxious odor associated with flatus," saying that "the charcoal cushion may improve patients' symptoms."[29] Taking charcoal internally will not do the trick.[30]

FLATUS WITH STATUS

Meanwhile, the soy industry has begun singing its version of the popular childhood song "The more you toot, the better you feel. Let's eat soy with every meal." Gas—they tell us—could be a good thing, and consumers might wish to reconsider their long-standing request for a new and improved "low gas" soy.

As Mark Messina, Ph.D., puts it, "there may be some beneficial effects associated with oligosaccharide consumption. Because of their growth-promoting effect on bifidobacteria, the oligosaccharides

---

GET WIND OF THIS!

Texas inventor Frank Lathrop has come up with the perfect solution for the soy gas problem – a seat cushion known as the "TooT TrappeR™" Billed as a "reverse whoopee cushion," it is packed with a carbon air filter that is guaranteed to absorb odors and stop toots in their tracks. The company also offers a panty liner made with the trademarked "Flatulence Filter.™" Both have been featured on *Regis and Kathie Lee*, in *Business Week*, and in at least two serious gastroenterology journals, *Gut* and *Treatment Options in Gastroenterology*. For more information: www.flatulence-filter.com.

might promote the health of the colon, increase longevity and decrease colon cancer risk."[31] This observation totally ignores research showing that the trypsin inhibitors present in soybeans adversely affect gut flora and allow more pathogenic strains to establish in the intestine[32] and confuses the nasty oligosaccharides in soy with another type of oligosaccharides known as the fructooligosaccharides that are being used effectively to feed friendly bacteria and promote gastrointestinal health. Despite considerable evidence to the contrary, Messina would prefer to believe that since soy is a good thing, then the soy constituents Raf and Stach help feed good (never bad) bacteria and produce only the finest, healthiest gas.

Should this news not inspire consumers to jump for soy, the industry still proposes to benefit. Japanese researchers have come up with a new miracle supplement—soybean oligosaccharides in powder form to be used as a substitute for table sugar and sprinkled directly on foods.[33]

Do hold your breath.

MELTDOWN AT EMISSION CONTROL

Soy eaters who complain that their favorite foods make them gain weight and pass gas at the same time will soon have their prayers answered with a hot, new product named Thermobean. It's a gas-suppressing legume-protein formula that's literally full of beans—*and* the galactosidase enzymes that will not only make those beans behave but go to work. Not to toot its horn, but Thermobean comes fully equipped with added antioxidants and other vitamins, the amino acid methionine, medium-chain fatty acids and flavor-rich spices. Everything needed to fuel a body generator, and provide for weight loss and energy needs.

SOURCE: New gas-suppressing legume protein formula named Thermobean. US Patents via NewsEdge Corporation, 2002.

part four
ANTINUTRIENTS IN SOYBEANS

16
PROTEASE INHIBITORS
tryping on soy

Protease inhibitors—sometimes called proteinase inhibitors —inhibit some of the key enzymes that help us digest protein. The most important of these is trypsin. Because early researchers knew only about the trypsin inhibitors, the terms trypsin inhibitors and protease inhibitors are often used interchangeably, albeit imprecisely. Protease inhibitors have been linked to malnutrition, pancreatic disease, intestinal disorders and even cancer, yet the industry now markets these same antinutrients as potential nutraceuticals that can prevent and even cure cancer.

Beans are the most famous of the foods containing protease inhibitors, but these antinutrients are also found in grains, nuts, seeds, vegetables of the nightshade family (potatoes, tomatoes and eggplant), egg whites, onions, garlic, bamboo, beets, broccoli, Brussels sprouts, turnips, rutabagas, buckwheat, lettuce, sweet potatoes, spinach, alfalfa, clover, apples, strawberries and grapes. Traditionally, few of these foods caused health problems because they were rarely eaten every day, and because cooking deactivates most of their protease inhibitors. The protease inhibitors in soybeans, however, are not only more numerous but more resistant to neutralization by cooking and processing than the inhibitors found in other commonly eaten foods.

For years, researchers put their efforts into finding safe and inexpensive ways to deactivate these troublesome components. They did not succeed completely, but as a result of their work, soy can now be used as an ingredient in many animal chows, although the percentage is restricted for most species, particularly growing animals. These animals achieve normal growth because high-temperature processing deactivates most of the inhibitors and because vitamins, minerals, amino acids and other nutrients are added to compensate for protease inhibitor-induced nutritional deficiencies. Even so, concerns about safety remain.

WASTE NOT, WANT NOT: THE ROLE OF COPROPHAGY IN THE PREVENTION OF TRYPSIN INHIBITOR-INDUCED AMINO ACID DEFICIENCIES

Nearly forty years ago, the rats in the laboratory at Cornell University came up with the perfect solution for the growth problem caused by trypsin inhibitors in soybeans. Their simple, if not elegant, solution involved the practice of coprophagy. In plain English, they dined on their own droppings.

The Ivy League rats' strategy was not a pathological aberration but a brilliant coping mechanism. The rats *knew* they couldn't get enough of the sulfur-containing amino acids methionine and cysteine from their diet, even when their lab masters gave them extra helpings in the form of supplements. What little they got was mostly tied up inside unusable trypsin produced by the pancreas or in the inhibitors from the soy itself. Unable to properly digest and absorb methionine and cys-

sixteen: protease inhibitors

THE EVOLUTION OF PROTEASE INHIBITORS

Evolutionists think that protease inhibitors developed as part of a defense system. Because plants wounded by microbes, insects or mammals produce additional inhibitors, predators will experience slowed growth and a diminished reproductive ability, thus saving the plant species. An even more widely held theory is that protease inhibitors protect the young bean or seed from sprouting before conditions are optimal.[1,2] When it comes to soybeans, the first theory seems more likely. Protease inhibitors isolated from soybean plants have proved incapable of inhibiting endogenous proteases from the same plant. Moreover, tests of the protease-inhibitor activity during germination have been inconsistent, sometimes showing no change in activity and other times showing an increase in activity followed by a decrease.[3,4]

---

teine, they could only pass them out of the body in the feces. What a waste!

Having nothing better to do than sit around and watch their own slow growth—or the scientists scratching their heads—the rats took matters into their own paws. As the researchers soon established, turd eating solved the problem, simply and economically. Whether the rats ate unheated soybeans or chow enhanced with cysteine, methionine or penicillin, those practicing coprophagy grew better than the aptly named "controls." (These rats were literally "controlled" from indulging by the wearing of fecal-collection cups.)

Why did the coprophagic rats benefit? Apparently their poop contained partially digested proteins rich in the sulfur-containing amino acids in the trypsin inhibitor complex that could be properly assimilated the second time around.

SOURCE: Barnes RH, Fiala G, Kwong E. Prevention of coprophagy in the rat and the growth-stimulating effects of methionine, cystine and penicillin when added to diets containing unheated soybeans. *J. Nutr*, 1965, 85, 127-131.

KUNITZ AND THE BBIs

Irvin E. Liener, Ph.D., tells us that soybeans contain two principal types of protease inhibitors—the Kunitz and the Bowman-Birk.[5] First described in 1945 by a researcher named Kunitz, the Kunitz inhibitor is a very reactive compound—at least when trypsin is involved. The Kunitz inhibitor is a big molecule with one active site—known as a "head"—that grabs trypsin, the object of its affection, so quickly and tightly that trypsin loses the freedom to do the one thing it does best—digest protein.

The second type of soybean protease inhibitor was discovered by Bowman in 1944 and described by Birk in 1961. The Bowman-Birk is a runt compared to the Kunitz type, but makes up for its small stature with a two-headed structure and a bit of a split personality, with one head indulging a taste for trypsin, the other for its cousin chymotrypsin. With the Bowman-Birk's two active sites, it is definitely a case of Dr. Jekyll and Mr. Hyde in that the chymotrypsin head is now being used to cure cancer while the trypsin head has been shown to cause it.

Soybeans also contain at least five other types of protease inhibitors with properties similar to the Bowman-Birk. One called the CII has the characteristic two heads, the first with the usual appetite for trypsin, the other preferring the pancreatic enzyme elastase. In the presence of trypsin, the elastase enzyme also helps digest protein. Though the trypsin head of this inhibitor has been shown to cause cancer, the elastase-inhibiting part may reduce painful inflammatory conditions.

Soybeans contain many different types of protease inhibitors because of genetic heterogeneity, with new strains of protease inhibitors emerging as a result of hybridization and genetic engineering. The relative numbers of the Kunitz versus the Bowman-Birk types and the strength of their inhibitory powers also vary widely from one breed of soybean to another.[6] In most soybeans, the Kunitzes outnumber the Bowman-Birks; the reverse occurs in chick peas, limas, azuki and mung beans.[7] The effect on different animal species differs strikingly as well[8] so it is no wonder that after decades of study, the field of protease inhibitors remains confusing, inconsistent and contradictory.

HOT, BUT NOT ALWAYS UNINHIBITED

Heat deactivates most—but not all—of the protease inhibitors in soy. The only way to come close to deactivating all of them is through the old-fashioned fermentation techniques used to make tempeh, miso and *natto*.[9] Otherwise some trypsin inhibitors *always* remain. Processed soybean products retain between 2.5 and 12.5 percent of the trypsin activity of the whole soybean. The average percentage of activity remaining in soymilk is 13 percent, in tofu 2.5 to 7.9 percent (depending upon the amount of remaining whey), miso 0.3 percent, *natto* 0.7 percent and soy sauce 0.8 percent.[10,11]

The heat, pressure and chemical treatments used by modern food processors kill off 80 to 90 percent of all the different protease inhibitors. This level of extermination would appear to be acceptable. Rats, after all, grow well if only 70 to 80 percent of the trypsin inhibitory activity is destroyed, and we know that rats are more easily harmed by trypsin inhibitors than humans.[12]

At best, this 80 to 90 percent success rate is a promise, not a guarantee. The numbers of live protease inhibitors remaining in soy products varies from batch to batch, and investigators have found unexpectedly high protease inhibitors present in soy foods, and startlingly high levels in some soy formulas and soy protein concentrates.[13-18]

BALANCING ACT

The obvious solution would seem to be to cook the trypsin inhibitors to death. Unfortunately, extra heating damages the structure of the essential amino acids methionine and lysine and in extreme cases damages the total protein so much that it is hard to digest, assimilate and utilize by the body. When alkaline solutions are used—as they are by modern food manufacturers—to speed things up, the essential amino acid lysine is transformed into the toxic lysinoalanine. This contributes further to the already imbalanced amino acid profile of soybeans and adds a toxin into the mix.[19,20] Consequently, overcooking soybeans is nearly as big a problem as undercooking. Although analytical methods are sometimes used to measure elimination of trypsin inhibitor activity, they provide a poor measurement of the effects of overheating on the other proteins.[21]

Given the varying levels of protease inhibitors in different strains of soybeans, the lack of rigorous quality control in soy processing plants, the pressure to keep costs down, the dearth of government regulation, and the failure by the soy industry to recognize that this issue should be taken seriously, the probability is high that soybean processing is imperfect and inconsistent. Thus we can count on finding some active protease inhibitors in all soyfoods.

A QUESTION OF DIGESTION

The question is whether there are enough of them to seriously impair digestion.

The answer is far from simple. Human trypsin exists in two forms. Between 80 and 90 percent exists in the cationic form, with a positively charged ion that is only weakly affected by trypsin inhibitors. The remaining 10 to 20 percent comes in the anionic form, with a negatively charged ion that is totally incapacitated.[22]

Thus it seems highly unlikely that protease inhibitors would harm human beings. Why worry when most trypsin inhibitors are deactivated by processing and those that remain bind only 10 to 20 percent of the trypsin in the body? Trypsin inhibitors would appear to be a non-issue, and have been roundly dismissed by pharmacist Earl Mindell, author of *Earl Mindell's Soy Miracle,* who says of the controversy, "It's stupid. Cooking eliminates the trypsin inhibitors entirely. No one, and I mean no one, ever eats raw soybeans."[23]

As we have seen, cooking does *not* eliminate the trypsin inhibitors entirely. Nor do pressure or chemical treatments. Complicating matters further, human gastric juice easily deactivates the Kunitz form but seems to have little effect on the Bowman-Birk.[24,25] And human chymotrypsin is inhibited to a much greater extent than the bovine trypsin used in many studies.[26]

And the human digestive system *is* affected. In addition to the 10 to 20 percent of the trypsin supply that is totally destroyed by the inhibitors, 80 to 90 percent is at least "weakly affected."

ADDING IT UP

For soy formula-fed infants, vegetarians and others who eat soy every day, the numbers add up. Most adults take in a lot less soy, yet even the small quantities used as extenders in meat products, bakery goods and other ordinary supermarket products can adversely affect people whose digestive capacities are already compromised by low hydrochloric acid levels, pancreatic insufficiency, bowel diseases and other health challenges. It may not be coincidental that these problems are on the rise even as "hidden" soy has been slipping into more and more food products.

Worse, the average American may be eating soy protein along with soy or corn oils, a deadly combination that has led to pancreatic cell proliferation and cancer in laboratory rats. Both have been shown to initiate or fuel cancers, and because of a synergistic effect, the danger appears to be greatest when the intake of both is high.[27,28]

MY SOY STORY: PANCREATITIS

Many articles and books praise tofu and other soybean products, and yet, so many of my friends who are vegan and who use tofu and soy milk as their main protein sources look so unhealthy. I have been a vegetarian for ten years and two years ago I tried to be a vegan. Whenever I significantly increased my tofu intake, I started to have problems with my liver and developed occasional pancreatitis.

M.L., Marshall, TX

Soy protein, soy oil and corn oil are all familiar ingredients in processed supermarket foods.

The amount of protein in the diet is yet another factor. Rats fed 0.6 percent trypsin inhibitor in a 10 percent casein diet scored poorly in protein efficiency ratio (PER) tests and had poorer weight gain than rats fed 14 percent casein. Simply increasing the quantity of casein protein by 4 percent prevented the protease inhibitors from blocking protein efficiency or growth. However, pancreatic hypertrophy—a problem to be discussed later in this chapter—occurred to all the rats fed the 0.6 percent trypsin inhibitors.[29]

As expected, some people are far more susceptible to these dangers than others. Animal studies show that a small proportion of calves, pigs and lambs react poorly even when eating perfectly prepared, properly heat-treated soybeans.[30] A good example is a long-term study involving a total of 26 Cebus monkeys, divided into groups of eight, ten, six and two. Low levels of protease inhibitors were fed to all four groups. After five years, there was no discernible pancreatic damage effect in monkeys in the first three groups, whose protein sources were lactalbumin, soy isolate and casein, respectively. One monkey in the fourth group, fed soy protein concentrate, however, was very badly affected, and was diagnosed with moderate diffuse acinar atrophy, moderate diffuse interstitial fibrosis and moderate chronic pancreatitis. In addition, the other showed some cell enlargement of lymphoid tissue.[31]

These and similar findings contradict claims that that low levels of soy protease inhibitors pose no threat to human health.

RAW DEAL

Earl Mindell's assurances to the contrary, people do occasionally eat raw or incompletely cooked soybeans. A few people exposed to high levels of trypsin inhibitors have been hospitalized. In one well-documented case, an individual suffered acute gastro-intestinal illness as a result of eating a tuna salad in which the tuna was "extended" with insufficiently processed textured vegetable protein

(TVP). The Kunitz trypsin inhibitor is a potent allergen, and such extreme reactions are almost always experienced by people who are allergic to soy.[32,33] (See Chapters 24 and 25.)

For most people, gastrointestinal distress from raw or undercooked soybeans is a miserable one-time event that comes from the bright idea of cooking soybeans from scratch at home. Whole soybeans can cook for hours and hours in home kitchens without softening, and readymade soy products sometimes enter the marketplace uncooked or partially cooked. Raw "enzymatically active" soy flour added to bread dough, cake batter and dry soup mixes are good examples. Because consumers who have tried such products rarely go back for seconds, few remain in the marketplace. Even so, some beans in every batch remain undercooked, making the many studies on raw soybeans and their connection to malnutrition, pancreatic disease and cancer highly relevant.

NO REST FOR THE WEARY PANCREAS

Since 1917, researchers have known that rats grow poorly on a raw soy diet, but grow normally if the soybeans are cooked for several hours. Since then, researchers have tested raw and cooked soybeans on a number of other animals and birds and reached the same conclusion. Until the trypsin inhibitor was discovered in the early 1940s, they blamed some unknown "antinutrient" in soy. Then they assumed simple cause and effect, with trypsin inhibitors interfering with protein digestion, leading to malnutrition and stunted growth.

Later they found that they could not blame growth problems on poor digestion and assimilation alone. Studies using predigested easy-to-assimilate soybean meal with added inhibitors showed that stunting still occurred. Researchers concluded that this was not the direct result of poorly assimilated protein but the indirect result of an enlarged, overworked and long-suffering pancreas.[34] Let's look at what happens.

When the level of trypsin in the small intestine is reduced—as is the case every time a serving of food with a load of trypsin inhibitors arrives—the hormone CCK (cholecystokinin) orders the pancreas to secrete and manufacture more digestive enzymes. When this occurs only occasionally, the pancreas responds to the crisis, rests and recovers. When it happens day after day, pancreatic hypertrophy (an enlargement of the pancreatic cells) and hyperplasia (an increase in the number of those cells) results.[35]

Growth depression occurs because the pancreas uses up amino acids that would ordinarily be used for growth and repair processes in order to produce extra digestive enzymes. Studies using radioactive methionine show an increased conversion of methionine to cystine occurring in the pancreas or blocking of the needed enzyme cystathione synthetase. This causes a shortage of the methionine needed for growth and repair. Part of the problem stems from the fact that most of the cystine in legumes is tied up in the protease inhibitors. Cystine tied up in protease inhibitors is not easily broken down by digestive enzymes and in chicks, at least, does not become available for growth.[36]

Trypsin inhibitors also affect other amino acids needed for health and growth, notably threonine and valine. Both are routinely added to rat and other animal chows to achieve proper growth. The extra amino acids, however, do not stop the damage to the pancreas, which continues to react with an immune system response that causes enlarged pancreatic cells.[37]

When the body runs out of trypsin, it must increase the number of pancreatic cells (hyperplasia)—not just their size (hypertrophy). This may occur because the zymogen granules—which contain the precursors of enzymes such as trypsin—are depleted. Trypsin and other digestive enzymes are produced in the pancreas as the inactive molecules known as zymogens to prevent self-digestion of the pancreas. Once activated in the small intestine, trypsin triggers the activation of other needed pancreatic enzymes such as chymotrypsin and elastase.[38]

The extent of pancreatic hypertrophy and hyperplasia varies widely from species to species in the animal kingdom. In some soy-fed animals the pancreas swells quickly, in others more slowly and in some not at all. Rats and chicks, which have large pancreases for their size, are the most likely to show changes in the organ as well as in their digestive capacities. Because their requirements for the sulfur-containing amino acids needed for the synthesis of pancreatic enzymes are higher than animals with a smaller pancreas (in proportion to their body weight), they are highly susceptible to trypsin-inhibitor damage.[39,40]

Though hypertrophy and hyperplasia are less likely to occur in calves, dogs, pigs and adult guinea pigs, these animals *do* suffer from the loss of their ability to secrete sufficient enzymes. For example, a study of calves showed that the weight of the pancreas of soy-fed animals was actually lower in the animals fed a soy diet compared to a milk diet. This was not good news, however, because the levels of trypsin and chymotrypsin were reduced by 43 and 38 percent respectively. Furthermore, the concentration of gastric inhibitory peptide (GIP) was lowered by 49 percent and secretin was 34 percent lower. These are significant percentages and suggest disruptive effects and imbalances throughout the digestive system.[41] Finally, pancreatic damage can be measured in levels of RNA and DNA. Increases in RNA and protein correspond with hypertrophy and increases in DNA with hyperplasia.[42]

Mark Messina, Ph.D., a spokesperson for the soy industry and organizer of five symposia on the role of soy in the prevention and treatment of chronic disease, claims that trypsin inhibitor studies are only relevant when done on "miniature swine because their digestive physiology and anatomy are similar to humans."[43] Messina cites two recently published studies by Larry H. Garthoff and other researchers at the FDA's Division of Toxicological Research and Nutritional Product Studies in Laurel, Maryland. According to Messina, these studies should put fears about trypsin inhibitors to rest because "dietary trypsin inhibitor at levels that once was shown to cause morbidity in swine and neoplasia in rats produced near-normal growth, health and behavior over a period of 39 weeks."

But Messina fails to mention that the supposedly happy little pigs experienced ongoing diarrhea and occasional vomiting and that the study—originally planned as a two-year study—was cut short at 39 weeks, long before precancerous or cancerous lesions would be likely to occur. Even so, there were changes in body weight, organ weights, pancreatic protein concentration and amylase activity. The researchers also chose to deemphasize adverse effects that showed up in the blood work such as evidence of macrocytic anemia. All these ill effects, however, are emphasized in the first version of this study for the FDA and obtained through the Freedom of Information Act. It is most interesting that this study was concluded in 1987, forgotten for more than a decade, and then reborn and published with a more favorable spin in 2002.[44-46]

PROMOTING AND/OR CAUSING CANCER

Whenever protease inhibitors cause cell proliferation (hyperplasia), cancer becomes a distinct possibility. Rapidly growing tissues are more susceptible to chemical carcinogens. Rats exposed to moderate levels of protease inhibitors in raw soy flour show increased susceptibility to cancer, while those subjected to high levels of the inhibitors suffer pancreatic cancer.[47]

Trypsin inhibitors potentiate two known pancreatic carcinogens, azaserine and nitrosamine. Though azaserine is a pancreatic cancer-causing chemical that is more likely to be found in the laboratory than in the average diet, nitrosamine is a byproduct of food processing found in most modern soybean products. Cancer also occurs in soy-fed animals that have not been exposed to known carcinogens. Trypsin inhibitors alone can cause adenomatous nodules on the pancreas of rats, with the cancer rates rising in step with the numbers of trypsin inhibitors.[48-56] Similar cancers, however, were not induced in mice and hamsters using the same strategies.[57,58]

Soybean proponents tend to blame the fat—either the soy oil in full-fat soy flour or added corn oil—but not the trypsin inhibitors in the soy protein.[59] This position ignores the fact that researchers at the USDA—as well as later researchers—tested these variables and found that the soy trypsin inhibitor concentrates had a significantly greater effect on the growth of azaserine-induced lesions than either soy or corn oil.[60-64]

CCK AND THE PANCREAS

The pancreas is not affected in isolation. The gallbladder contracts and secretes bile within 30 minutes of a trypsin-inhibitor-rich soy meal at the very time when the pancreas secretes compensatory enzymes. This suggests an important role for cholecystokinin (CCK), and in rats we know that trypsin inhibitors significantly increase the circulating level of CCK and cause pancreatic enlargement. In addition, the numbers of rat CCK receptors increase with age along with pancreatic hypertrophy.[65-67] Pharmaceutical doses of CCK antagonists have also stopped trypsin inhibitor-induced enlargement of the pancreas.[68] Most importantly, cancer researchers widely acknowledge a link between raised levels of the hormone CCK in blood and the development of cancer.[69,70]

As yet, human studies do not clearly connect soy protease inhibitors to pancreatic cancer. However, short-term studies on human subjects show that protease inhibitors stimulate pancreatic secretions, suggesting that long-term ingestion might lead to the development of lesions of the pancreas similar to those observed with rats.[71-74] And premature infants fed soy formula show increased levels of digestive enzymes compared to dairy formula-fed babies, indicating low digestibility of the soy formula and stress on the pancreas.[75]

FROM FIVE TO FOUR

It may not be coincidental that pancreatic cancer recently moved up to fourth place as a cause of cancer deaths in men and women in the United States.[76] In the 1970s and 1980s, researchers studying protease-inhibitor damage on the pancreas noted that pancreatic cancer had then moved up to fifth place and wondered whether there might be a soybean-protease inhibitor connection.[77-79] The fact that this ongoing rise has occurred along with a rise in the human consumption of soybeans does not prove cause and effect. However, the concurrent increase in pancreatic cancer cases alongside pertinent animal studies is suggestive—and sobering.

Researchers who toe the industry line say that soybeans are the cure—not the cause—of cancer. They roundly dismiss the protease inhibitor-pancreatic cancer connection by pointing out that we are not rats and that protease inhibitors stimulate acinar cell proliferation in animals but that human pancreatic cancer is ductal in origin.[80] This response is simplistic. During embryonic development of the pancreas, all exocrine and endocrine cells derive from common precursor cells, the stem cells. Recent studies suggest that acinar, ductal and islet cells are all highly plastic and able to transdifferentiate or change their phenotype from one type to another. In terms of determining the origin of any pancreatic cancer, all pancreatic cells could be considered potential facultative stem cells.[81]

BETTER SAFE THAN SORRY

Clearly, we must be cautious in extrapolating the results from animal studies to humans. Different animals react differently to feeds containing protease inhibitors, and no animal provides a completely appropriate model for humans. Rats have different growth requirements and growth patterns. Pigs have similar digestive tracts but different growth rates, size at maturity and life span. Primates are closest to humans in terms of growth, life span, reproduction, digestion and teeth, but are furry, mostly vegetarian and able to take food from spoon to stool in a mere five to six hours.[82] Nonetheless, protease inhibitors have adversely affected either the growth and/or the pancreas of every mammal and bird species tested. Whether protease inhibitors alone or some other soybean factor (such as lectins) must share the blame, the human animal appears to be at risk. Safety has yet to be proven.

sixteen: protease inhibitors

No one appreciates the safety issues better than Irvin E. Liener, Ph.D., the world's leading expert on protease inhibitors. In 1998, he pulled no punches when he wrote to the FDA: "Soybean trypsin inhibitors do in fact pose a potential risk to humans when soy protein is incorporated into the diet."[83]

INDUSTRY TRYPING

For years the soy industry took the trypsin inhibitor problem very seriously. Processors tested heat, pressure, microwaving, chemicals and combinations thereof in the hope that the trypsin and other protease inhibitors could be completely deactivated.

Having failed to disarm the trypsin arsenal, the soy industry has regrouped to turn devils into angels. This began when protease inhibitors and other known "antinutrients" were re-labeled as "nonnutritive dietary compounds."[84] This phrase suggested an absence of bad effects—harmless fodder with possible positive effects that had yet to be identified. From there, the industry made its move to support research studies "proving" that trypsin inhibitors and other protease inhibitors have anti-carcinogenic activity.

To date, most of this work has involved the Bowman-Birk inhibitor (BBI). A great deal of publicity has greeted announcements of its possible anticarcinogenic effect on colon, liver, lung, and mouth cancers. BBI supposedly prevents the extension and metastasis of induced cancers and tumors even in animals that are genetically susceptible to cancer. BBIs may even reverse the initiation of cells, a talent possessed by few other anti-carcinogenic agents. This has occurred both *in vitro* and *in vivo*; that is, in test tubes and in the animals. The soy-derived product used in most of these studies is known as Bowman-Birk Inhibitor Concentrate (BBIC) and it has achieved Investigational New Drug status by the FDA.

One woman is behind most of these studies—Ann R. Kennedy, D.Sc., of the University of Pennsylvania Medical School. In 1998 she published "The Bowman-Birk Inhibitor from Soybeans as an Anticarcinogenic Agent," in a special supplement of the *American*

Journal of Clinical Nutrition.[85] The article summarizes the BBI work through 1998 and is extensively referenced with 75 citations, of which 43 refer back to her own work.

Kennedy summarily dismisses research showing that protease inhibitors are toxic agents that inhibit the growth of young animals and contribute to the development of pancreatic cancer. She also ignores the fact that Liener and other investigators have demonstrated in *human* subjects that the Bowman-Birk inhibitor does in fact stimulate the pancreatic secretion of digestive enzymes.[86-87]

She then writes, "Many investigators now recognize that the soybean protease inhibitors are not responsible for the growth-suppressing effects of raw soybean products in young animals. The effect on the promotion of atypical growth in rat pancreata, which was previously associated with the soybean protease inhibitors, is not expected to occur in humans." Most interesting here is her reference to "many investigators" since Liener has gone on record disagreeing with this position.[88] Indeed since Kennedy herself was involved in every one of the six investigative studies she cites, the identity of at least three of those "many investigators" would appear to be "me, myself and I."

Left out of the abstract but appearing in Kennedy's text is the statement that only one of the BBI's two gluttonous heads—the one that inhibits chymotrypsin—might prevent cancer. By her own admission, the trypsin-inhibiting head does induce cancer. Because these two heads are distant from each other in the BBI molecule, it is possible to separate them in the laboratory. The pharmaceutical product that results—known as BBIC (Bowman-Birk Inhibitor Concentrate)—contains a greatly reduced number of trypsin inhibitors and increased numbers of chymotrypsin inhibitors.[89] Whether its safety and efficacy will pan out over the long run is unknown. What's not in doubt is that the BBIC is very different from the two-headed parent molecules that live in soy foods.

Kennedy acknowledges this fact. "There are many reasons for using a BBI-containing preparation rather than the whole soybeans as an anticarcinogenic agent: There are several agents in soybeans, soybean flour, and various commercial preparations of soybeans that can enhance the development of cancer. These compounds are removed from BBIC . . . Normally, there is far more trypsin inhibitor activity than chymotrypsin inhibitor activity in raw soybeans. . . The very low trypsin inhibitor activity in BBIC is presumably the reason that even very high doses have not resulted in histopathologic alterations in rat pancreata in the Kennedy laboratory or at SRI."[90]

In other words, do not eat soyfoods if you want to keep a healthy pancreas and reduce your risk of cancer! Yet one paragraph later Kennedy states that "the amount of protease inhibitor activity from soybeans in the traditional Japanese diet could account for a decreased cancer risk" and helpfully cites levels of protease inhibitor activity in tofu and other soyfoods.[91] And so she goes, courting and kowtowing to an industry that sells soyfoods now, but which hopes to profit mightily from a patented soy-derived drug in the future. That the one could be touted to cure the cancer caused by the other is unstated but obvious.

BBIC may or may not prove to be a useful drug. BBI as it exists in tofu and other soyfoods is *not* a viable cancer-preventing nutraceutical. Such claims represent wishful thinking, gullibility, ignorance or—deception.

THEY CAN'T BE DIFFERENT, THEY SHOULDN'T BE DIFFERENT

Monsanto claims that its Roundup Ready GM soybean is substantially equivalent to the conventional soybean—hence safe. In fact, tests showed that concentrations of trypsin inhibitors and lectins (another antinutrient) were significantly higher in the toasted GM soybean. And unlike the antinutrients in the conventional soybean, those in the GM strain were stubbornly resistant to deactivation by a heat treatment known as "toasting."

Monsanto took this bad news to mean that the GM beans had not been properly cooked and asked for retreatment of the sample. Further heating, however, widened the difference even more. The logical conclusion would be that substantial difference exists between the GM and conventional soybeans and that the GM soybean is more likely to cause digestive distress and growth problems in humans and animals. Monsanto, however, concluded that the second toasting was still not enough and toasted twice further until they got the result they wanted, namely that *all* proteins were denatured and inactivated. At this point, most of the soy's protein value was also destroyed, but it gave Monsanto the proof it needed to conclude that where trypsin inhibitors and lectins were concerned, GM and normal soybeans were equivalent.

SOURCE: Kawata, Masaharu. Monsanto's dangerous logic as seen in the application documents submitted to the Health Ministry of Japan. Third World Biosafety Information Service, July 28, 2003. www.organicconsumers.org.

17

PHYTATES
ties that bind

Phytates are natural compounds found in beans, grains and other seeds that serve two primary functions: they prevent premature germination and they store the phosphorous that a plant needs to grow when the seed begins to sprout. Because phytates stop oxidative damage such as discoloration and decomposition, food processing companies use them as preservatives.[1-4]

Phytates are valuable plant components that allow humans to store seeds safely over the winter, but a potential problem if you want to eat those seeds, grains and beans. Also known as phytic acid or inositol hexaphosphate (IP6), phytates incapacitate the life force by binding tightly with minerals such as iron, zinc, calcium and magnesium.

In the human body, this means good news and bad. Phytates tie up toxic metals such as cadmium, but also needed ones like zinc and calcium. Iron is a special case, essential for health and growth, but toxic in excess. Phytates are a leading cause of poor growth, anemia, immune system incompetence and other health woes in Third World countries where plant-based diets are the norm and mineral deficiencies common but have potential health benefits for well-fed omnivores when used for short-term detoxification.[5-8]

Finally, phytates constitute the main source of phosphorous in grains and beans. Although it is widely assumed that these plant foods contain plenty of phosphorous for growth, anywhere from 50 to 75 percent is bound up in the phytates and not readily bioavailable.[9] Inefficient utilization can result in serious nutritional and environmental consequences. Farmers raising animals on corn and soybean-based diets must give them phosphate supplements to ensure they grow properly. Meanwhile, the undigested phytate excreted in the manure can result in serious waste disposal problems. Excess phosphorous will accumulate in the soil if manure from factory-fed animals is applied repeatedly as a fertilizer while runoff from pastures and croplands with elevated soil phosphorous levels can contaminate surface water, lakes and streams.[10,11]

PROCESSING MATTERS

The phytates in soybeans are plentiful and hardy—more so than in any other legumes. Soybeans contain three times the level of phytates as mung beans and four times more than chickpeas,[12] and can withstand heat, harsh field conditions, transportation and storage environments.[13] They can be rendered relatively harmless *only* by old-fashioned soaking and fermenting processes that enlist the enzyme phytase and replicate what happens when seeds are planted in warm, moist soil. Miso cultured for a year or more loses nearly all its phytate content, but tempeh, which is fermented over a much shorter period, only reduces its phytates by about half. Heat, pressure cooking and home cooking are far less effective and likely to kill the food before the phytates. Tofu, soymilk and all the modern soyfoods such as soy protein isolate (SPI) and textured vegetable protein (TVP) carry their baggage of phytates mostly intact, putting formula-fed infants, vegetarians and other high consumers of soybeans at risk for mineral deficiencies.[14-19]

Although modern soy processing techniques do not remove

phytates, the technology *does* exist to remove the phytates from these products. Accordingly, leading scientists have strongly recommended that soy infant formula be cleared of all phytates.[20] Several technologies are available, including using the enzyme phytase to hydrolyze the phytate, ultrafiltration techniques and ion-exchange chromatography.[21,22] Instead, the soy industry prefers the cheaper solution of stemming the damage by loading up their products with cheap forms of zinc, iron and calcium as a compensatory measure. They are required to do this by law for soy formula, and are doing so voluntarily for soymilk and some other products as well. The addition of calcium has immeasurably helped the marketing of soy milk as a "calcium-rich" replacement for cow's milk. This fortification tacitly acknowledges the inadequate nutritional profile of natural soy products as well as the seriousness of the phytate problem.

IRON-POOR BLOOD

Phytates cause iron deficiencies. Without iron, the hemoglobin in our blood cannot adequately carry oxygen, leading to anemia. This is a major global problem both in Third World countries where people do not have enough meat to eat and in western countries where more and more people are choosing not to eat it. Even minor iron deficiencies can lead to fatigue, lethargy, poor athletic performance, a weakened immune system and learning disabilities. Iron deficiencies also affect the thyroid by reducing the output of thyroid hormone, which in turn leads to lower body temperature, lethargy and weight gain. Soy foods also contain goitrogens, dishing a double whammy to the thyroid (see Chapter 27).

The natural amount of phytate found in soy protein is 4.9 to 8.4 mg per gram. These phytates are so strong that they dramatically inhibit iron absorption as long as phytates levels remain above 0.3 mg per gram. Reduced to less than 0.01 mg per gram, iron absorption increases four to five times. Even with that tiny bit of phytate remaining, iron absorption from soy protein is only half of that of egg whites.[23]

Iron absorption from regular soy infant formula is 27 percent compared to 65 percent from human milk, 60 percent from whey formula and 46 percent from casein formula. Phytate content must be reduced by at least 83 percent for iron absorption to increase significantly and must be removed completely for a pronounced effect.[24] Bioavailability of iron also improves if ascorbic acid levels are increased in the formula.[25]

Although meat eaters would not expect to have difficulties absorbing iron, people who eat hamburgers made with textured soy protein extenders at ratios of 3:1 and 2:1 lose 61 percent and 53 percent respectively of their ability to absorb iron.[26] Most fast food hamburgers and some supermarket frozen and canned meat products contain such extenders.

The risks for vegetarians are higher. A study carried out in China compared Buddhist vegetarians who ate soyfoods as their main source of protein to controls who ate meat. The amount of iron in both diets was similar and even higher among the female vegetarians, but the soy-eating vegetarians assimilated their iron poorly. Although the men did not suffer from iron deficiency, the women did. Thirty percent were diagnosed as anemic, and 50 percent as iron deficient—twice the levels of the non-vegetarian women. The researchers concluded that a "diet rich in soy and restricted in animal foods is limited in bioavailable iron" and "promotes iron deficiency."[27] Summing up this study in the *Townsend Letter for Doctors and Patients*, Alan Gaby, M.D., advised vegetarians who eat a lot of soy to "be screened for iron deficiency and given iron supplements or dietary recommendations when necessary."[28]

Had those soy foods been fermented, the phytates might have had a minimal effect. A Chinese study of 437 children carried out over a period of six months found that the incidence of iron deficiency anemia decreased from 21.7 to 1.25 percent after switching to old-fashioned fermented forms of soy.[29]

In addition to causing fatigue and other typical problems, iron deficiencies may lead to increased absorption of the heavy metal lead which, in turn, interferes with brain and nervous system function.[30] Making matters worse, phytates also latch onto zinc and other essential brain minerals. Because deficiencies of any of these minerals facilitate displacement by toxic metals—iron by lead, zinc by cadmium[31]—it is most interesting that phytates, which are a major cause of the problem, are now being used to chelate unwanted minerals out of the body.

SINKING ZINC

Infants and adults also suffer when phytates block the absorption of zinc. Growth, immune system functioning, wound healing, mental health, intelligence, digestion, blood sugar regulation, thyroid function, weight, sex hormones, and skin are all adversely affected by zinc deficiency. As a component of more than 300 enzymes, zinc affects every function in the body. Infants who need zinc for proper growth and brain development are particularly susceptible.

Zinc is far more easily absorbed from the newer soy-protein-based infant formulas than in the old soy flour formulas, but markedly less than from breast milk or cow's milk formulas. However, when phytates are removed from the soy formula, zinc absorption shoots up an impressive 47 percent. Bo Lonnerdal, Ph.D., of the University of California at Davis, a leading expert on mineral absorption, concludes, "We would suggest that rather than substantially increasing zinc supplementation for soy formula, reduction of phytate content using new technological processes may be preferable." The cheaper, easier solution of adding more zinc has a downside because too much zinc interferes the absorption of other needed trace minerals such as iron and copper.[32]

Researchers have found victims of zinc deficiency among preschoolers in China who were raised on diets rich in phytic acid and fiber. Though their diets were marginal in zinc, poor absorption aggravated matters considerably, leading to stunted growth, poor appetite, pica (a tendency to eat dirt) and other complaints.[33]

Defenders of phytates suggest that fiber, not the phytates, ought to take the rap, but research does not support this contention. A 63-day study of young men confined to a metabolic ward—so that the types and quantities of food they ate could be strictly controlled—showed that the average zinc absorption rate was 33.8 percent, and this absorption was not affected by cellulose, a source of fiber. The same men absorbed only half as much zinc or 17.5 percent when phytate was added to their diets. The researchers concluded, "Daily intake of a high level of phytate could result in zinc deficiency despite recommended intake of dietary zinc."[34] This is true of rats and other animals as well. Chicken meal and other animal protein sources consistently and significantly out-perform soy feeds in terms of zinc absorption. When phytate is removed, however, zinc and copper absorption both improve.[35,36] Similarly, the addition of phytase (the enzyme that digests phytates) to soy feed enhances the assimilation of zinc.[37]

Phytates form tight complexes with zinc in the upper GI tract. These are virtually insoluble at a pH of 6, which is the approximate pH of the duodenum and the upper jejunum of the small intestine.[38] Matters improve when animal protein, particularly beef, is added to high-phytate soy meals. Meat somehow acts as an "antiphytate," perhaps because of the presence of sulfur-containing amino acids, which are in notably short supply in soy. Absorption decreases when soy protein extenders are added to hamburgers, although soy added to chicken seems to have little effect. When soy flour is added to white bread, zinc absorption goes down. Soy flour has no effect when added to whole wheat bread, which itself contains phytates that inhibit zinc absorption.[39,40]

The fact that soy protein is difficult to digest may be another confounding factor. Infant monkeys find it easier to absorb zinc from soy formulas in which the soy protein has been hydrolyzed (partially digested).[41] Modern processing methods may also deserve some of the blame. The Maillard reaction—the browning that occurs when protein and sugar combinations are subjected to intense heat treatment—can also inhibit zinc.[42]

Studies indicate that zinc absorption from soy foods worsens when calcium is present. To compensate, extra zinc must be added.[43,44] Thus, calcium-enriched soy infant formulas and soy milks sold in supermarkets and health food stores might worsen the health of people who already have marginal zinc status. However, researchers at the Fomon Infant Nutrition Unit at Iowa State University disagree, positing that high levels of added calcium will keep the phytates sufficiently distracted so that some of the zinc can be absorbed.[45]

CALCIUM AND OTHER MINERALS

Phytates take their toll on other minerals as well, as shown by a study of breastfeeding mothers in the Kathmandu region of Nepal. Although these women took in more copper, similar amounts of zinc, less iron, and less selenium than American lactating women, their stores of copper, zinc, iron and selenium were *all* markedly lower. High levels of phytates from whole wheat bread in the Nepalese diet took the blame.[46] This study also makes it apparent that while foods high in phytate are often high in zinc, the levels of zinc rarely suffice to offset the decrease in absorption.

Calcium too is affected by phytates. Although the soy industry promotes soy milk as an excellent source of calcium, even spokesperson Mark Messina, Ph.D., agrees that the calcium is less bioavailable than in milk and green leafy vegetables.[47] Calcium absorption from fortified soy milk is about 75 percent compared to cow's milk.[48]

Not all the studies agree that phytate results in loss of calcium availability. Rats absorb calcium well from soy flour, but humans are different. Rats produce phytase, an enzyme that hydrolyzes phytates to inositol and phosphoric acid, thereby removing the chelating properties of phytates.[49] Calcium levels may also be lower in soy products because phytates are especially likely to form complexes with calcium and magnesium during processing at alkaline pHs.[50]

Curiously, most of the studies on calcium and phytates concern its effect on zinc, with some researchers concluding that calcium is absorbed at the expense of zinc and others saying that it sacrifices itself to prevent zinc deficiencies.[51,52] Whether calcium dominates or submits to phytate abuse, one thing is clear—at least one important mineral is tied up in knots.

PHY FUTURES

Phytates fascinate biochemists and cell biologists. Once scorned as potent antinutrients that should be eliminated at all costs, phytates now receive praise as "highly charged antioxidants" able to scavenge free radicals and chelate unwanted metals such as iron, cadmium, zinc and calcium.[53-57] Curiously, most of this recent pro-phytate literature claims that phytates were once thought to be "inert." "Inertia" hardly describes the activity seen in scores of studies carried out over the past century showing that phytates actively bind needed minerals thereby contributing to malnutrition and disease. Perhaps "inertia" is perceived by the soy industry as a necessary, intermediate and neutral stage between the phytate's earlier reputation as an actively bad antinutrient and its recent rebirth as a metabolically active, powerful, "all natural," safe and profitable pharmaceutical.

To date, most of the research has centered on the phytate as a chelator of excess iron. The problem with unusable iron is that it doesn't just passively wait for the right opportunity to serve, but causes oxidizing, a form of "rusting" in the body. When phytates grab this iron and usher it out of the body, they serve useful functions as "antioxidants" that may serve in the fight against cancer, heart disease, diabetes and neurogenerative diseases such as Alzheimer's disease, ALS and Parkinson's disease.

PHYT-ING CANCER

Phytates protect the body from iron-induced as well as other causes of cell injury, which, in turn could lead to DNA damage, cell proliferation and cancer. As cancer fighters, phytates have decreased cell proliferation, brought about cell differentiation, increased natural killer (NK) cell activity and diminished a variety of experimental tumors in the laboratory. No single mechanism has been found. The data point towards the involvement of signal transduction pathways, cell cycle regulatory genes, differentiation genes, oncogenes and perhaps, tumor suppressor genes. Hormones do not appear to be involved.[58-61]

Working under the assumption that excess iron promotes DNA damage in the colon and may cause colon cancer, researchers damaged the colons, livers and small intestines of pigs by feeding them

PHYTATES AND TRADITION

Traditional preparation of grains, legumes and other seeds involves sprouting, soaking and long sourdough leavening, methods that get rid of phytates and other antinutrients in grains. At least one culture follows a tradition that seems to recognize both the dangers and the benefits of phytates—that is the Hebrew culture.

The Hebrews ate leavened bread most of the year. But during the period preceding the feast of Passover, they removed all the leaven from their houses and ate only phytate-rich unleavened bread. The period before feast days, especially in the early spring, was a natural time for fasting, a practice that encourages detoxification. The addition of unleavened bread to the diet at such a time might have been a very effective way to rid the body of any heavy metals through the action of phytic acid.

But unleavened bread was only consumed for a short period of time. Most of the year, the Hebrews consumed naturally leavened (fermented) bread with the phytate content removed, so that deficiencies of beneficial minerals would not occur.

high-iron diets. They then gave the pigs phytates and proved that phytates could indeed take care of the acute iron overload.[62] Phytates have also been used to prevent the type of damage to the crypts of cells that have been identified as intermediate biomarkers for colon cancer.[63,64] Similar experiments on rats and mice suggest that phytates might also lower breast cancer risk or reverse it, at least in the early stages.[65,66] Cancers of the liver, blood, lung, skin and soft tissue have also responded in various degrees to phytate therapy.[67-72]

Although most researchers have credited the phytates' antioxidant and iron-binding ability, phytates might also fight cancer by binding the zinc and magnesium needed for cell proliferation, leading to decreased tumor sizes and a slowing down or even halting of cancerous growth.[73,74] Common sense suggests that this would appear to be a short-term, short-sighted solution in that zinc and magnesium deficiencies are epidemic in America and both minerals are vital for normal body function.

Phytates have performed impressively in many studies, but not all. A Japanese team, for example, found that phytates showed no inhibitory effect on the initiation of cancer.[75]

PHYT-ING HEART DISEASE

Excess iron also plays a role in the oxidation of LDL-cholesterol and has been associated with heart attacks and strokes. Phytate may stem such oxidative damage. It may inhibit the platelet clotting that is a key factor in thrombosis and atherosclerosis, protect the myocardium of the heart from ischemic damage and reperfusion injury, help cure hyperlipidemia and diabetes, and contribute to the lowering of cholesterol.[76-78]

PUMPING IRON

Although toxic iron loads can contribute to many diseases, the problem of iron overload does not come from eating meat, which is rich in the absorbable, useful form known as heme iron, but from the non-heme iron in "enriched" flour, cereals, fortified soy foods and most vitamin and mineral supplements. Synthetic, inorganic non-heme iron is poorly utilized and accumulates in the body, contributing to cancer, heart disease, neurodegenerative diseases, infections and other ailments. Men begin accumulating non-heme forms of iron shortly after puberty. Women rarely start accumulating it until they stop menstruating.[79]

CASTING STONES

Finally, phytates may be used to treat hypercalciuria—the dumping of calcium in the urine—a condition associated with kidney stone formation.[80] Phytates are certainly skilled at reducing the intestinal absorption of calcium, but the phytates had best not come from soy foods, which are sky high in oxalates, themselves a risk factor for kidney stones (see Chapter 20). Phytates may actually be a very poor food for the kidneys. Even low doses of a Japanese soy-based "natural food additive" called *daiichi* caused calcification and necrosis of the renal papillae, which are the pointy tips of the pyramidal structures of the brown, inner region of the kidney known as the medulla.[81]

SCI-PHY

The soy industry has heavily publicized the most promising of the phytate studies, and although the phytates in wheat, rice or other beans would do as well, has urged consumers to eat lots of soy foods. Inositol hexaphosphate—a ten-dollar word for phytic acid, the active ingredient of phytates—is a hot new over-the-counter health food store supplement said to reduce cell proliferation, increase differentiation of malignant cells and induce their return to normal.

Such products may have valid pharmaceutical applications, but should never be used casually or for long periods of time. Researchers who have compared purified phytates to phytates in foods such as bran or beans have found that the foods do not have the same beneficial effects.[82] As A.M. Shamsuddin, Ph.D., of the University of Maryland, puts it, "For cancer prevention, prophylactic intake of

IP6 (phytate) may be not only more effective, but more practical than gorging on large quantities of fiber."[83]

The laboratory scientists who have achieved promising results preventing and curing cancer and other diseases using phytates have almost always worked with carefully measured doses of purified phytates. They administer these purified phytates by tube feeding, injection or in drinking water to ensure better control over the levels of metabolically active phytates, to speed up the rate of absorption, and to increase the likelihood that the right toxic minerals will be bound and removed from the body. Otherwise phytates form insoluble complexes with many needed minerals.[84,85]

Without tight levels of control, faith in phytates as the cure-all for cancer and other disease is unwarranted and represents wishful thinking. Decades of research on the phytates in real foods have shown that phytates are antinutrients—more likely to contribute to disease than prevent it.

MY SOY STORY: PHYT-ING OSTEOPOROSIS

I had an interesting experience with soy overconsumption. I am a 47-year-old male. I have always thought of myself as being in excellent health. I'm a vegetarian who occasionally eats fish and eggs and I also get a lot of exercise, both aerobic and strength training. Several years ago, I began to consume huge quantities of soy and soy products: soy beans, soy meat substitutes, soy milk, the whole thing.

Recently, I had an extensive series of blood tests, just out of curiosity. I was shocked to find out that my parathyroid hormone (PTH) level was 274.0 (the normal range was 12.0-72.0). My doctor told me to stop eating soy and to take calcium supplements with vitamin D. I retested several months later and my PTH was back to normal.

I can only conclude that all the soy I was consuming was interfering with my calcium absorption and that my parathyroid glands were telling my body to extract calcium from my bones so that there would be enough calcium in my blood. Also, on these tests my levels of T3 and T4 were on the low end of "normal."

It seems frightening that we are exposed to so much pro-soy propaganda. I certainly fell for it. If I hadn't had those blood tests, I'd still be practically living on soy, and I'd be well on my way to developing osteoporosis.

G.S., Seattle, WA

18
LECTINS
glutins for punishment

Lectins are proteins with a "sweet tooth." Found in beans, grains and other foods, they bite into carbohydrates, particularly sugars, often causing immune system reactions and blood clotting. Because they agglutinate blood—glue it up—lectins are also known as hemagglutins, hemagglutinins and phytohemagglutins.

Soybean lectins have two main functions. First, they react with the carbohydrate component of cell membranes, causing cell injuries and deaths. As this damage accumulates, it adversely affects the gastrointestinal, immune and other systems of humans and other animal species. Second, they exist in a symbiotic relationship with *Rhizobium* bacteria. By fixating atmospheric nitrogen in the roots of the soybean plant, the lectin-bacteria team supports the miracle bean's traditional, historical use as a fertilizer and crop rotator.[1]

PROCESSING MATTERS

In ideal circumstances, soybean lectins would not be a problem in human nutrition. They would be incapacitated before they

227

even entered the human mouth, either by enzymes—such as those that are abundantly present in fermented soyfoods—or by heat, as in processing and cooking.

Most of the negative findings on soy lectins have occurred after feeding uncooked soy-based chow to rats and other animals. Scientists have found that both lectins and trypsin inhibitors (see Chapter 16) are responsible for poor growth, pancreatic enlargement and digestive distress. But because soy lectins are far easier to deactivate by cooking and gastric digestion than trypsin inhibitors, researchers once assumed that soy lectins were safe so long as the soybeans were well cooked.[2-6]

This conclusion was premature, given our still incomplete knowledge of the toxicology of soy lectins. Subtle effects can be easily missed if the degree of toxicity is low, if the negative effects accumulate slowly over time, or if a toxin studied in isolation becomes more toxic in the presence of other toxins. In addition, an absence of toxic manifestations in one animal species does not preclude possible toxic effects in others. Although lectins have proved toxic to all animal species studied, including human beings, vulnerability varies.[7]

In 1999, researchers reported that conventionally processed defatted soy proteins retained significant levels of lectins, but that most of their capacity to cause clotting was destroyed during processing. All seemed well until the researchers also found that "soybean meals can, on occasion, retain functional lectins at levels that may be detrimental to the animal's health and productivity."[8] Soy protein intended for human consumption has consistently contained low levels of functionally intact lectins.[9] However, the many studies indicating a wide range of protease inhibitor levels in processed food (see Chapter 16) make it reasonable to assume that erratic and improper processing conditions will sometimes leave the lectin count at unacceptable levels.

Whether it is high levels found "on occasion" or low levels found in soy foods eaten in large quantities on a regular basis, soy lectins are more than capable of perturbing digestive, absorptive, protective and secretory functions throughout the gastrointestinal tract. As Arpad Pusztai, Ph.D., author of *Plant Lectins* puts it, lectins "can have serious consequences for growth and health."[10]

GUT REACTION

Lectins that have not been successfully cooked away are unlikely to succumb to normal digestive processes. Unlike ordinary food proteins, lectins strongly resist breakdown by enzymes in the gut. At least 60 percent remain biologically active and immunologically intact, a combination that can represent a time bomb in the digestive tract.[11,12]

Soybean lectins bind to the villi and crypt cells of the small intestine. The villi are tiny fingerlike projections that increase the surface area available for absorption. The crypt cells hide in the pits, where they are involved in cell reproduction. Under a microscope, the villi display an edge that looks like a brush and that is sometimes called the "brush border." Lectin binding contributes to cell death, a shortening of the villi, a diminished capacity for digestion and absorption, cell proliferation in the crypt cells, interference with hormone and growth factor signaling and unfavorable population shifts among the microbial flora.[13-15]

NOT BY LECTINS ALONE: SAPONINS AND SOYATOXINS

Lectins gain strength in the company of other soybean antinutrients, particularly saponins. Lectins or saponins tested alone in amounts comparable to those likely to be found in foods cause only mild damage to the jejunum (the mid section) of the small intestine of rabbits, but they are 100 times more potent when tested together. The damage is not additive but synergistic.[16]

Yet another factor confounding our understanding of lectins is the recent discovery of a toxic protein called soyatoxin. Soyatoxin causes clotting like a lectin; it can be separated from lectins using modern purification techniques in the laboratory. Soybean meals used in early studies undoubtedly contained both lectins and soyatoxin, suggesting that lectins were once unfairly blamed for the dastardly deeds of soyatoxins.

Soyatoxin has proved lethal to mice, causing breathing difficulties, convulsions and partial paralysis prior to death. Ilka Vasconcelos, Ph.D., lead scientist of the team that discovered soyatoxin, concluded her report by stating that it seemed "important to gather more information concerning its nutritional value, and to develop ways to counteract any detrimental effects."[17,18] As yet no one has funded these important studies, although it is not too farfetched to assume that a toxic agent that acts so much like botulism might be formulated into an "all natural" soy-based injectable to compete with the wrinkle-removing paralytic Botox.

ENLARGING THE SMALL INTESTINE

Lectin-induced cell deaths lead to increased cell turnover and a greatly increased requirement for protein needed for DNA and RNA synthesis. The intestinal villi shrink from the combination of premature cell death and replacement by immature cells, changes that alter both form and function. Meanwhile, the deeper so-called "crypt" cells speed up the production of new cells, producing them at such a prodigious rate that hyperplasia results. As a result, the wall of the small intestine thickens and the organ gains weight.[19,20] Enlargement of the pancreas may also occur, a condition generally blamed on protease inhibitors but strong evidence suggests that lectins should share the blame.[21]

IMMUNE REACTIONS

Lectin damage is not confined to the gut. As the body attempts to maintain the integrity of the small intestinal lining at all costs, proteins that would ordinarily be used for normal growth and repair elsewhere may be appropriated instead for emergency repairs in the intestinal tract. Furthermore, lectins consumed with the diet may travel through the damaged "leaky gut" into general circulation, provoking allergic reactions and immune system disruption.[22,23] Infants allergic to soy formula have suffered grievous damage to the small intestine similar to but not precisely identical to that caused by lectins, perhaps because the lectins are doing double duty as allergenic proteins. Certainly research to date suggests that *all* lectins of either plant or microbial origin provoke allergic reactions in the gut, usually of the delayed hypersensitivity type IgG.[24-26]

Lectins are three to four times more likely to move into the bloodstream through the "leaky gut" than other food proteins and the amounts absorbed into the system may be as high as 15 percent. The antibody response to lectins is similar whether they have been eaten or injected. In contrast, food proteins or lectins that have been denatured by chemicals or cooking trigger allergic responses only when injected. This tells us that maintaining the integrity of the gut lining is crucial to keeping undigested and partially digested food proteins, lectins and environmental toxins out of the bloodstream.

Finally, lectins can cause shifts in the gut flora, including overgrowth by *E. coli*, streptococcus and lactobacillus bacteria; fortunately, when lectins are removed from the diet conditions generally revert to control levels within 48 hours.[27,28] Although most of these studies were done using highly toxic kidney bean lectin known as PHA, soybean lectins act similarly, though less strongly. Pusztai explains: "Despite a general interest in lectins, most of our understanding of their toxic, gastroenterological effects in diets is the result of studies carried out with PHA. However, the results of more fragmentary studies with other dietary lectins largely support the findings obtained with PHA and the basic features of the interactions between different lectins and the digestive system are sufficiently similar as to allow us to draw some generalized conclusions."[29]

POPULATIONS AT RISK

Damage from soybean lectins is most likely to occur in people who consume large quantities of soy foods on a regular basis. In one study, rats put on rotation diets showed significantly less damage from lectins than rats fed soy proteins continuously. Because the rats did nearly as well with the rotation diet as they did on a steady diet of high quality low-lectin feed, the authors proposed this as a "novel method" that is "cheap," makes processing "unnecessary" and could be "easily adapted for the use of soyabean whey, regarded as a waste product."[30] A "cheap" feeding method that would allow slow poisoning of animals with waste products so long as the consequences are not immediately felt cannot be recommended ethically for either animals or humans. The study does, however, suggest the importance of rotating foods in the diet so as to reduce repeated exposure to all lectin-rich legumes, especially soybeans and kidney beans.

Infants fed soy formula and vegans who regularly eat a lot of soy-based meat and dairy replacements do not experience sufficient variety in their diets and so are especially vulnerable. In the average adult with "leaky gut" and other GI tract problems, soy foods are likely to be one factor among many, with cumulative damage coming from food allergies and intolerances, antibiotics, aspirin, ibuprofen and other NSAID drugs, heavy metal contamination, alcoholism and other factors.[31]

MORE THAN CORPUSCLE PUNISHMENT

The 1948 discovery that plant lectins are specific to blood types has created a thriving multidisciplinary research industry and led to the 1996 bestselling book *Eat Right 4 Your Type* by Peter J. D'Adamo, N.D.[32]

According to Dr. D'Adamo, lectins in foods only prove troublesome when they are incompatible with the person's blood type. When these lectins bite into intestinal cells or leak into the bloodstream, they may be attacked as foreign antigens and become part of a network of antibodies bound to antigens that are known as "immune complexes." These can clot and block blood flow or lodge in organs of the body where they interfere with key processes related to digestion, absorption, insulin utilization and a host of other vital functions. As incompatible lectins cause the immune system to react and overreact, the stage is set for autoimmune diseases. Permeability of the intestinal lining correlates with numerous disorders, including food and environmental allergies; bowel problems such as IBS, Crohn's disease and celiac disease; inflammatory joint diseases such as rheumatoid arthritis; dermatological diseases such as psoriasis, and many forms of cancer.

If Dr. D'Adamo's theory were correct, it would make good sense to "eat right for your type." However, when we take a careful look at the theory, it appears a bit "sticky." A healthy body with full digestive and assimilative capabilities is capable of handling a variety of food lectins. However, regular assaults by large servings of lectin-rich soybeans, kidney beans, wheat or other foods will breach the integrity of the intestinal lining, allowing lectins and incompletely digested food proteins and other toxins to move into the bloodstream.

The probable reason that so many people benefit from Dr. D'Adamo's diet plans is that he urges people with Type O blood to reject vegetarian diets containing large amounts of lectin-rich plant foods and soy foods and advises them to eat low-lectin meats instead. In addition, he tells Types O, A and B to "just say no" to "wheat" and flour products such as breads, bagels, muffins, flours, cakes, cookies, pastas and cereals. In addition to the wheat germ lectin, wheat contains gluten and gliadin, two proteins that bind to the human intestinal mucus lining much like lectins. Indeed, ever increasing amounts of wheat and gluten in the modern diet have been associated with rising rates of a gut disorder known as celiac disease.[33,34] Since people with Type O blood represent 45 percent of the white and 46 percent of the black population and that people of Type O, A and B blood types represent 96 percent of whites and 93 percent of blacks,[35] it is obvious why Dr. D'Adamo's basic recommendations have had a positive effect.

NOT SO SWEET

Soy lectins may contribute to Type 1 juvenile onset diabetes by destroying the cells in the pancreas responsible for the secretion of insulin. In one study of diabetic children, nearly twice as many received soy formula during infancy compared to nondiabetic controls.[36] The soy lectin-diabetes connection has received little publicity; instead much fanfare attended the announcement that dairy lectins may cause this autoimmune disorder.[37,38]

SHOCK OF THE NEW

Lectins play a role in allergic reactions. As we have already discussed, they are themselves allergenic proteins and cause damage to the intestinal mucosa, increasing vulnerability to both food and environmental allergies. Allergic reactions may dramatically increase in the future because of the insertion of lectins into genetically engineered foods. For example, a lectin that causes many people to experience allergic reactions to latex was engineered into GM tomatoes in order to improve its anti-fungal properties. As a result, we may start hearing about latex-sensitive individuals coming down with "tomato allergies."[39]

In 1998, Pusztai set off a furor regarding the safety of genetically modified foods when he disclosed that rats fed GM potatoes containing a lectin from a snowdrop plant suffered depressed immune systems and damage to the kidney, stomach, spleen and brain. The snowdrop lectin had been inserted into the potato because it is a naturally occurring insecticide. Pusztai's testimony made a mockery of claims to safety put forth by Monsanto and other biotechnology giants that stand to profit mightily from GM crops and within four days, the distinguished researcher was forced to retire from a job he had held for 36 years at the Rowett Research Institute in Aberdeen, Scotland. The pretext was that he had muddled his findings. More likely greed led the Institute to kowtow to Monsanto, which had given a $230,000 (U.S. dollars) research grant to the institute. Although 20 scientists including toxicologists, genetic engineers and medical experts from 13 countries examined Pusztai's work and found that his conclusions were warranted, the once widely respected researcher is now considered "controversial."[40,41]

HANNIBAL LECTINS

Scientists have high hopes for lectins from soy and other foods. The word "lectin" means "to choose," and lectins may prove useful pharmaceutically because they are biologically active *and* able to discriminate. Lectins of the future may be sent into the body to grab onto specific sugars that coat body cells, microbes and proteins. Because these sugars change throughout the ordinary life cycles of the cell and change radically during pre-disease and disease states, doctors of the future may be able to treat cancer and infectious disease by sending in lectin troops to disrupt or destroy the enemy's essential sugar coatings. With apologies to Mary Poppins, lectins may prove to be the spoonful of medicine with which the sugar goes down.[42]

Used in cancer treatment, specific lectins could move in on early mutated cells and sweep them from the system, leaving normal cells alone. This, according to researchers, could stop cancer in its tracks at a very early stage. Soy lectins have already been used to remove cancerous breast cells from harvested bone marrow before it is reintroduced into patients. As diagnostic tools, lectins may facilitate early detection not only of cancer but also of arthritis and infectious diseases by monitoring changes in cells.[43,44]

Surprisingly, lectins are also being touted for cancer treatment because of their ability to spur hyperplastic growth of the gut. Despite the fact that cell proliferation is itself a precursor of cancer, researchers believe that the growth of the tumor will slow down once it has to compete with the proliferating small intestinal lining for the large amounts of the polyamines putrescine, spermidine and spermine needed to sustain that growth. Studies using mice have shown an initial low level of tumor growth under these conditions.[45,46]

Lectins are of particular interest to researchers studying the small

and large intestines. Areas of investigation include the characterization of normal and abnormal intestinal mucus, epithelial cell changes
associated with differentiation and maturation, and the relationships between secretory IgA, gut microrganisms and immune response. Most of the studies have involved the small intestine, but
similar binding occurs throughout the GI tract. Currently there is
much speculation about the possibilities of matching the right lectins
to the right regions and to pharmaceutically "engineer" the digestive tract for improved physiological performance and bacterial ecol-
ogy.[47-50]

These are exciting developments, but they are not an argument
for eating soy foods. Soy lectins and other food lectins used in this
medicine of the future will be used precisely and pharmaceutically.
The same benefits are highly unlikely to come from simply eating
the foods. For starters, there's no way to accurately gauge the numbers of lectins that would survive food processing, cooking and digestion. More important, soyfoods always enter the body carrying
their cargo of other anti-nutritional factors—saponins, soyatoxin,
phytates, protease inhibitors, oxalates, goitrogens and estrogens, all
of which have shown the potential to cause harm.

In short, those who eat soyfoods in the hope of gaining benefits from the lectins are "glutins for punishment."

MY SOY STORY: THE LECTIN CONNECTION

I was a healthy, active 45-year-old woman when I suffered a bout of deep vein thrombosis (DVT) and pulmonary embolism. I ended up in the hospital with a heparin drip and am now on lifelong Coumadin therapy. Because I had no family history of this condition, they gave me numerous blood tests at the hospital to find a cause. Because nothing surfaced, I started thinking about what I had changed in my diet. The only thing I could come up with was that I had started eating a lot of soy and was using a soy protein supplement, having heard that this "natural hormone" would help me transition into menopause.

I spent a great deal of time researching this subject to see whether I could find a connection between soy and DVT before I learned that soy contains lectins, which I understand are clot-promoting substances that cause red blood cells to clump together. I learned that years ago researchers discovered that clots from lectins have killed rabbits. Yet no one sees fit to warn consumers that soy can kill us in the same way.

K.G., Nashville, TN

19
SAPONINS
soap in your mouth

Saponins are bitter, biologically active components in plant foods that foam up like soap suds in water and that break down red blood cells. Researchers have isolated and characterized three main types and many subtypes in soy. For years saponins kept company with protease inhibitors, phytates and lectins and other undesirable antinutrients in soy, all of which seem to have evolved to help plants defend themselves against microbes, insects and animal predators.

Now scientists are seeking new uses for saponins. Saponins from alfalfa, a cover crop similar to soy, have been used by farmers to decrease root rot from fungi and bacteria, soy saponins have aided the growth of lettuce and mung beans, and researchers see a grand future for soy saponins as natural herbicides.[1-3]

Although ingestion of saponins has been linked to poor growth, bloat and other problems in animals, studies conducted thirty years ago found that chicks, rats and mice grew well even when fed massive doses from soy. These findings were neither consistent nor conclusive, but they were sufficiently soothing to mitigate any worry scientists might have had about saponins and to create the impression that the levels in soybeans pose little threat to human health.[4-6]

Little evidence of harm, however, is not the same as none, and growth is only one of many saponin-related health issues.

A KICK IN THE GUT

The main concern with soy saponins today is not growth inhibition but damage to the mucosa of the intestines. This occurs when saponins bind with cholesterol, causing injuries that result in increased permeability, a condition popularly known as "leaky gut."[7-9] Although researchers think this effect is "weak," soy allergens and lectins cause similar damage, suggesting a cumulative risk.

Non-soy saponins have a bad reputation for breaking red blood cells in a process known as hemolysis. Although soybean saponins bind readily to cell membranes, most researchers report that they are either not hemolytic or only weakly so.[10,11] However, the body's ability to resist this type of damage from saponins decreases with age, along with an age-related decline in the quality of red cell membranes.[12]

Saponins also inhibit important enzymes. One is succinate dehydrogenase, a key player in the citric acid cycle of the body, which must function properly if we are to properly absorb nutrients, heal and grow.[13] Digestive enzymes that are disturbed by saponins include trypsin and chymotrypsin, which may be why some of the problems associated with protease inhibitors remain even when they are totally removed by cooking or processing.[14] (See Chapter 16.) Finally, saponins may be goitrogenic. Although the best known goitrogens in soy are the isoflavones, the Japanese researcher Shuichi Kimura discovered back in the mid-1970s that saponins can also spur enlargement of the thyroid.[15]

NOT A WASH OUT

Saponin content in soybean products is rather high—5.6 percent in whole soy beans, 2.2 percent in defatted soy flour and 2.2 percent in tofu.[16] It's a tough job ridding soyfoods of saponins. Cooking and most food processing methods (such as steaming or boiling) don't faze them. Only alcohol extraction removes them. When soy protein is separated from the oil, saponins stick with the protein, making them an unavoidable constant in every soy product except oil and lecithin.[17,18] Soy protein isolates contain the highest levels of saponins of any soy product. Fewer saponins are found in the old-fashioned fermented "good old soys" miso and tempeh, or in okara, the dregs left over after preparation of soy milk. *Aspergillus oryzae* used in the fermentation of miso and soy sauce produces an enzyme known as soybean saponin hydrolase, which is capable of hydrolyzing (breaking down) soybean saponins.[19] While it is true that saponins are metabolized by bacterial enzymes, this does not occur in the human body until they have scrubbed their way around the many twisting loops of the small intestine to arrive in the large intestine.

SPIN CONTROL: THE CLEAN, NEW IMAGE

The soy industry once tried to develop strains of soybeans low in saponins and to find processing methods that could remove them. The emphasis today is on publicizing a squeaky clean, new image. Although electron microscopy studies suggest that soy saponins do less damage to cell membranes than herbal varieties and are not dose dependent,[20] the cholesterol-binding mechanism that causes the damage gets credit for lowering blood and liver cholesterol and preventing and reversing colon cancer.[21]

CHOLESTEROL DOWNER

Saponins do lower cholesterol. Their ability to bind with cholesterol and with bile decreases absorption by the intestines and increases elimination in the feces.[22-25] However soy protein rat feed has sometimes been found to greatly suppress the effects of soy saponins.[26] And when cholesterol lowering does occur, it may result in a decrease in the important ratio of the amino acids lysine to arginine, itself a risk factor for heart disease.[27] Saponins may be marketed someday as cholesterol drugs and used in the production of cholesterol-free dairy products.[28,29]

CANCER ANSWER?

High hopes for saponins also include cancer prevention and reversal. This possibility hinges on two ideas: that saponins bind with bile and that bile acids poison the cells and so promote tumors. By reducing the absorption of bile through the cell membrane, precancerous epithelial cell proliferation in the colon is thought to be less likely. The theory is that cancer cell membranes contain more cholesterol than normal cell membranes and that saponins bind more easily to them, thus triggering their destruction, a phenomenon that has been observed in cancer-stricken mice.[30] However, destruction occurs in normal cells as well (albeit at lower levels), making soy saponins a poor choice for cancer prevention. After all, "leaky gut," with its attendant malabsorption, dysbiosis and other problems, increases the risk of cancer.[31]

IMMUNE SYSTEM IRRITANT

Yet another possible role for saponins is as an immune-system stimulant,[32] which might be a plus where cancer is concerned, but actually functions as a doubled-edged sword. Some people need immune system stimulation, but others with autoimmune diseases need modulation. Saponins contribute to "leaky gut" syndrome, which has been associated with autoimmune disorders, including allergies and asthma.[33] Higher levels of hemoglobin in the body—one sure effect of saponins—are found in people afflicted with respiratory diseases such as asthma.[34] Asthma is also found more often in children who have been fed soy formula than those fed breast milk or milk-based formulas (see Chapter 24.)

nineteen: saponins

SOY FUNGICIDE

Most saponins are toxic to fungi and yeast—at least to those that contain ergosterol and zymosterol in their cell membranes. The more sterols, the more quickly the membrane is penetrated, with a spilling of the cell guts and cell death.[35]

Pharmacists point out that the antifungal drugs nystatin and amphotericin-B behave like saponins, binding to the fungal cell membranes, causing increased permeability and the leakage of potassium and other essential components of the cell interior.[36] Commonly prescribed to wipe out yeast infections, these drugs achieve that goal at a steep price. Side effects include pronounced damage to the patient's own cell membranes, with users complaining of gas, diarrhea, nausea and stomach pain.[37] Not incidentally, these are some of the most common unwanted side effects of soybean consumption.

SOAP FUTURES

Despite these clear warnings, saponins represent one of the soy industry's rising stars, with a promising pharmaceutical future. In addition to marketing them as cholesterol reducers, bile binders and cancer preventers, the pharmaceutical industry has singled out saponins for their ability to increase the body's level of immune response. This has led some researchers to propose adding saponins to vaccines.[38]

Finally, there may be big profits to be made in using saponins as a component of spermicides. Hemolysis damages the mucosa of the vagina, providing an inhospitable environment for sperm.[39] An interesting prospect, given the rising rates of infertility already associated with soy consumption. Eat your soy, douche with soy—the "soy natural" approach to birth control.

20
OXALATES
casting stones

O xalates are indigestible compounds in foods that prevent the proper absorption of calcium. Contrary to popular belief, oxalates are not significantly neutralized by cooking. In addition to contributing to deficiencies of calcium, they may lead to two painful conditions—kidney stones and vulvodynia.

SPINACH, RHUBARB, PEANUTS. . . and SOY

The foods highest in oxalates are spinach and rhubarb. These rarely pose a problem since few people other than Popeye eat much spinach and fewer still eat rhubarb. More likely to be troublesome are oxalate-containing foods that are habit forming, if not addictive. The best known of these are chocolate and peanuts. The least known is soy.

Soy foods are high in oxalates.

Researchers from Washington State University in Spokane recently tested 11 varieties of soybeans and 13 types of soy foods for total oxalates and found to their surprise that the total amounts ranged from 16 to 638 mg per serving.[1] These levels totally eclipse the American Dietetic Association's recommendation of no more than 10 mg of oxalate per serving for patients prone to kidney stones.[2]

The highest amount was found in textured soy protein, which contains a whopping 638 mg of oxalate per 85 gram serving, more than 60 times the ADA recommended amount. Soy cheese, the soyfood with the lowest oxalate content, was still high at 16 mg per serving. By comparison, spinach—the best known oxalate-containing food of all—has approximately 543 mg per one cup (2 ounces fresh) serving. Peanut butter comes in at 197, refried beans at 193 and lentils at 100 mg of total oxalate per serving. "Under these guidelines, no soybean or soy based food tested could be recommended for consumption by patients with a personal history of kidney stones," warns Washington State's Linda Massey, Ph.D.[3]

NO KIDDING: OXALATES AND KIDNEY STONES

It is a mystery why kidney stones crop up in some individuals but not others, but we do know that high levels of oxalate in the diet increase the risk. In healthy individuals, oxalates bind with calcium in the gut to be excreted in the feces. In individuals troubled by the fat malabsorption problem known as steatorrhea, the calcium binds instead with fats. As a result, free oxalates are absorbed through the intestinal wall into the bloodstream. Inflammatory bowel disease also increases the rate of oxalate absorption. Before passing out of the body through the urine, oxalates may precipitate with calcium to form kidney stones.

Doctors diagnosed kidney stones in more than a million people in the United States in 1996, the most recent available data from the National Institutes of Health. An estimated 10 percent of the U.S. population, mostly men, will develop a kidney stone at some point in their lives, and the numbers of cases of kidney stones have been increasing over the past few decades.[4] Yet the FDA recommends that these same men lower their cholesterol by eating 25 grams of soy protein every day. Unhappily, this amount could lead to excruciatingly painful kidney stones.

Clearly, soy should be eliminated from the diet of people

who either have experienced kidney stones or who have a family history of it.

ECSTASY TO AGONY: OXALATES AND VULVODYNIA

Women too are at risk. Though less likely than men to develop kidney stones, more and more women are experiencing an agonizing condition known as vulvodynia. As its Greek name suggests, it refers to pain of the vulva, the external female genitalia. Symptoms include burning, stinging, itching, swelling and painful sex. Some women afflicted with this condition are so hypersensitive that they cannot wear underwear and can barely walk.

Clive C. Solomons, Ph.D., former Director of Research at the University of Colorado Health Sciences Center and now an independent consultant to the Vulvar Pain Foundation, reports that oxalate is an irritant that causes the release of histamine and the burning of tissues in women. These women excrete higher-than-normal concentrations of oxalate in their urine at certain times of day and experience the most intense pain during these peak periods.[5]

According to Joanne Yount, Executive Director of the VP Foundation in Graham, North Carolina, some women report relief from an oxalate-reduced diet alone. "For others, treatment consists of supporting connective tissue metabolism and reducing inflammation."[6,7] Research as to how to best achieve these objectives is underway at SCI-CON, Solomons' laboratory in Denver. As many sufferers also experience irritable bowel, interstitial cystitis, chronic fatigue, fibromyalgia, muscle and joint paint, burning mouth and tongue, allergies, headaches, dryness in the eyes and mouth and rectal itching, many health practitioners advise a whole-body wellness program. Solomons has no doubt that for some women foods and beverages high in oxalate such as soyfoods "add fuel to the flames."[8]

THE CALCIUM FACTOR

People not afflicted with or at risk for kidney stones or vulvar pain should still take their oxalate consumption seriously because oxalates bind with calcium, preventing its absorption. (The reverse is also true and calcium citrate has been recommended as a treatment for patients with hyperoxaluria or high levels of oxalates in their urine.[9]) Although studies with rice, wheat, rye and soy indicate that phytates cause more calcium binding than oxalates, soy is burdened with both (see Chapter 17). Increased calcium excretion and increased oxalic acid excretion ride tandem and have been linked to osteoporosis.[10]

Massey concluded her study by recommending that the soy industry "find soybean cultivars lower in oxalate, which will have lower risk for kidney stone formation after human consumption." Alternatively, she recommended the development of a processing method capable of removing the compound.[11] As yet, neither has occurred. This bad news came out just recently, in 2001, so the soy industry has yet to put a positive spin on the oxalate problem.

LOW-CARB PROFITS

"Soy and low-carb mania may prove to be good for each other since some sectors of the soy industry appear to be plateauing, and since soy protein provides a healthful alternative to taxing your kidneys with a lot of animal protein," says Peter Golbitz, president of Soyatech. "Soy protein with isoflavones has been shown to be rather helpful in slowing the progression of risk factors associated with kidney failure," agrees Debra Miller, Director of Nutrition Communication for the Solae Company. Forget that the oxalate connection is a proven danger. Say that soy protein could help prevent kidney failure though that's based less on science than speculation. Soy can be helpful right now in preventing that worst of all soy industry problems—plateauing profits.

SOURCE: Low carb mania: Has soy found another wave to ride? www.soyatech.com. Posted 5/21/2004.

part five
HEAVY METALS

21
MANGANESE TOXICITY
ADD-ing it up

Manganese is a vital trace mineral, needed for growth, reproduction, wound healing, brain function, thyroid and adrenal health and proper metabolism of sugars, insulin and cholesterol. Its name comes from the Greek word for "magic," and clinical nutritionists sometimes see magical results when giving it to manganese-deficient patients suffering from diabetes, heart disease, bone problems, joint disease or neurological disorders. Scientists also refer to manganese as the "maternal mineral" because mothers who are manganese deficient are more likely to neglect their young.[1-3]

Soybeans naturally contain manganese as well as other needed macro and trace minerals. For years, investigators had concerns that the phytates in soy would block absorption of its manganese, much as it blocks zinc, iron, calcium and copper. In fact, manganese absorption from soy formula is substantially lower than from breast milk or dairy formula.[4,5] In this case the phytates do the infant a service—but not well enough. Infants fed soy formula take in as much as 75 to 80 times more manganese per day than infants who are breastfed. Per liter, breast milk contains 3 to 10 ug manganese, cow's milk formula 30 to 50 ug, and soy formula a whopping 200 to 300 ug.[6-8]

MAD SCIENTISTS

At a conference held in September 2000 at the University of California at Irvine, leading nutritionists, pediatricians and toxicologists warned that newborns exposed to the levels of manganese present in soy formula risk brain damage in infancy that could lead to learning disabilities, attention deficit and other behavioral disorders, and even violent tendencies.[9]

Although healthy toddlers, children and adults who ingest excess manganese can usually eliminate most of it, infants cannot because their immature livers are not fully functional. At the same time, their growing brains and other organs are more susceptible to manganese damage. Even tiny doses of excess manganese are dangerous when stored long term in the body and brain where they do not belong.[10] Hair mineral analysis tests of children with learning and attention deficits have revealed elevated levels of manganese compared to normal youngsters. Youths convicted of felonies are also much more likely to show elevated hair levels. Although few infants are chronically exposed to high levels of manganese from industrial sources, many are exposed to toxic levels through soy infant formula. Indeed, hair mineral analysis tests on infants using soy formula reveal high levels of manganese in their scalp hair, a clear indicator of manganese toxicity.[11-14]

Scientists have known about manganese toxicity for years. In 1980, the U.S. government set permissible manganese levels at 2.5 to 3.0 mg per day for adults; 1.0 to 1.5 mg per day for toddlers; and 0.5 to 1.0 mg per day for infants.[15] The calculations for the "safe" levels set for infants seem to have been based on their smaller size alone and did not take into account the fact that infants with immature livers cannot successfully metabolize excess manganese. As it happened, the soy industry put little or no effort into keeping manganese under the permissible—but still unacceptable—levels.[16] Soy formulas on the shelves in the early 1980s contained anywhere from 0.2 to 2.2 mg of manganese per quart; during that same period, scientists confirmed the likelihood of risk to newborns from manganese storage in the brain.[17-20] In 1983, Phillip J. Collipp, M.D., a pediatrician at Nassau County Medical Center, confirmed a correlation of high manganese levels with childhood learning disabilities and speculated that soy-based infant formula might determine a child's likelihood of developing Attention Deficit Disorder (ADD) or Attention Deficit Hyperactivity Disorder (ADHD) later in life. [21]

Despite the alarming and consistent results of these studies, few people have ever heard of the link between soy infant formula and manganese toxicity. Now teams of scientists have moved from speculation about a probable connection to ADD/ADHD and other behavioral and learning problems to studies using rats, monkeys and human subjects designed to fully elucidate cause and effect.[22]

TRIPLE THREAT MAN

Manganese toxicity is a problem for people and animals of all ages, but represents a triple threat for infants. Newborns absorb more manganese because of their immature and permeable intestines, fail to eliminate excess manganese because of their immature livers, and are extremely vulnerable to manganese damage because their brains and other organs are still growing. By eight months of age, an infant on soy formula absorbs 1.1 mg of manganese per day above its metabolic needs and deposits about eight percent of that in the basal ganglia cells of the brain. Years later, this manganese may impair the brain's ability to make the neurotransmitter dopamine and trigger behavioral problems ranging from ADD and ADHD to violent and sociopathic behavior.[23,24] Bo Lonnerdal, Ph.D., of the University of California at Davis pulls no punches when he says, "Ingestion of soy-based formula in infancy could impair brain development."[25]

Animals fed even small excesses of manganese during the first weeks of life have shown biochemical abnormalities followed by lesions in the substantia nigra, caudate, putamen and globus pallidus areas of the brain. These areas all depend upon dopamine production for proper function and relate to our abilities to think clearly and flexibly, focus, complete tasks and perform well under stress.[26,27]

Trinh Tran, Ph.D., who worked with Lonnerdal at UC Davis, found that baby rats given manganese chloride supplements at levels comparable to the manganese in soy-formula-fed infants showed no adverse effects until reaching adolescence. At that point in their development, they displayed a range of behavioral and brain disorders, including poor performance on burrowing, detour and shock-avoidance tests. Because rats cannot survive without maternal breast milk, investigators fed the animals manganese supplements, not soy formula.[28] Studies on rhesus monkeys fed with soy formula showed higher-than-normal tissue manganese absorption. Whether the higher tissue levels will result in lowered dopamine levels and behavioral deficits later in life is the subject of current research. This group of researchers also plans two prospective studies with human newborns on soy formula, which will chart manganese levels and behavior as they grow up.[29]

In a separate study, rat pups fed manganese at levels found in breast milk grew up as healthy as controls. However, if given five times more manganese, they showed a 48 percent decline in levels of basal ganglia dopamine. Given ten times the appropriate amount, they suffered a 63 percent decline.[30] These results are particularly sobering when we consider the fact that levels of manganese in soy infant formula are 75 to 80 times higher than those in breast milk.

Francis Crinella, Ph.D., of the University of California Irvine Child Development Center, notes that "Most behaviorists assume that cognitive benefits of breastfeeding are associated with mother-child intimacy," and then asks, "Could another advantage be that the child is also protected against over-absorption of manganese?"[31]

MAD BEAN DISEASE

Whether manganese enters the body by the mouth, lungs or

injection, the metal lodges in the basal ganglia. Neurology and toxicology textbooks have reported disorders known as "manganese madness" and "manganism" since the turn of the century. Until soy formula entered the picture, most cases involved miners exposed to manganese dust or people who breathed in high amounts of tetraethyl lead in the emissions from tail pipes or methylcyclopentadienyl manganese tricarbonyl from gasoline. Symptoms of manganism include instability, impulsivity, irrationality and hallucinations, or, with chronic exposure, the *paralysis agitans* of Parkinson's disease.[32-35] The area of the brain most affected in Parkinson's is the dopamine system, the very part of the brain now associated with ADD and ADHD.[36]

According to toxicologists, "manganese toxicity arising from excessive intakes of the elements in foods was never reported" and "virtually impossible except where industrial contamination has occurred."[37] In the past few decades, cases *have* begun to emerge, with the most frightening reports of manganese poisoning happening to very sick babies and other patients receiving parenteral nutrition.[38]

Manganese toxicity rarely exists in isolation. Fluoride—found in high levels in soy formula (see Chapter 22) and in most of the tap water used to mix soy formula—can increase manganese absorption.[39-41] Zinc, calcium and iron deficiencies can also push manganese absorption up to toxic levels.[42-44] Animal studies suggest that an infant born to a woman with low calcium and/or iron status is more susceptible to the negative effects of manganese.[45] Sub-optimal liver function can also contribute to manganese toxicity. These and other indications of higher manganese consumption and accumulation in the brain have spurred some scientists to study more thoroughly the impact of low-level manganese-induced neurotoxicity on the rate of aging.[46]

Manganese deficiency is commonly associated with hypothyroidism, but excess manganese may be a problem to the endocrine system as well. To date, scientists have linked toxic levels of manganese to goiter in female and castrated male mice. Castrated male mice treated with ordinary levels of testosterone, however, did not form goiters,[47] suggesting that testosterone confers some protection. As we shall see in Chapter 23, testosterone levels are lowered by soybean estrogens, causing emasculation. Altered T4, T3 and thyroid stimulating hormone (TSH) levels have been linked to manganese accumulations in the pituitary gland.[48] Finally, manganese-related auto-antibodies have been found in patients with Graves' disease.[49] These studies are particularly interesting in the light of reports of damage to the thyroid caused by soy infant formula and other soy foods over the past 60 years. Clearly manganese deserves to join the list of soy goitrogens, the best known of which are the isoflavones and saponins (see Chapters 19 and 26).

USDA researchers J.W. Finley and C.D. Davis at the Grand Forks Human Nutrition Research Center in North Dakota have expressed concern about the potential for manganese toxicity in the growing ranks of vegetarians. Vegetarians eat more manganese because plant foods contain far more than animal foods. Vegetarians are also more likely to absorb more manganese because of zinc, calcium and iron deficiencies.[50,51] Low-protein diets also contribute to manganese toxicity.[52] All of these risk factors, of course, co-exist in people who eat a lot of soy.

The soy industry is mostly in denial about the manganese problem in soy formula. When interviewed by David Goodman, Ph.D., an expert on neurological disorders, John Lasekan, Ph.D., of Abbott Laboratories shifted the focus from manganese toxicity to manganese's role as a trace metal essential for life and claimed that deficiencies are the problem—at least for premature and low birth weight babies.[53] Because babies are not able to store manganese until they are born, premies need manganese, but at the minuscule, appropriate levels found in breast milk, not high levels that put the neonatal brain and other organs at risk.[54] Mardi Mountford, a spokesperson for the International Formula Council, told Goodman that there are "no reports of manganese toxicity in healthy infants fed soy formula."[55] This may very well be the case. Healthy infants—by definition—don't manifest manganese toxicity early in life although they can fall prey to negative effects at a later age.

Researcher Tran—who has done much to bring public awareness of manganese toxicity to the forefront—is appalled that some hospitals feed premature babies soy formula, and asks, "Can you imagine the effects of the soy formulas on these underdeveloped organs?"[56] One industry supporter has faced the facts: Greg Caton, of Lumen Foods, has decided that the evidence is sufficiently damning to post a manganese toxicity warning on his cartons of soy milk.[57]

Robert Presley, former California state senator and former secretary of the California Adult and Juvenile Corrections Agency, the world's largest prison system, is also convinced, stating, "Somewhere in the soy formula story may lie the answer to a lot of crime."[58]

SOYMILK WARNING

Lumen Foods, a manufacturer of soy-based foods, has posted the following warning label on its soymilk cartons:

WARNING: Soymilk may be detrimental to infants under 6 months of age. It contains manganese at levels important to human nutrition but over 50 times the level found in mother's breast milk.

Company president George Ackerson noted that he has two concerns: "First that there is mounting evidence of a correlation between manganese in soymilk (including soy-based infant formula) and neurotoxicity in small infants, and secondly that if we know that credible research exists and we don't act responsibly, we could be held liable."

SOURCE: Lumen Foods adds infant warning label to soymilk. PR Newswire via NewsEdge Corporation 6/18/01. www.soyatech.com.

Everett L. "Red" Hodges, founder of the Violence Research Foundation, agrees. On November 17, 2004, Hodges set up an informational hearing in Sacramento before the California Public Safety Committee. Scientists who have recently conducted animal research testified on the dangers of soy formula and the growing evidence that the high manganese content of soy formula is contributing to behavioral disorders and violent crime.[59] If Hodges succeeds, California in 2005 will become the first state to make it illegal for soy formula to be given to infants under six months of age.

22
FLUORIDE TOXICITY
dental and mental fluorosis

Fluorine is a pale yellow, highly toxic, extremely reactive and corrosive gas. In nature, fluorine is found combined with minerals and known as fluoride. Commercial production of fluorine began after World War II, prompted by the requirements of the atomic bomb. The U.S. Agency for Toxic Substances and Disease Registry lists fluoride as among the top 20 of 275 substances that pose the most significant threat to human health.[1-3]

Yet fluoride is promoted as a healthy mineral needed to prevent cavities. The evidence for this is mixed, at best, with mounting evidence that fluoride actually causes a condition known as fluorosis, an unsightly mottling or discoloring of the teeth.[4-6] Fluorosis is not just a cosmetic defect but a sign of pathological, poorly mineralized and porous teeth. In severe cases, the teeth crumble like chalk.

Although toothpaste tubes carry warnings that little children should not use more than a "pea-sized" amount and not swallow the toothpaste, toothpaste alone cannot take the blame for mounting rates of fluorosis. Half of all U.S. municipal water supplies are fluoridated, most commercial foods are grown with pesticides containing fluoride, and nearly all bottled sodas, drinks, canned foods, baby foods and formulas are processed with fluoridated water.[7-16]

As we shall soon establish, soy foods naturally contain fluoride and processed soy foods contain a lot of it.

If the fluoride danger is dose related—a point on which nearly all health professionals agree—then the widespread presence of fluoride in soy products, other processed foods and our drinking water supply cannot fail to contribute to health problems.

GOING WITH THE FLUO

Soy foods obtain their fluoride content in two ways. First, soybeans—like most plants—pull fluoride from the soil and from commercial fertilizers. Stored in warehouses, the beans can also take in fluoride from hydrogen fluoride gas, used as a pesticide.[17-19]

A 1972 article in *Prevention* magazine reported that soybean plants are also adept at taking industrial fluorides from the air and converting them into the toxic organic forms. Leonard H. Weinstein, Ph.D., of Cornell University, coauthor of *Fluorides in the Environment: Effects on Plants and Animals* (2004) says that the *Prevention* article was "essentially, completely wrong." Although several papers published in the late 1960s and early 1970s alleged that soybeans synthesized monofluorocitrate and monofluoroacetate from inorganic, airborne fluoride, the researchers had made a serious error. Weinstein explains: "If soybean was capable of synthesizing these highly toxic compounds, the amount was below any concentration that would be toxic to man or animals."[20]

But the main reason that levels of fluoride are high in many soy products is that soybeans go to the food processing factory where tap water—which almost always has been fluoridated—is used both in processing treatments and as an ingredient in products such as soy milk and soy ice cream. Finally, most parents who use powdered soy formulas reconstitute them with tap water.

twenty-two: fluoride toxicity

FORMULA FOR DISASTER

The fluoride content of both soy and dairy formulas is substantially higher than that of breast milk, but only soy formulas exceed safe limits when reconstituted with non-fluoridated distilled water. The levels increase considerably when formulas are reconstituted with fluoridated tap water.[21-28] Making matters worse, soy formula is not only high in fluoride but also in aluminum (see Chapter 23) and cadmium. Cadmium levels in soy formula are six times higher than those in milk formula, according to one study, and 8 to 15 times higher according to another.[29,30] Cadmium is a toxic metal that contributes to heart disease, cancer, diabetes and reproductive ills.[31]

In the United States, a team of investigators compared cases of mild to moderate fluorosis with levels of exposure during early childhood. They found that soy formula put children at risk for fluorosis of the enamel surfaces of their teeth if used during the first year, but not when used later, when consumption would normally decline or cease. At that point, fluoridated drinking water, toothpaste, supplements and fluoride containing foods became the key factors in fluorosis.[32]

In communities where the drinking water is fluoridated, ingestion can easily exceed levels that even fluoridation supporters consider "optimal." Samuel J. Fomon, M.D., Department of Pediatrics, University of Iowa, and the lead researcher on hundreds of studies concerning infant formula, concedes, "Prolonged exposure to high intakes of fluoride during infancy is much more common now than in the past."[33]

Hardy Limeback, Ph.D., D.D.S., of the Department of Preventive Dentistry at the University of Toronto and president of the Canadian Association for Dental Research, goes a step further, warning that "Children under three should never use fluoridated toothpaste or drink fluoridated water. And baby formula must never be made up using Toronto (fluoridated) tap water. Never." Once Canada's most prominent fluoride promoter, Dr. Limeback reversed his position in 1999, publicly apologized to patients, and acknowledged the sound-

261

ness of toxicology studies going back more than 50 years.[34]

BONING UP

Although the maximum contaminant level for fluoride in U.S. drinking water has been set by the Surgeon General at 4 ppm, much higher levels have occurred due to the failure of municipal water authorities to maintain proper quality control.[35] Even at lower—supposedly safe—levels fluoride accumulates in the human body over time and can lead to bone abnormalities including skeletal fluorosis. Such bones are abnormally weak, brittle and prone to fracture, and new data suggest links between fluoridated water supplies and fluoride supplements with increased levels of fractures.[36-39] A National Academy of Science textbook reports three stages in the development of bone fluorosis: chemical fluorosis, bone mottling and abnormal bone.[40]

Cause and effect will be harder to establish with soy formula, soy milk and other foods high in fluoride, but people who consume such products regularly would be prudent to consider them when calculating probable exposure levels.

NOT THINKING STRAIGHT

Before it shows up as tooth mottling or skeletal fluorosis, fluoride exposure affects the nervous system. In fact, fluoride may play a role in the epidemic of ADD, ADHD, learning disabilities and other brain dysfunctions so prevalent today.[41-46]

Because the blood-brain barriers of fetuses and newborns are permeable and their brains still developing and growing, they are particularly vulnerable to fluoride toxicity. Brain tissue acquired from aborted fetuses in high fluoride areas of China has shown poor differentiation of brain nerve cells and delayed brain development. Researchers have also found that the IQs of children in such areas are lower.[47,48] Cretinism is especially likely in low-iodine and high-fluoride areas such as the region of Xinjiang in China.[49] Many of the symptoms of thyroid dysfunction resemble those of fluoride poisoning. An organization called Parents of Fluoride-Poisoned Children hosts a website that lists more than 150 matching symptoms backed by 173 references from medical journals.[50] Because the soybean naturally contains goitrogens, fluoride added through processing further contributes to the likelihood of thyroid problems (see Chapter 27).

Fluoride may also contribute to memory loss, a side effect common to almost all the fluoridated drugs listed in the *Physician's Desk Reference*. These drugs include Fenfluoramine (a weight-loss drug), fluoridated corticosteroids, antidepressants such as Prozac and the date-rape drug Rohypnol.[51]

Finally, fluoride synergizes and potentiates the actions of many neurotoxins. This fact is well known to toxicologists and pharmacists, yet few studies have considered the combined impact of fluoride with lead, mercury, aluminum, manganese and other neurotoxins commonly found in the environment and food supply on the brain and other organs.[52,53] Soy not only contains fluoride but manganese, aluminum and the plant estrogens known as isoflavones, which share some of the known neurotoxic effects of estrogens (see Chapters 21, 23 and 26-30).

Fluoride has also been linked to cancer (particularly osteosarcoma), infertility, reproductive problems, skin eruptions, gastric distress, thyroid disturbances, immune system breakdown and other woes.[54,55] Indeed fluoride would appear to be a contributor to the entire litany of problems caused or worsened by soy's antinutrients, toxins, goitrogens and other plant hormones.

As Andreas Schuld, Director of Parents of Fluoride-Poisoned Children, puts it, "It is of utmost urgency that public health officials cease promoting fluoride as beneficial to our health and address instead the issue of its toxicity."[56]

MY SOY STORY: FLUORIDE POISONING

In 1962, when my son Joey, slightly over a year old, was diagnosed with a lactose intolerance, the doctor prescribed soy-based (Neo-Mulsoy) infant formula. Within a week, he was vomiting and had severe diarrhea. I changed his bedding and diapers about five times during the night. The next morning I awoke, shocked to find him sitting up in the crib with a dead expression on his face. He looked like a frail little old man because he had lost most of his body fluids. Terrified, I called the doctor who immediately admitted him to the hospital. My baby was so dehydrated they strapped him to a wooden board, put intravenous needles into his arms and legs, and fed him fluids and nutrients. The pediatrician realized that my son had suffered a reaction to the soy formula and recommended a diet consisting of only mashed bananas. After another week, he was well enough to come home. The diagnosis was gastroenteritis.

It was only years later, in 1989, that I learned that fluoride concentrations in soy-based infant formula were consistently higher than in milk-based products. I realized that my son exhibited classic indicators of severe fluoride poisoning. We never used fluoride toothpaste, tap water or fluoride sealants so it must have been the fluoride in the soy formula that later caused the stains on my son's teeth. I remember walking into the bathroom and watching Joey trying to scrape the stains off his teeth with a sewing needle. People asked him whether he ever brushed his teeth. The children at school ridiculed him about his teeth. My son, who nearly died in infancy after being fed soy infant formula for one week, will carry a legacy of fluoride toxicity throughout his life—dental fluorosis, severe and chronic gastroenteritis and bone problems.

R.L., San Diego, CA

23
ALUMINUM TOXICITY
foil-ing health

Aluminum—the most abundant metal in the earth's crust—is distributed all over the world, but has no known useful biological function and is toxic to most plants and animals. Aluminum interferes with cellular and metabolic processes in the nervous system and other tissues, and has been linked to dementia, memory loss, confusion, disorientation, loss of coordination and digestive problems including colic.[1,2]

Humans beings are exposed to aluminum from drinking water, aluminum foil, food and drinks in aluminum cans and containers, aluminum cooking pans (including high-end products such as Calphalon), antacids and other medications, antiperspirants and tap water. Many cities add aluminum to the public water supply. If the water is fluoridated as well, the fluoride will increase the leaching of aluminum from aluminum pots, pans and foils.[3,4]

The most common food sources of aluminum are baking powders, drying agents added to table salt and other products, processed cheese, bleached flour, and foods, drinks or sodas made with tap water[5,6] . . . and soy.

AL AND THE BEANSTALK

Soy gets its aluminum both naturally and unnaturally. The soy plant's deep roots suck up aluminum from the soil, with the amount varying according to the soil content and its pH. Far more aluminum is added when "natural" soy products undergo food processing. Aluminum contamination comes from food additives (such as baking powder), additives that increase aluminum absorption (such as iron, fluoride, calcium citrate or potassium citrate); tap water used as part of the manufacturing process; aluminum vats and storage containers at the factory; and leaching from foil, cartons and cans used in consumer packaging. Finally, the aluminum burden increases with the tap water added at home to reconstitute soy formula from powder. [7-10]

CALLING AL FORMULAS

The aluminum levels of all infant formulas are much, much higher than those of breast milk, with the very highest levels found in soy formulas made with soy protein isolate. Soy infant formulas contain 100 times the aluminum found in breast milk. When it comes to manufacturing infant formulas, the more high-tech, industrial processes are used, the more aluminum appears in the final product. Thus, minimally processed cow's milk formulas contain less aluminum than whey formulas, but casein hydrolysate and soy protein isolate formulas contain very high levels of aluminum. [11-14]

AL AND THE BRAIN

Aluminum toxicity is a problem for people of all ages, but especially for infants because their immature gastrointestinal tracts and blood-brain barriers are more permeable to all toxins, including aluminum. Growing animals administered aluminum have developed neurological abnormalities. In humans, the evidence for neural damage is less clear, with aluminum damage most evident in patients with renal failure on dialysis and tube feeding. The evidence that aluminum causes Alzheimer's disease is inconsistent and contradictory.[15-21] Aluminum is probably most dangerous in conjunction with other neurotoxins such as fluoride, manganese and estrogens, all of which are also found in soy foods.[22]

AL DEM BONES

When the body absorbs more than it can dispose of, aluminum is deposited in bone. High aluminum exposure in adults and children leads to microcytic (iron-deficient) anemia, osteomalacia, rickets and bone fractures. Aluminum toxicity disturbs both calcium and phosphorous metabolism, causing decreased bone mineral content, as determined by photo absorptiometry, and smaller carpal bones. High-aluminum formulas are also associated with higher rates of rickets. However, because these effects can be modified by increasing calcium and phosphorous intake, the exact role of aluminum in the development of fractures, rickets and bone disease remains unknown.[23-25]

SAFE . . . OR SORRY?

The Food and Agricultural Organization of the United Nations and the World Health Organization have set a tolerable intake of aluminum at 1 mg per kg per day,[26] an amount that is double the 0.5 mg per kg per day received by infants on soy formulas. The American Academy of Pediatrics accepts these levels for full-term infants, but thinks it "prudent to seek further reduction in the aluminum levels of infant formulas and to investigate whether aluminum accumulates in the tissue of premature infants fed formula."[27]

Many leading scientists have stated that these recommendations are not prudent enough.

Winston Koo, M.D., Department of Pediatrics, University of Alberta, Canada, points out that it is difficult if not impossible to recommend a "safe" aluminum load from infant formulas because the amounts that affect bone metabolism are not known.[28] Furthermore, intake is only one consideration. Levels of aluminum stored in the body are better markers of toxicity. Unfortunately, levels can be difficult to ascertain because aluminum is tightly bound within body tissues such as the bone. Blood tests are notoriously inaccurate because the body quickly moves aluminum out of the blood into the tissues. Tissue mineral analysis—often called hair mineral analysis —is a far better indicator of aluminum toxicity, but aluminum will sometimes not move from the bone out into the hair until chelation therapies have been carried on for some months.[29]

Until more is known, it is logical to assume that infants on soy formula are at risk. Dr. Koo warns that it "would seem prudent to minimize the tissue accumulation of this known toxin, especially during infancy, a period of rapid growth which theoretically could potentiate the toxic effect of aluminum."[30] Of the "safe" limits set by WHO and accepted by the American Academy of Pediatrics, Nicole M. Hawkins of the Institute of Child Health in London, adds: "We cannot assume that infants are not at risk of toxicity when consuming lower intakes since they are considerably higher than intakes from either human milk or whey-based infant formulae. The fate of this extra aluminum load remains to be determined, and long term effects of early exposure to high concentrations of aluminum need to be monitored."[31]

part six
SOY ALLERGENS
shock of the new

24
THE RISE IN SOY ALLERGIES

n the 1980s, Stuart Berger, M.D., labeled soy one of the seven top allergens—one of the "sinister seven." At the time, most experts listed soy around tenth or eleventh. Bad enough, but way behind peanuts, tree nuts, milk, eggs, shellfish, fin fish and wheat. Today soy is widely accepted as one of "the big eight" that cause immediate hypersensitivity reactions.[1-4]

Food allergies are abnormal inflammatory responses of the immune system to dust, pollen, a food or some other substance. Those that involve an antibody called immunoglobulin E (IgE) occur immediately or within an hour. Reactions may include coughing, sneezing, runny nose, hives, diarrhea, facial swelling, shortness of breath, a swollen tongue, difficulty swallowing, lowered blood pressure, excessive perspiration, fainting, anaphylactic shock and even death.[4-9]

Delayed allergic responses to soy are less dramatic, but more common. These are caused by antibodies known as immunoglobulins A, G or M (IgA, IgG or IgM) and occur anywhere from two hours to days after the food is eaten. These have been linked to sleep disturbances, bedwetting, sinus and ear infections, crankiness, joint pain, chronic fatigue, gastrointestinal woes and other mysterious symptoms.[4-9]

Food "intolerances," "sensitivities" and "idiosyncrasies" to soy are commonly called "food allergies," but differ from true allergies in that they are not caused by immune system reactions but by little-understood or unknown metabolic mechanisms.[7-9] Strictly speaking, gas and bloating, common reactions to soy and other beans are not true allergic responses. However, they might serve as warnings of the possibility of a larger clinical picture involving allergen-related gastrointestinal damage.

PROFIT vs RISK

The soybean industry knows that some people experience severe allergic reactions to its products. In a recent petition to the Food and Drug Administration (FDA), Protein Technologies International (PTI) identified "allergenicity" as one of the "most likely potential adverse effects associated with ingestion of large amounts of soy products." Yet PTI somehow concluded that "the data do not support that they would pose a substantial threat to the health of the U.S. population."[10]

This statement is hardly reassuring to the many children and adults who suffer allergies to soy products. And it ignores a substantial body of evidence published during the 1990s showing that some of these people learn for the first time about their soy allergies after experiencing an unexpectedly severe or even life-threatening reaction. Although severe reactions to soy are rare compared to reactions to peanuts, tree nuts, fish and shellfish, Swedish researchers recently concluded, "Soy has been underestimated as a cause of food anaphylaxis."[11]

A BAD HAMBURGER

The Swedes began looking into a possible soybean connection when a young girl suffered an asthma attack and died after eating a hamburger that contained only 2.2 percent soy protein. A team of researchers collected data on all fatal and life-threatening reactions caused by food between 1993 and 1996 in Sweden and found that the soy-in-the-hamburger case was not a fluke, and that soy was indeed the culprit. They evaluated 61 cases of severe reactions to food, of which five were fatal, and found that peanuts, soy and tree nuts caused 45 of the 61 reactions. Of the five deaths, four were attributed to soy.

The four children who died from soy had known allergies to peanuts but not to soy. The amount of soy eaten ranged from one to ten grams—typical of the low levels found when soy protein is used as a meat-extending additive in readymade foods such as hamburgers, meatballs, spaghetti sauces, kebabs, sausages, bread and pastries.

When soy is "hidden" in hamburgers and other "regular" foods, people often miss the soy connection. And allergic reactions to soy do not always occur immediately, making cause and effect even harder to establish. As reported in the Swedish study, no symptoms—or only very mild symptoms—occurred for 30 to 90 minutes after the consumption of the food containing soy. Then, the children suffered fatal asthma attacks. All had been able to eat soy without any adverse reactions right up until the dinner that caused their deaths.

The Swedish study was not the first to report life-threatening events after eating soy. Food anaphylaxis is most often associated with reactions to peanuts, tree nuts, shellfish—occasionally fish or milk—but soy has its own rap sheet. Anaphylactic reactions to bread, pizzas or sausage extended with soy protein date back at least to 1961. Subsequent studies have confirmed that the risk may be rare but is very real.[12-20]

The increasing amount of "hidden" soy in the food supply is undoubtedly responsible for triggering many allergic reactions not attributed to soy. French researchers who studied the frequency of anaphylactic shocks caused by foods reported that the food allergen remained unknown in 25 percent of cases. They noted the prevalence of "hidden" and "masked" food allergens and stated that they saw "a strikingly increased prevalence of food-induced anaphylactic shock in 1995 compared to a previous study from 1982."[21] This period coincided with a huge increase in the amount of soy protein added to processed foods.

None of these studies has attracted much media attention. Nor have health agencies issued alerts. For example, Ingrid Malmheden Yman, Ph.D, of the Swedish National Food Administration and co-author of the study, wrote to the Ministry of Health in New Zealand at the request of an allergy sufferer. Two years before the article—first published in Swedish—came out in English, she informed the agency that children with severe allergy to peanuts should avoid intake of soy protein. To be on the safe side, she further advised parents to make an effort to "avoid sensitization" by limiting both peanuts and soybeans during the third trimester of pregnancy, dur-

---

PARENT WARNING:
HIDDEN SOY—HIDDEN SOY ALLERGIES

If your child is allergic to peanuts, you must eliminate all soy as well as all peanuts from your child's diet. Your child's life may depend upon it.

Take care even if your child has never reacted poorly to soy in the past. Some sensitive children have "hidden" soy allergies that manifest for the first time with a severe—even fatal—reaction to even the low levels of "hidden" soy commonly found in processed food products. Those at the highest risk suffer from asthma as well as peanut allergy. Other risk factors are other food allergies; a family history of peanut or soy allergies; a diagnosis of asthma, rhinitis or eczema; or a family history of these diseases.

SOURCE: Swedish National Food Administration.

ing breast feeding, and by avoiding the use of soy formula.[22]

Controversy has raged since the 1920s as to whether or not babies could be sensitized to allergens while still *in utero*. In 1976, researchers learned that the fetus is capable of producing IgE antibodies against soy protein during early gestation and newborns can be so sensitized through the breast milk of the mother that they later react to foods they've "never eaten."[23,24] Families who need to take these precautions seriously include those with known peanut and/or soy allergies, vegetarians who would otherwise eat a lot of soy foods during pregnancy or breastfeeding and parents considering the use of soy infant formula.

Because the numbers of children with allergies to peanuts are increasing, we can expect to see greater numbers of children and adults reacting severely to soy. Peanuts and soybeans are members of the same botanical family, the grain-legume type—and scientists have known for years that people allergic to one are often allergic to the other. Other children at risk for an undetected but potentially life-threatening soy allergy include those with allergies to peas, lima beans or other beans, a diagnosis of asthma, rhinitis, eczema or dermatitis, or family members with a history of any of those diseases. Reactions to foods in the same botanical family can be cumulative, resulting in symptoms far more severe than either alone.[25-32]

SOY'S ALLERGENIC PROTEINS

Scientists are not completely certain which components of soy cause allergic reactions. They have found at least 16 allergenic proteins, and some researchers pinpoint as many as 30. Laboratories report immune system responses to multiple fractions of the soy protein, with no fraction the most consistently antigenic.[33-36]

Some of the most allergenic fractions appear to be the Kunitz and Bowman-Birk trypsin inhibitors. As we saw in Chapter 16, food processors have tried in vain to completely deactivate these troublesome proteins without irreparably damaging the remainder of the proteins in soy. Although extremely rare, near deaths from allergic reaction to trypsin inhibitor has been a matter of public record since the *New England Journal of Medicine* carried a report in 1980.[37,38] The Kunitz trypsin inhibitor has been identified as one of three allergic components in soy lecithin, a soy product considered hypoallergenic because it is not supposed to include any soy protein, but which invariably contains trace amounts.[39]

The soybean lectin—another antinutrient—has also been identified as an allergen.[40] As discussed in Chapter 18 , whenever there is a damaged intestinal lining or "leaky gut," soy lectins can easily pass into the bloodstream, triggering allergic reactions. Indeed, this is very likely because both soy allergens and saponins (an antinutrient discussed in Chapter 19) can damage the intestines.

Histamine toxicity can also resemble allergic reactions. In allergic persons, mast cells release histamine, causing a response that strongly resembles an allergic reaction to food. In cases of histamine toxicity, the histamine comes ready-made in the food. This is most often associated with reactions to cheese and fish, but soy sauce also contains high levels of histamine. Researchers who have calculated the histamine content of foods consumed in a typical Asian meal report that histamine intake may easily approach toxic levels.[41]

CLEARING THE AIR

Allergic reactions occur not only from eating soy but also from inhaling soybean flour or dust. Among epidemiologists, soybean dust is known as an "epidemic asthma agent." From 1981-1987, soy dust from grain silo unloading in the harbor of Barcelona, Spain, caused 26 epidemics of asthma, seriously jeopardizing 687 people and leading to 1,155 hospitalizations. No further epidemics occurred after filters were installed, but a minor outbreak in 1994 established the need for diligent monitoring of preventive measures.[42,43]

Reports of the epidemic in Barcelona led epidemiologists in New Orleans to investigate cases of epidemic asthma that occurred from 1957-1968 when more than 200 people sought treatment at Charity Hospital. Investigations of weather patterns and cargo data from the New Orleans harbor identified soy dust from ships carrying soybeans as the probable cause. No association was found between asthma-epidemic days and the presence of wheat or corn in ships in the harbor. The researchers concluded: "The results of this analysis provide further evidence that ambient soy dust is very asthmogenic and that asthma morbidity in a community can be influenced by exposures in the ambient atmosphere."[44]

The first report of "occupational asthma" appeared in the *Journal of Allergy* in 1934. W. W. Duke described six persons whose asthma was triggered by dust from a nearby soybean mill and predicted that soy could become a major cause of allergy in the future.[45] Today it is well established that soybean dust poses an occupational hazard for those working in bakeries, animal feed factories, food processing plants and health food stores and co-ops with bulk bins. Dust explosions are a safety hazard at soybean processing plants.[46-49]

Most victims develop their "occupational asthma" over a period of time. In one well-documented case, a 43-year-old woman spent six years working in a food processing plant in which soybean flour was used as a meat extender before developing asthma. Symptoms of sneezing, coughing and wheezing would begin within minutes of exposure to soy flour and resolve two hours after the exposure ceased.[50]

Rare reactions to soy have also occurred in asthmatic patients using inhalers with bronchodilators containing soy-derived excipients. Bronchospasms with laryngospasms and cutaneous rash have occurred even in patients who were otherwise not affected by soy allergy.[51]

SOY INFANT FORMULA

For years, the soy industry billed soy formula as "hypoallergenic." Herman Frederic Meyer, M.D., Department of Pediatrics, Northwestern University Medical School, categorized soy formulas as "hypo-allergic preparations" in his 1960 textbook *Infant Foods and Feeding Practice* and named Mull Soy, Sobee, Soyalac and

Soyola products as good examples.[52]

Over the years the soy industry has promoted this and similar misinformation in advertising, labels and educational literature by ignoring relevant studies in favor of largely irrelevant studies based on guinea pigs.[53,54] As late as 1989, John Erdman, Ph.D. —a researcher honored in 2001 by the soy industry for his "outstanding contributions to increasing understanding and awareness of the health benefits of soy foods and soybean constituents"—claimed "hypoallergenicity" for soy in the *American Journal of Clinical Nutrition*. In a follow-up Letter to the Editor, another researcher corrected his misinformation.[55,56]

FUDGING STATISTICS

The soy industry today has shifted from claiming hypoallergenicity for soy to minimizing its extent. That has been fairly easy because no one seems to know just how many sufferers there are. Estimates are rough at best because diagnoses of allergy include anything from parental complaints of spitting, fussiness, colic and vomiting to laboratory provings using RAST and ELISA tests, to clinical challenges and elimination diets. Because the tests are not completely reliable and anecdotal evidence tends to be taken lightly, many cases are not counted. The figures cited most often delineate 0.3 to 7.5 percent of the population as allergic to cow's milk and 0.5 to 1.1 percent as allergic to soy. However, evidence suggests that soy protein is at least as antigenic as milk protein, especially when gastrointestinal complaints and delayed hypersensitivity (non-IgE) reactions are taken into account.[57-62]

On the soy-industry website "Soy and Human Health," Clare Hasler, Ph.D., formerly of the University of Illinois Urbana-Champaign, now executive director of the Robert Mondavi Institute for Wine and Food Science at the University of California Davis, picks the low 0.5 percent figure and claims that soy protein is rated 11th among foods in terms of allergenicity.[63] This may have been true in the 1970s (her source is dated 1979), but soy is widely acknowledged as one of the "big eight" today. Indeed, one prominent researcher puts soy in the "top six" and another in the "top four" foods causing hypersensitivity reactions in children.[64,65]

Soy formula is a far-from-optimal solution for bottle-fed infants who are allergic to dairy formulas. As we will see in Chapters 27 and 28, the plant estrogens in soy can interfere with proper development of the infant's thyroid gland, brain and reproductive systems. Soy formula also falls short as a solution to cow's milk allergy.

Symptoms such as diarrhea, bloating, vomiting and skin rashes sometimes go away when infants are switched from dairy formula to soy, but the relief is usually only temporary. In many infants they return with a vengeance within a week or two. As Stefano Guandalini, M.D., Department of Pediatrics, University of Chicago, writes, "A significant number of children with cow's milk protein intolerance develop soy–protein intolerance when soy milk is used in dietary management."[66] Interestingly enough, researchers recently detected and identified a soy protein component that cross reacts with caseins from cow's milk.[67] Cross reactions occur when foods are chemically related to each other.

Adverse reactions caused by soybean formulas occur in at least 14 to 35 percent of infants allergic to cow's milk, according to Matthias Besler, Ph.D., of Hamburg, Germany, and the international team of allergy specialists that help him with the informative website www.allergens.de.[68]

Dr. Guandalini's helpful allergy website www.emedicine.com reports the results of an unpublished study of 2,108 infants and toddlers in Italy, of which 53 percent of the babies under three months old who had reacted poorly to dairy formula also reacted adversely to soy formula. Although experts generally attribute this high level of reactivity to the immature—hence vulnerable—digestive tract of infants, this study showed that 35 percent of the children over one year old who were allergic to cow's milk protein also developed an allergy to soy protein. In all, 47 percent had to discontinue soy formula.[69]

Infants who are allergic to dairy formulas are allergic to soy formulas so often that researchers have begun advising pediatricians to stop recommending soy and start prescribing hypoallergenic hydrolyzed casein or whey formulas. A study of 216 infants at high risk for developing allergies revealed comparable levels of eczema and asthma whether they were drinking cow's milk formula or the more "hypoallergenic" soy formula. Upon conclusion of the study, the message was clear. Only "exclusive breast feeding or feeding with a partial whey hydrolysate formula is associated with the lower incidence of atopic disease and food allergy. This is a cost-effective approach to the prevention of allergic disease in children."[70]

Scientists can no longer argue that soy formula is hypoallergenic, but many still say that its soy proteins may be less sensitizing than cow's milk proteins. When babies develop soy intolerance, the blame tends to go to earlier damage done to the intestines by cow's milk protein.[71] This has led some physicians to recommend starting infants off from birth on soy formula. However, this practice does *not* stop a tendency to develop food allergies. As the late Charles D. May, M.D., Department of Pediatrics, National Jewish Hospital and Research Center in Denver, put it: "Feeding a soy product from birth for 112 days did not prevent a brisk antibody response to cow milk introduced subsequently, comparable to or greater than the antibody response seen when cow milk products were fed from birth."[72]

BOWELED OVER

People diagnosed with "allergic colitis" suffer from bloody diarrhea, ulcerations and tissue damage, particularly to the sigmoid area of the descending colon. The leading cause in infants is cow's milk allergy, but 47 to 60 percent of those infants react the same way to soy formula. Curiously, inflammatory changes in the mucus lining of the intestines appear even in infants who seem to be tolerating soy—no diarrhea, hives, blood in the stool or other obvious allergic signs. One study showed that clinical reactions occurred in 16 percent of the children on soy formula, but that histological and

FORMULA FOR DISASTER:
AROUND THE WORLD WITH SOY ALLERGIES

Allergic reactions occur to soy formula in children all over the world, particularly those affected by other allergies.

- San Diego, USA. Soybean allergies found in 25 percent of infants sensitive to cow's milk.
- Bangkok, Thailand. Soybean allergies in 17 percent of children sensitive to cow's milk.
- Malmo, Sweden. Soybean allergies in 35 percent of infants with cow's milk allergies.
- Victoria, Australia. Soy milk allergies in 47 percent of 97 children with cow's milk allergies.
- Berlin, Germany. Soybean allergies in 16 percent of children with atopic dermatitis.
- Bonn, Germany. Soybean allergies in 10 percent of children with suspected food allergy.
- Milan, Italy. Soybean allergies in 17 percent of children with food intolerance.
- Milan, Italy. Soybean allergies in 21 percent of 704 atopic children.
- Rome, Italy. Soy allergies found in 22 percent of 371 children with food allergy.
- Thailand. Soy allergies in 4 percent of 100 asthmatic children.
- New Haven, CT, U.S.A. Soy and milk allergies found in 62 percent and soy and gluten allergies found in 35 percent of infants and children with multiple gastrointestinal allergies.
- Ohio, USA. Sensitivity to soy formula found in five percent of 148 children with respiratory allergies.

SOURCE: Literature review on Dr. Matthias Besler's website www.allergens.de For full citations, see Endnotes to this chapter #110-121.

enzymologic intestinal damage occurred in an additional 38 percent of the children. This second group showed damage to the intestinal cells and tissues as viewed under a microscope and through blood tests indicating increased levels of xylose, an indigestible sugar used to diagnose "leaky gut" and other intestinal disorders. The researchers also found depleted levels of sucrase, lactase, maltase and alkaline phosphatase—evidence that the infants' digestive capacity was compromised, their stress levels increased and immune systems challenged.[73]

Most gastrointestinal problems connected to soy formula involve non-IgE delayed immune reactions.[74] However, local IgE reactions may contribute to these problems by triggering the formation of immune complexes that alter the permeability of the gut mucosa. As C. Carini, the lead author in an *Annals of Allergy* study, wrote, "The resultant delayed onset symptoms could be viewed as a form of serum sickness with few or many target organs affected."[75]

The baby's small intestine is at special risk. Scanning electron microscopy and biopsies have revealed severe damage to the small intestine, including flattening and wasting away of the projections (known as villi) and cellular overgrowth of the pits (known as crypts). Allergic reaction may not be the sole cause here as the observed destruction dovetails with that caused by the soy antinutrients lectins and saponins, with the lectins possibly doing double duty as allergic proteins (see Chapters 18 and 19). Flattening and atrophy of the villi lead to malnutrition and failure to thrive, with a clinical picture very similar to that found in children and adults afflicted with celiac disease.[76-78]

Celiac disease is a serious malabsorption syndrome most commonly associated with gluten (a protein fraction found in wheat and some other grains) and dairy intolerance. Few people realize that there is also a connection with soy. Some adults with celiac disease experience diarrhea, headache, nausea and flatulence even on a gluten-free diet when they eat a tiny amount of soy. And a study of 98 infants and children with multiple gastrointestinal allergies revealed that 62 percent had both soy and milk allergies and 35 percent both soy and gluten.[79,80]

OUTGROWING SOY ALLERGIES

Allergy specialists say that "most" young children "outgrow" their sensitivities.[81] This makes sense— to a point. If infants develop soy allergies because of immature digestive tracts and immune systems, the risk of developing a soy allergy would decrease with age and many children would outgrow their soy allergies. Yet other studies—even by the same authors—reveal that only a minority of subjects outgrow them.

One study showed that only 26 percent of children suffering from soy, egg, milk, wheat and peanut allergies lose their hypersensitivity after one year. While peanut—soy's even more allergenic relative—may have skewed those results, another study found that only two out of eight infants outgrew soy allergies after 25 months.[82-84] And many children who "successfully" outgrow food allergies develop respiratory allergies. A study of 322 children showed that only six percent still experienced food sensitivity after five years, but 40 percent of those children "grew into" respiratory allergies. This was true of milk, egg, chocolate, soy and cereals, in that order.[85] Yet this study is often cited as proof that most children "successfully" outgrow their allergies.

Children are more likely to outgrow allergies to cow's milk or soy than allergies to peanuts, fish or shrimp, but will continue to react to them if they eat these foods often enough. And treatment of these allergies requires total exclusion of the offending food. Soy-induced enterocolitis, for example, will resolve after six months to two years of strictly avoiding soy.[86] As families of allergic youngsters know, keeping soy off the dinner table and out of meals and snacks provided at daycare centers and schools can be a serious challenge. Even in non-vegetarian families, soy is ubiquitous in processed and fast foods. As a result, sensitization to soy has increased, is not necessarily outgrown, and can either reemerge or develop later in life.

FRANKENSOY'S MONSTER

Soy allergies may also be on the rise because of genetically modified (GM) soybeans. The York Nutritional Laboratories in England—one of Europe's leading laboratories specializing in food sensitivity—found a 50 percent increase in soy allergies in 1998, the same year in which genetically engineered beans were introduced to the world market. York's researchers noted that one of the 16 proteins in soybeans most likely to cause allergic reactions was found in concentrations higher by 30 percent or more in Monsanto's GM soybeans.

The York researchers sent their findings to British Health Secretary Frank Dobson, urging the government to act on the information and impose an instant ban on GM food pending further safety tests. Michael Antoniou, M.D., a molecular geneticist at Guy's Hospital, Central London, observed, "This is a very interesting if slightly worrying development. It points to the fact that far more work is needed to assess their safety. At the moment, no allergy tests are carried out before GM foods are marketed and that also needs to be looked at."[87,88]

People allergic to GM soybeans may not even be allergic to soy. The culprit can be foreign proteins introduced into the soybean. People allergic to Brazil nuts but not to soy have shown allergies to GM soybeans in which Brazil nut proteins were inserted to increase the level of methionine and improve the overall amino acid profile of soy.[89] Scientists say that such problems can be prevented by doing IgE-binding studies, by accounting for physico-chemical characteristics of proteins and referring to known allergen databases. That might have identified the Brazil nut problem, but there is no way to assess the risk of *de novo* sensitization, which happens when experiments generate new allergens.[90]

THE MARGARINE CONNECTION

Allergies to pollen, dust, dander and foods are on the increase wherever margarine replaces butter.

That's the conclusion of Finnish researchers who found that children who developed allergies ate less butter and more margarine compared with children who did not develop allergies. Nearly all commercially marketed margarines are made with soy oil.

The study showed that children with eczema, dermatitis and other itchy skin conditions consumed an average of 8 grams of margarine for every 1000 calories compared to 6 grams among children without allergies, and 9 grams of butter compared to 11 grams of butter or more among the children without the allergies.

Lab testing revealed that the allergic children had a higher ratio of polyunsaturated to saturated fat and lower percentage of myristic acid (an indicator of saturated fat intake) than children without allergies. They also showed lower levels of the very unsaturated EPA and DHA fatty acids found in fish.

The inescapable conclusion: Butter is better.

SOURCE: Dunder T, Kuikka L et al. Diet, serum fatty acids and atopic diseases in childhood. *Allergy*, 2001, 56, 5, 425-428.

MY SOY STORY: FEELING BAD

I finally deduced that the "peri-menopause" symptoms I was having (migraines, photophobia, brain fog, fatigue, hair loss, heavy periods and more) were actually from the soy that I was eating. I am not a vegan, but because of a blood sugar issue, I had a high protein diet. I tried to balance meats with soy because of the risks of too much meat. So I wasn't even in the high soy intake levels. But even after the banning of soy from my diet, I would feel bad. Mayo was one of the things that slipped my scrutiny. I remember when Best Foods made their mayo with some other oil but now they use soy oil. Well, I have been fine for several months until the other day, when I ate a snack that contained soy (labeled as "latticing"). It was within 24 hours and I was down for 3 days! Migraine, unbearable weakness, joint pain, eye twitching, vertigo and general feeling of BAD that just angered me to no end. How and what did I miss the soy in? Please, people! Don't stop with spouting these horrors!!! The world has got to WAKE UP!

R.C., Boca Raton, LA

latticing

25
THE SOY-FREE CHALLENGE

The ways that the soybean is grown, harvested, processed, stored and prepared in the kitchen can all affect its allergenicity.

PROCESSING MATTERS

Raw soybeans are the most allergenic while old-fashioned, fermented products (miso, tempeh, *natto*, *shoyu* and tamari) are the least. Modern soy protein products processed by heat, pressure and chemical solvents lose some of their allergenicity, but not all. Foods like partially hydrolyzed proteins or soy sprouts, which are quickly or minimally processed, remain highly allergenic.[1,2]

An industry newsletter *The Soy Connection* states that highly refined oils and lecithin "are safe for the soy-allergic consumer."[3] Unfortunately, many allergic persons who put their trust in such reassurances have ended up in the hospital. Highly susceptible people cannot use either safely. Adverse reactions to soy oils—taken either by mouth as food or via tube feeding—range from the nuisance of sneezing to the life-threatening danger of anaphylactic shock.[4-10]

If soy oil and lecithin were 100 percent free of soy protein, they would not provoke allergic symptoms. Variable conditions, quality control and processing methods used when the vegetable oil industry separates soybean protein from the oil make the presence of at least trace amounts of soy protein possible, even likely. Although healthier in many respects, the cold-pressed soy oils sold in health food stores can be deadly for the allergic consumer. They may contain as much as 100 times more than the trace protein found in the highly refined soy oils sold in supermarkets.[11,12]

Soy protein is a standard ingredient in margarines and spreads. Above and beyond any stray protein that remains after the processing of the soy oil, food manufacturers commonly use soy protein isolates or concentrates to improve the texture or spreadability. This occurs most often in low-fat or "low *trans*" products (see Chapter 9).

HIDDEN DANGER

People allergic to soy protein face danger 24/7. Hidden soy exists in thousands of everyday foods, cosmetics and industrial products such as inks, cardboards, paints, cars and mattresses. The four Swedish fatalities documented in Chapter 24 are only the best known of thousands of reported cases of people who experienced severe

MY SOY STORY: SOY MILK SHOCK

Our neighbor is a doctor who was on night duty at the Los Angeles County Hospital and saved a boy's life. The boy was allergic to peanuts and went into shock when his parents gave him a glass of soy milk. Bob said he could hear him dying on the R/T and the ambulance was still 30 minutes away. He directed the paramedic to give him an adrenaline injection and he recovered immediately. The ambulance took him home instead of to the morgue. We often wonder how many are not so lucky.   G.S., Los Angeles, CA allergic reactions to soy after inadvertently eating foods that contained soybean proteins.[13-15]

Of 659 food products recalled by the U.S. Food and Drug Administration (FDA) in 1999, 236 (36 percent) were taken off the market because of undeclared allergens. The three factors responsible for the undeclared allergens were: omissions and errors on labels (51 percent), cross contamination of manufacturing equipment (40 percent), and errors made by suppliers of ingredients (5 percent). It wasn't inspectors, however, but ticked off U.S. consumers who fingered 56 percent of the undeclared allergens.[16]

During 2002, the Canadian Food Inspection agency (CFIA), which takes soy allergies seriously, recalled bagels, donuts, rolls, pizza and other items containing undeclared soy protein.[17] Although agencies in many countries claim to be stepping up efforts to enforce labeling laws, enforcement is difficult even when officials make it a priority. The chief problem is that few methods reliably detect and quantify minute amounts of allergens in foods.[18]

INFORMATION GAP

Even when soy-containing ingredients are accurately listed on food labels, many consumers miss the soy connection. A study of 91 parents of children allergic to peanuts, milk, egg, soy, and/or wheat revealed that most parents failed to correctly identify allergenic food ingredients, and that milk and soy presented the most problems. Only 22 percent of the parents with soy allergies correctly identified soy protein in seven products. The researchers concluded: "These results strongly support the need for improved labeling with plain-English terminology and allergen warnings as well as the need for diligent education of patients reading labels."[19]

Help for the consumer comes in January 2006 when the Food Allergen Labeling and Consumer Protection Act (S. 741) goes into effect. The law requires food manufacturers to clearly state whether a product contains milk, eggs, peanuts, tree nuts, fish, shellfish, wheat or soy, and requires the FDA to conduct inspections to ensure that manufacturers comply with practices to reduce or eliminate cross-contamination with any major food allergens that are not intentional ingredients of a food. The law represents a major victory for the Food Allergy Initiative, a New York-based nonprofit organization that has supported public policy initiatives intended to create a safer environment for students and other Americans suffering from food allergies who are in danger of dying from anaphylactic shock.[20]

WHERE THE SOYS ARE

Those who are allergic to soy must exclude *all* soy from their diets. This can be a challenge. Soy lurks in nearly everything these days, even in products where we would not reasonably expect it. It's in Bumblebee canned tuna, Chef Boyardee Ravioli, Hershey's chocolate, Baskin Robbins ice cream, McDonald's and other fast food burgers, Pizza Hut pizza, many luncheon meats, most bread, muffins, donuts, lemonade mixes, hot chocolate, some baby foods, and tens of thousands of other popular products.

If you absolutely must keep soy out of your life or that of your children, memorize the following:

+ SOY GOES BY MANY ALIASES. Food processors are less likely to list the three letter word "soy" than a technical term such as "textured vegetable protein (TVP)," "textured plant protein," "hydrolyzed vegetable protein (HVP)," "vegetable protein concentrate," "vegetable oil" or "MSG (monosodium glutamate)." Ingredient lists also include words such as "lecithin," "vegetable oil," "vegetable broth," "boullion," "natural flavor" or "mono-diglyceride" that do not necessarily come from soy, but are likely to.

twenty-five: the soy-free challenge

- FOOD LABELS AND INGREDIENT LISTS CHANGE. Check them every single time. Manufacturers can switch the ingredients used in food products without warning. Allergic consumers need to check the labels every time they make a purchase and ask about ingredients every time they eat at restaurants or purchase food at a deli. To make things easier, many allergic people carry cards listing foods on their "no" lists.

- PRODUCTS MAY BE MISLABELED OR CONTAIN UNDECLARED SOY. The only solution here is to hope, pray and make your own food from scratch using known ingredients.

- CROSS CONTAMINATION OCCURS. Improperly cleaned pans, plates, utensils, cutting boards at restaurant or delis, bins at health food stores, or vats at the factory can contaminate food with traces of soy. All it takes is a bit of old soy oil or soy protein residue to trigger severe reactions in people who are highly susceptible.

- SOY MAY BE IN THE PACKAGE AS WELL AS ITS CONTENTS. Soy protein isolate used in the manufacture of paperboard boxes can flake off and migrate into food. Some foods may be shrink wrapped in an edible soy-based plastic.

- SOY CAN BE BREATHED AS WELL AS EATEN. Expect soy dust in some bakeries, shipyards and the bulk bin aisle of your health food stores.

- SOY MAY BE IN YOUR PILLS. Vitamins, over-the-counter drugs and prescriptions may contain an unwanted dose of soy. Beware of pills with soy oil bases, vitamin E derived from soy oil, and soy components such as isoflavones The inhaler Atrovent is just one of many drug-store products containing unexpected soy. A new type of aspirin called "aspirin cocholeates" made with "all natural" soy-derived phospholipids will soon be on drugstore shelves.

- SOY IS THE LATEST THING IN JUST ABOUT EVERYTHING. Soy inks, paints, plastics, carpets, mattresses, cars, etc. are just a few of the industrial products that may be green for the environment but deadly for highly allergic persons.

- KISS WITH CARE. Finally, someone who is exquisitely sensitive to soy could die from contact with the lips of someone who has just eaten soy. Unlikely as this might seem, it has happened with peanuts, soy's even more allergenic relative.

part seven
SOY ESTROGENS
hormone havoc

26
PHYTOESTROGENS
food's fifth column

Phytoestrogens are plant estrogens. Although they are not true hormones, they are similar enough structurally to act like hormones and bind with estrogen-receptor sites throughout the body. This is possible because receptor sites are so flexible. The fact that phytoestrogens can take the place of "real" estrogens in the human body has led many researchers to propose that they be used for "natural" hormone replacement therapies, cholesterol lowering, and cancer prevention and cures. Efficacy and safety, however, have yet to be proven.[1-3]

THE BIG THREE

The top three phytoestrogens found in foods are isoflavones, coumestans and lignans. Isoflavones exist in more than 70 plants with the highest concentrations found in soybeans. Coumestans occur in young sprouting legumes such as soy, clover and alfalfa sprouts. Lignans are present in flaxseeds.[4-6]

Now that pharmaceutical firms see future profits in phytoestrogens, they have developed sensitive and accurate analytical methods to measure these compounds. The most widely used techniques are reversed-phase high-performance liquid chromatography with ultraviolet detection; gas chromatography with mass spectrometric detection; and liquid chromatography with mass spectrometric detection. These techniques allow scientists to measure phytoestrogens in foodstuffs and biological samples down to concentrations of parts per billion.[7]

Predicting isoflavone content in any given food, however, remains elusive. Levels in soybeans are influenced by many factors including crop year, geographical location, number of daylight hours, temperature, humidity, rain, fertilizers, types of pathogens and the plant's response to attack or disease. American varieties of soybeans have significantly higher total isoflavone content than Japanese breeds. This uncertainty frustrates manufacturers who would like to advertise the levels of the supposedly beneficial isoflavones contained in their products and stymies consumers who would like to monitor their consumption.

Although it is difficult to predict the quantities of isoflavones

ISOFLAVONE BASE CAMP

Want to know the level of isoflavones in a soy food? Go to www.nal.usda.gov. In 1999, the USDA and Iowa State University, with partial funding from the U.S. Army, established a database of isoflavone concentrations in foods. The database gives best guestimates for the major isoflavones in 128 soy foods and ingredients and even lists some brand names. Relying heavily on analyses by Patricia Murphy, Ph.D., of Iowa State University, scientists evaluated and compiled some 30 scientific reports on isoflavone content. Before new information is added to the database, workers evaluate the analytical methodology and compare it to a reference. A confidence code is assigned to indicate the data quality with a grade A signifying reliability.

SOURCE: www.ars.usda.gov

in any given bean, the order of the three highest types of soy isoflavones remains consistent, with genistein first, followed by daidzein, with glycitein a distant third.[8,9] Conceivably scientists could breed and cultivate plants to achieve the most beneficial mix but no one has yet determined what that mix might be.[10]

Isoflavones in the soybean exist primarily in the glucoside forms of genistein, daidzein and glycitein, but must be converted to the aglucone forms of genistin, daidzin and glycitin to be absorbed. The fact that the glucoside forms have not been found in plasma indicates that they cannot be transported intact across the gut mucosa. To be absorbed, an enzyme known as beta-glycosidase must first chip off a sugar. This generally occurs in the small intestine or the liver.[11]

ALL THINGS EQUOL

High-carbohydrate diets cause increased fermentation in the gut, resulting in greater production of an estrogenically active metabolite of daidzein known as equol. Kenneth D.R. Setchell, Ph.D., explains: "The estrogenic potency of equol is an order of magnitude higher than that of its plant precursor, daidzein. The importance of the microflora in the metabolic handling of isoflavones is well illustrated from observations that antibiotic administration blocks metabolism, germfree animals do not excrete the metabolites, and infants fed soy infant formulas in the first four months of life cannot form appreciable amounts of equol."[12]

This last is cited as evidence of soy formula's safety for infants although Setchell's own work has shown that infants can and will absorb other forms of isoflavones.[13] Though less metabolically active than equol, they nonetheless have the power to perturb the endocrine system and adversely affect reproductive development (see Chapters 28 and 29).

Interestingly, some people are equol producers while others are not. It seems that different people excrete different phytoestrogen metabolites even when the quality and quantity of soy food eaten is tightly controlled. Retests tend to be consistent in individuals. Populations of gut flora are highly individual and seem to play key roles in the metabolism and bioavailability of isoflavones. Antibiotics, dysbiosis or bowel disease also modify isoflavone metabolism.[14]

Isoflavones have been found in most body fluids—urine, plasma, feces, prostatic fluid, semen, bile, saliva, breast milk, breast aspirate and cyst fluid. Isoflavones can cross the blood-brain barrier in rats and pass through the placenta to the fetus.[15] This property of isoflavones is of great interest to pharmaceutical companies and a

ESTIMATED ISOFLAVONE CONTENT OF COMMON FOODS

Isoflavone intake in Asia ranges from 3 mg per person per day (China) to a high of 28 (Japan).

Bread with added soy flour, 2 slices	4 mg
Meatless chicken nuggets, 1/2 cup	15 mg
Soy hot dog	15 mg
Green soybeans, raw, 1/2 cup	20 mg
Miso, 1/4 cup	21 mg
Tofu, 1/2 cup	28 mg
Dr. Soy candy bar	30 mg
Soy cheese, 1/2 cup	31 mg
Soy milk, 1 cup	45 mg
Soymilk skin or film , cooked, 1/2 cup	51 mg
Tempeh, cooked, 1/2 cup	53 mg
Soybean chips, 1/2 cup	54 mg
Mature soybeans, cooked, 1/2 cup	55 mg
French Meadow Bakery Women's Bread, slice	80 mg
Dry roasted soybeans, 1/2 cup	128 mg
Revival soy-based meal replacement, 1 serving	160 mg

SOURCE: www.nal.usda.gov

reason to be concerned about the isoflavones naturally found in soy foods.

HALF LIVES

In general, concentrations of daidzein and genistein in the blood peak within six to eight hours after eating. Plasma concentrations begin to rise within two hours but can occur within 15 minutes

MY SOY STORY: EARLY ALZHEIMER'S

I am an executive secretary but almost lost my job during my mid-50s because I developed Alzheimer-like symptoms. I became extremely forgetful, to the point of not knowing what to do or say when I answered the phone. I once found myself walking across the street with heavy traffic coming towards me and not knowing how I got there. I did not eat soy, just a typical western diet. However, in order to lose weight, I went on a diet and stopped eating bread. My forgetfulness and brain fog cleared up mysteriously. When I went off the diet, the symptoms returned.

I have long had a thyroid problem for which I take medication. When our office got connected to the internet, I went online to learn about thyroid health and learned that soy depresses thyroid function. Then I started reading labels and found that soy is added in small amounts to all commercial bread. Since that time I have religiously avoided all products containing soy (very hard to do these days). I make my own bread now and have never had any further problems with forgetfulness or similar symptoms. Just the small levels of isoflavones in the soy flour added to commercial bread were enough to cause serious symptoms in someone like myself, with a pre-existing thyroid problem.

J.S., Auckland, New Zealand

after eating. Many individuals exhibit more than one plasma peak, which probably reflects circulation of the isoflavones back and forth between the liver and intestines.[16,17]

The majority of isoflavones are excreted in the urine, with only a small percentage of absorbed isoflavones ending up in the feces. Yet human and animal studies indicate that no more than 50 percent of the isoflavones ingested end up in the urine. This frustrates researchers, who would like to know why so many of the isoflavones go missing. Setchell speculates that gut flora metabolize these into metabolites that are either not yet known or not being measured by investigators. This, of course, raises the question of whether the level of isoflavones excreted in the urine should be considered a reliable indicator of dietary intake.[18] It also suggests that more research is needed before the soy industry advises people to eat more of these hormonally active substances.

PROCESSING MATTERS

Soy foods with the highest levels of isoflavones are soy flours, grits, nuts, soy protein isolates and textured vegetable proteins. Within these categories, isoflavone content varies depending upon the variety and growing conditions of the soybean. Fermented soybeans, tofu, soymilk and soy yogurt contain middling levels. Second generation American soy foods such as soy hot dogs and burgers contain the least because the soy is diluted with other ingredients. Cooking and processing will sometimes reduce phytoestrogen concentrations and alter the chemical form of the phytoestrogens present in foods but it will not eliminate the isoflavones. Only alcohol extraction at the processing plant can do that.[19-21]

Which forms of isoflavones are the most bioavailable? No one knows for sure. The old-fashioned fermented soy products miso and tempeh contain lower levels of isoflavones than modern products, but contain the more absorbable form.[22,23] A few researchers, however, report that the bioavailability of the isoflavones in fermented and modern products is about the same, although absorption takes place faster with the fermented soy products.[24]

Setchell believes the glycoside forms are the most potent because they stay in the system longer and undergo multiple passes through the enterohepatic system. People eating the glucoside forms of soy found in modern soy products tend to show several plasma peaks, which indicate that the soy estrogens are recirculating.[25] "Clinical efficacy of isoflavones is almost certainly related to the plasma circulating concentration," writes Setchell, "and it is this endpoint that is likely to be the most reliable one to measure in clinical studies."[26] A believer in the benefits of soy, he recommends eating small amounts of soy throughout the day to best achieve "steady-state plasma concentrations."

Setchell notes that adults who consume modest quantities of soy foods containing about 50 mg per day of total isoflavones will achieve plasma concentrations of 50 to 800 ng/L. These values are similar to those of Japanese people consuming soy as a condiment in their traditional diet but far less than the quantities consumed by many vegetarians and others who regularly include soy products to their diet. Setchell concedes that plasma concentrations are much higher in infants fed soy formula and can far exceed normal plasma

---

DRUNK ON SOY

Consumers can now get their daily fix of soy estrogens by swigging water. Soy20—pronounced "soy two oh"—is a fruit-flavored water that contains 20 mg of soy in every 12-ounce bottle. Just two bottles a day will exceed the amount that caused thyroid damage in only three months in healthy Japanese adults. Best of all, this "crisp and clear" new product is said to deliver the goods without the "taste, appearance and odor of soy."

SOURCE: Leading Brands Inc announces launch of blend of fruit-flavored water and natural soy isoflavones called Soy20™ Vancouver, BC, October 14, 2003. www.thesoydailyclub.com.

estradiol concentrations: "It was this early observation that led us to the hypothesis that with such disproportional levels one could anticipate hormonal effects from phytoestrogens."[27] In fact, the risks to infants are considerable and discussed in depth in Chapter 28.

POTENCIES

Phytoestrogens exert estrogenic effects directly and indirectly: directly by binding with estrogen receptors and indirectly by interfering with estrogen production. Measurements of estrogenic potency, however, are notoriously inconsistent, depending upon the assay used.[28] This poses a huge problem for researchers testing isoflavones and is one more reason the results of studies are so inconsistent and contradictory.

To date, most of the research on the estrogenic effects of isoflavones has been carried out using rodents. Different animal species differ in their absorption, distribution, metabolism and excretion as well as in the timing of their fetal, neonatal and pubertal development, endocrine physiology and function.[29,30] These differences must be recognized and taken into account when extrapolating experimental findings to humans. Otherwise it is all too easy for soybean enthusiasts to discount the adverse effects that have appeared in animals—calling them irrelevant—but to quickly publicize the benefits—in the hope and belief that they are significant.

The route of administration must also be noted. Oral administration—eating—is most important in considering soy foods, but injections could be useful pharmacologically. Multiple doses of a soy compound may exert greater or longer term estrogenic effects than a single exposure—or vice versa.[31] Finally, synergy with other estrogens and toxins should be taken into account. This is especially true in light of the many antinutrients and toxins that occur either naturally in the soybean or as the result of modern processing.

WINDOWS OF VULNERABILITY

The timing of exposure to estrogens is critical. The safe, intelligent use of soy isoflavones as food or supplements demands sure knowledge of windows of vulnerability—or opportunity—as found *in utero*, during infancy, before puberty, during puberty, the reproductive years or beyond. Phytoestrogens exert their influence throughout the body in many different ways. While this fact assures a future for these compounds in nutraceutical and pharmaceutical products, it definitely presents a case of "buyer beware." Like steroidal estrogens, plant estrogens have the potential to exert adverse as well as beneficial actions.[32] The idea that they are "natural," hence safe, is wishful thinking.

THE ISOFLAVONE CHALLENGE

Patricia Whitten, Ph.D., of Emory University in Atlanta, Georgia warns us that the isoflavonoids and other estrogenic plant chemicals are generally lumped together under the general rubric of phytoestrogen, but that they are actually a diverse group with a variety of biological properties. Each type needs to be characterized in terms of its sites of action, properties, potency, and short-term and long-term effects.[33] In general, she sees three roles for phytoestrogens, all of which have a potential for good or for evil.

- Estrogen agonists (competitors) whose actions might benefit postmenopausal women but might also contribute to cancer.
- Antiestrogens or antiproliferative agents that could help prevent estrogen-dependent cancers, but also contribute to infertility by suppressing normal reproductive function.
- Developmental toxins that could disrupt sexual differentiation in infants by altering sex-specific patterns of development, but which might provide protection against environmental estrogens by altering steroid response thresholds.

Only one thing is clear: soy estrogens are not weak. Yet popular health writers continually repeat the misinformation that soy

HAELAN: PERKING PROFITS

An exorbitantly priced soy supplement known as Haelan 951 presents itself as "a novel fermented soy beverage" and the nutritional cure all for terminal cancer, AIDS and the nausea, vomiting and other side effects of chemotherapy. Even people who are wise to the health problems caused by modern soy products have fallen for the health claims made for this product. Supposedly, this high-isoflavone concentrate offers all the cancer-curing attributes of soy but with the safety of the traditionally fermented soy products miso, *natto* and tempeh. Truth is there's nothing traditional about the manufacturing process.

The product is made by condensing 25 pounds of "phytochemically-rich hand-picked soybeans grown in the People's Republic of China into an 8-ounce bottle and then fermenting it with *Azotobacter vinelandii*." The proprietary "nitrogenation process" hydrolyzes soybean proteins and concentrates isoflavones as well as other antinutrients such as saponins, protease inhibitors and phytates. High price to the contrary, hydrolyzing is a fast, cheap and highly profitable process. In contrast, the old-fashioned time-consuming fermentation methods lower the levels of antinutrients and toxins. Although the Haelan process could create a potent and possibly useful soy drug, the drink is sold as a safe and natural super food. As the company puts it, "Soybean phytochemicals are food micronutrients required for optimal health" and "health problems are directly related to these nutrient deficiencies." Yup, and depression is a Prozac-deficiency disease.

SOURCES: Nair, Vijaya. Hernandez V. Fermented soy: an aid to cancer prevention and therapy. *Well Being Journal*, 2002, 11, 6, and Haelan product literature.

phytoestrogens are safe, useful and effective because, unlike other estrogens, they are "weak" estrogens.

Archer Daniels Midland (ADM), Protein Technologies International (PTI), Nestlé and many corporate researchers have all fostered this impression. Spokespersons routinely claim that their phytoestrogens are 10,000 to 1,000,000 times less potent than the human estrogen estradiol. These unsubstantiated figures are then duly repeated by the mass media.

NESTLE CRUNCHES THE NUMBERS – Ph.D. FLUNKS MATH

The correct figure is 1,200 times less potent, according to studies by Markiewicz and others published in 1993.[34] That figure was agreed upon by participants at the Third International Conference on Phytoestrogens in Little Rock, Arkansas, in December 1995.[35] Although the figure of 1/1,200 might seem "weak," isoflavones are potent endocrine disrupters when consumed in sufficient quantities. How the soy industry came up with the much weaker figures of 10,000, 100,000, and even 500,000 or 1,000,000 times less potent is most instructive.

The erroneous figure of 1/10,000 appeared for the first time in a report made by Anthony C. Hugget, Ph.D., a scientist at the Nestlé

GENISTEIN AND THE HEART

The FDA allows products containing soy protein to carry a claim stating that they protect against heart disease. But the isoflavone genistein, the principle isoflavone in soy protein, has been shown to cause heart arrhythmias. Researchers have found that genistein interfers with potassium in the heart "suggesting the potential for soy isoflavones to cause heart arrhythmias."

SOURCE: Chaing CE et al. Genistein inhibits the inward rectifying potassium currents in guinea pig ventricular myocytes. *J Biomed Sci*, 2002, 9, 321-326.

Research Centre in Lausanne, Switzerland, in 1994. Making some calculations based on figures in the 1993 Markiewicz study, Hugget misplaced a decimal point turning 0.00l into .000l. Although Environmental scientist Mike Fitzpatrick, Ph.D., pointed out this error to Hugget on a visit to Lausanne in September 1994, the 1/10,000 figure lived on in Nestlé's communications.[36] For example, it was used to establish the probable safety of soy formula in a report dated December 14, 1994 that was furnished by Nestlé to the World Health Organization (WHO) and forwarded by them to the New Zealand Ministry of Health. Whether the inclusion of the 1/10,000 figure was a deliberate attempt to deceive or simple negligence is unknown. What is known is that Nestlé is a major manufacturer of soy infant formula.

So is Wyeth-Ayerst, the maker of the soy infant formula Infasoy. New Zealand's Soy Information Network reports that in a press release sent out during the same period, Wyeth-Ayerst claimed that soy phytoestrogens "exhibit very weak biological activity: 1/1000 to 1/100,000 that of estradiol." Subsequently, other soy companies repeated these figures.[37]

Most revealing is a "Technical Brief" provided by Protein Technologies International (PTI) of St. Louis, Missouri, that was also sent to the New Zealand Ministry of Health on January 26, 1995. In this document, PTI states that the soy phytoestrogens "exhibit very weak biological activity: 1/1000 to 1/1,000,000 of the activity of estradiol." The writer cited two scientific papers in support of these figures.[38] Dave Woodhams, Ph.D., tracked down the papers that PTI cited and found that in the first study genistein (the principal soy phytoestrogen) was compared to the synthetic estrogen diethylstilbestrol (DES), not to estradiol, as was claimed by PTI. DES is 100 times as strong as estradiol. In that soy infant formula is supposed to simulate human milk, the comparison to DES was both irrelevant and dishonest. The second paper by Mark Messina, Ph.D., stated that genistein exerts "an estrogenic effect ranging from approximately 1×10^{-3} to 1×10^{-5} that of diethylstilbestrol (DES) or estra-

TOFU
AND THE INCREDIBLE SHRINKING BRAIN

Men and women who eat two or more servings of tofu per week in midlife are more likely to experience cognitive decline, senile dementia and brain atrophy later in life than those who eat little or none. This startling announcement sent shock waves through the soy industry when announced at the Third International Symposium on the Role of Soy in the Prevention and Treatment of Chronic Disease in Washington, DC, in 1999.[40]

Lon R. White, M.D., a neuro-epidemiologist with the Pacific Health Institute in Honolulu, procured his initial data from a group of 8,006 Japanese-American men born between 1900 and 1910. All had been enrolled in the Honolulu Heart Project, a longitudinal study established in 1965 for research on heart disease and stroke. Researchers carried out standardized interviews in 1965-67 and again in 1971-74 to learn details about their diets in mid-life.

From 1991 to 1993 Dr. White and his team completed cognitive testing on 3,734 men, magnetic resonance imaging on 574 and autopsies on 290. They also analyzed cognitive test data for 502 wives on the assumption that they had eaten the same meals as their husbands. The results? Men and women who ate tofu at least twice per week experienced accelerated brain aging, diminished cognitive ability and were more than twice as likely to be clinically diagnosed with Alzheimer's disease. MRI scans showed enlarged ventricles while autopsies revealed atrophied brains with lower weights. Subjectively, the researchers couldn't help but notice that by age 75 to 80 the tofu eaters looked about five years older than those who abstained.[41-43]

The industry claims "the tofu effect" is just a fluke but the statistical probability of the results being true varied from

95 to 99.9 percent, depending upon the particular brain aging endpoint. The investigators also searched for—but failed to find—confounding factors such as age, education, obesity or other food and drinks. Although the tofu eaters were more likely to have been born in Japan, nothing about their early upbringing such as diet or education could explain the finding. Both miso and tofu correlated with measures of senility, but the miso effect shrank into statistical insignificance while the tofu effect remained strong. Indeed the more tofu eaten the more cognitive impairment and/or brain atrophy.[44]

The study has earned high marks from researchers not on the soy industry's payroll, including Dan Sheehan, Ph.D., and Daniel Doerge, Ph.D., at the FDA's National Laboratory for Toxicological Research: "Given the great difficulty in discerning the relationship between exposures and long latency adverse effects in the human population, and the potential mechanistic explanation for the epidemiological findings, this is an important study. It is one of the more robust, well-designed prospective epidemiological studies generally available."[45]

Dr. White hypothesizes that it is the isoflavones in tofu and other soy foods that cause so many adverse effects in the brain. Numerous animal studies show that soy isoflavones interfere with an enzyme called tyrosine kinase in the hippocampus, a brain region involved with learning and memory.[46,47] Elevated levels of phytoestrogens in the brain also cause decreases in brain calcium-binding protein (needed for protection against neurodegenerative diseases) and in brain-derived neurotrophic factor (essential for the survival and genesis of brain cells).[48,49] Finally, genistein reduces DNA synthesis in the brain, reducing the birth of new brain cells and promoting apoptosis and cell death.[50]

Of soy phytoestrogens, Dr. White says, "The bottom line is these are not nutrients. They are drugs."[51]

diol." In plain English, that means 1/1,000 to 1/100,000.

In a letter to the Assistant Director General of Health, Woodhams criticized Messina's figures with the words: "Comparing the strength of one thing to that of two other substances that themselves differ in strength by a factor of 100 is nonsense. Messina's statement is the same as saying that a 'rat is 1/1,000 to 1/100,000 times the size of a man or an elephant.'"[39] How PTI managed to turn Messina's already inaccurate 1/100,000 figure into the flagrantly erroneous 1/1,000,000 is an unsolved mystery.

MY SOY STORY: MEMORY LOSS

I heard that isoflavones were good for prostate health so I bought a bottle of 50 mg tablets. Within a few hours of taking two tablets I found that it was difficult to speak and I nearly got into a serious accident due to impairment in judging the speed of a car. I definitely had serious mental impairment which I attributed to the isoflavone supplement. (This was gone by the next day.) I don't think it was due to an allergic reaction or mini-stroke. Once before I had similar difficulty in speech when a doctor gave me an atropine-like medicine. Atropine antagonizes acetylcholine action, which triggers some of the nerves involved in memory. Memory is an essential component of speech!

Previously I had thought (based on ignorance) that isoflavones in soy probably had insignificant health effects. After the reaction to the isoflavones, I starting searching *Bioabstracts* for studies on soy isoflavones (I am a biochemist). I quickly learned that genistein is a potent inhibitor of tyrosine kinase, a key enzyme in mediating cell responses to our natural cell growth factors. (It had been used for this purpose in over 1000 research studies!) That did not sound like something I wanted in my body! Furthermore, I found several studies that showed that tyrosine kinase is also involved in triggering of nerves involved in memory, and this is blocked by genistein! My memory was flaky enough already so I quit eating all soy products.

Besides inhibition of tyrosine kinase, adverse cognitive effects of soymilk could also be due to anti-estrogenic actions (estrogens are important for speech and memory in both males and females) or to anti-thyroid action. Or maybe to all three!

G.T, Beltsville, MD

310

27
SOY AND THE THYROID
a pain in the neck

Soybeans contain goitrogens.[1] Goitrogens are substances that block the synthesis of thyroid hormones. As their name suggests, they can cause goiter, which is a pronounced swelling in the neck caused by an enlarged thyroid gland.

Unfortunately, the problems caused by goitrogens aren't always as plain as a swelling on the neck. People without goiters can have malfunctioning thyroids while people with goiters sometimes show normal levels of thyroid hormones. While this paradox has made it difficult to predict exactly what kind of damage soy goitrogens might cause, endocrine disruption is certain. Given that thyroid health affects the function of every cell in the body and that babies, children and adolescents depend on optimal secretion of thyroid hormone for normal growth and development, no one should make casual claims about the safety of soy.

GOITROGENS IN THE FOOD SUPPLY

Soy is not the only goitrogenic food. Broccoli, cabbage, Brussels sprouts, cassava, rapeseed, turnips, mustard, radish, peanuts and millet also contain goitrogens. However, few adults—and even fewer children—eat these foods to excess.[2] Furthermore, the goitrogens in most of these foods are easily neutralized by cooking or fermentation.

Soy foods are different. The principal goitrogens in soybeans are the estrogenic plant hormones known as isoflavones. The antinutrients known as saponins in soy may also be goitrogens (see Chapter 19). Cooking and processing methods using heat, pressure and alkaline solutions will neither deactivate nor remove isoflavones or saponins. Only solvent extraction can do that.[3,4] So far, the soy industry has resisted using these processes—even for soy destined for babies, who are highly vulnerable to their estrogenic and goitrogenic effects.

AN EPIDEMIC OF THYROID TROUBLES

America is plagued by an epidemic of thyroid disorders. The Colorado Thyroid Disease Prevalence Study showed that thyroid dysfunction is common, that it often goes undetected, and it is associated with myriad health problems. Researchers enlisted subjects at a statewide health fair; measured levels of thyroid stimulating hormone (TSH), total thyroxine (T4) concentrations and lipid levels; and tallied the answers to a questionnaire. They not only found hypothyroidism in 9.5 percent of the population (nearly double the numbers diagnosed by doctors) but also discovered that more than 40 percent of those patients taking prescription thyroid medications still had abnormal TSH levels.[5]

Patient advocate and thyroid patient Mary J. Shomon, author of *Living Well with Hypothyroidism* (2000), editor of the newsletter *Sticking Our Necks Out* and director of the excellent thyroid website http://thyroid.about.com, has found evidence that 13 million Americans suffer from low thyroid function, many of whom have been misdiagnosed, undiagnosed and poorly treated.[6] Ridha Arem, M.D., an endocrinologist at Baylor College of Medicine in Houston and author of *The Thyroid Solution* (1999), goes even further, identifying a "hidden epidemic" in which one in ten Americans—more than 20 million people, most of them women—have a thyroid disorder.[7,8]

Symptoms of low thyroid (hypothyroidism) include sluggishness, chills, brain fog (short-term memory deficits), attention-deficit disorders, hypoglycemia, depression, dementia, emotional instability, dry skin, thinning hair and weight gain. The autoimmune form of hypothyroidism is known as Hashimoto's thyroiditis.

An overactive hyper-thyroid gland results in anxiety, restlessness, irritability, panic attacks, attention deficit and hyperactivity disorders, heart palpitations, tremors, sweating, bulging eyes and even sudden death. The autoimmune form is known as Graves' disease. In some cases, acute hyperthyroidism will exhaust the thyroid gland, bringing on chronic hypothyroidism.[9-12] There are also growing numbers of reports of people exposed to thyroid toxins—including soy—who experience wildly fluctuating levels of thyroid hormone. They may go from the "thyroid storms" of heart palpitations and sweats one day to lethargy and cold limbs the next. [13]

Thyroid cancer statistics are also sobering. The American Cancer Society reports that overall thyroid cancer incidence across all ages and races is now increasing at 1.4 percent per year and that incidences rose 42.1 percent between 1975 and 1996, with the largest increases among women. Thyroid carcinoma is one of the most common cancers among U.S. children and adolescents, with approximately 75 percent occurring in adolescents between the ages of 15 and 19. The National Cancer Institute (NCI) comments that "the preponderance of thyroid cancer in females suggests that hormonal factors may mediate disease occurrence."[14]

Other "hormonal factors" could include plant estrogens. It may not be coincidental that soy infant formula consumption took off during this very time period and is currently given to nearly 25 percent of bottle-fed infants in the United States, a higher percentage than anywhere else in the world.[15]

The causes of so much thyroid disease appear to be many and synergistic. Radiation, mercury, fluoride, plastics, pesticides, dioxins, solvents and estrogens (and estrogen mimickers) found in commercial meats, plastics and hormone replacement therapies (HRT) have all been implicated.[16,17] And so has soy.

The United Kingdom's Committee on Toxicity (COT) has identified several populations at special risk for soy-induced thyroid disease—infants on soy formula, vegans who use soy as their principal meat and dairy replacements, and men and women who are self medicating with soy foods and/or isoflavone supplements in an attempt to prevent or reverse menopausal symptoms, cancer or high cholesterol. As early as 1980, British government researchers pointed out that soy-consuming vegans were at risk.[18,19]

BELOW THE BELT

Despite credible laboratory, clinical and epidemiological studies that link soy with thyroid disease, soy proponents scoff at the notion that soy causes thyroid problems because, they say, goiter is not a problem in Asia.[20,21] In fact, the *New York Times* has reported an epidemic of cretinism in impoverished rural areas of China where iodine deficiency is widespread and poverty forces people to eat more soy than the small quantities that are the norm.[22] (See "Is Soy a Staple?" page 12.) In Japan, where soy consumption is the highest of any country in Asia, thyroid disease is widespread. After all, Hashimoto's thyroiditis, the autoimmune form of hypothyroidism, was first detected in Japan, and the prevalence there of thyroid disease has motivated Japanese researchers to undertake important studies proving the adverse effects of soy foods on the thyroid gland.

Goiter is most common in areas of the world known as "goiter belts" where iodine is deficient in the soil. Iodine—a mineral common in the sea but rare on land—is essential for the manufacture of thyroid hormones. Tri-iodothyronine (T3) and thyroxine (T4) are synthesized in the gland from iodine and the amino acid tyrosine. The abbreviations T3 and T4 indicate the number of iodine atoms in each molecule of thyroid hormone. Insufficient levels of iodine in the diet will reduce the levels of thyroid hormone, causing a compensatory increase in thyroid stimulating hormone (TSH), often leading to goiter.[23] Although iodine deficiency increases the antithyroid effects of goitrogenic foods, iodine sufficiency does not offer complete protection in the face of high soy consumption.

THE IODINE FACTOR

The first report in medical journals of enlarged thyroid glands in rats and chickens fed soybean rations appeared in the 1930s.[24-26] In 1961, researchers discovered that spiking the chow with iodine could prevent goiter.[27] But this quick-fix solution to a serious problem turned out to be simplistic. Rats and chickens fed soybean-based chows required twice as much iodine to prevent thyroid enlargement as animals fed soy-free diets. Even then, their thyroid glands showed abnormal cell proliferation.[28] When iodine is largely absent, soy can provoke malignant hyperplastic goiter.[29]

Dr. Mieko Kimura of Kyoto University writes: "It is well known that a goiter is induced by simple iodine deficiency, but it was noteworthy that hyperplastic goiters can be induced in rats in a high percentage by the administration of soybean factor(s) under iodine-deficient conditions, together with accurate signs of malignancy such as invasiveness and metastasis formation in the lungs." Further studies are needed to clarify whether the component that Dr. Kimura calls "the soybean factor(s)" promotes changes induced by iodine deficiency or is carcinogenic in and of itself.[30]

Taking extra iodine above and beyond the recommended daily allowance can prevent symptoms, but carries its own risks. The epidemic of autoimmune thyroid disease in western countries may be due to excess iodine in the diet. Both the United States (where people eat iodized salt) and Japan (where people eat a lot of iodine-rich seaweed) have high incidences of autoimmune thyroid disease. Iodine concentrations at 30 times the RDA prevent thyroxine production by inhibiting thyroid peroxidase (TPO), an enzyme involved in hormone biosynthesis.[31]

THE ESTROGEN FACTOR

Women naturally have larger thyroid glands than men and produce more thyroid hormone, because estrogen partially blocks the efficiency of T3 and T4. Physicians often recommend that women who take Synthroid or other thyroxine-replacement medications increase their dosage if they start taking birth control pills or hormone replacement therapy (HRT).

Likewise, the soy estrogens known as the isoflavones can inhibit the action of thyroid drugs. To ensure their efficacy, many health professionals recommend that they not be taken at the same time as foods or supplements high in soy.[32-34] Christiane Northrup, M.D., bestselling author of *Women's Bodies, Women's Wisdom,* dispenses this advice to her patients and follows it herself.[35] Dr. Northrup's recent diagnosis of hypothyroidism is not surprising given her avowed consumption of the very high-isoflavone soy product known as Revival, a product for which she is a spokesperson.

PUSH ME, PULL ME:
SOY AND THYROID DRUGS

Boosting the thyroid with drugs like Synthroid, then depressing it with thyroid inhibitors like soy foods or isoflavone supplements can put extreme stress on the thyroid. Environmental scientist Mike Fitzpatrick, Ph.D., points out that this is the classic way that researchers induce thyroid tumors in laboratory animals. The fact that soy is "natural" does not make it safe or weak. A serving of soy food provides up to three times the goitrogenic potency of the pharmaceutical thyroid-inhibiting drugs methimazole and 6-propylthiouracil.

SOURCE: Fitzpatrick, Mike. Soy formulas and the effects of isoflavones on the thyroid. *NZ Med J,* 2000, 113, 1103, 24-26.

twenty-seven: soy and the thyroid

MECHANISMS OF ACTION

Plant estrogens interact with the thyroid gland in several ways. Genistein and daidzein (the key isoflavones in soy) and biochanin A (found in clover and alfalfa) are potent inhibitors of thyroid peroxidase (TPO), an enzyme involved in the synthesis of T3 and T4. *In vitro* experiments have shown that soy isoflavone's inhibition of thyroid peroxidase interferes with a critical stage in thyroid hormone production—the iodinization of the amino acid tyrosine.

This interference occurs whether or not sufficient or extra iodine is present. As a result, the body produces useless mono-, di- and tri-iodoisoflavones and not the mono, di and tri and quarto forms of thyroid hormone. In the human body, this interference can cause a drop in thyroid hormone levels, an increase in thyroid stimulating hormone and stress on the thyroid gland.

Rao L. Divi, Ph.D., and Daniel R. Doerge, Ph.D., top scientists with National Center for Toxicological Research, Jefferson, AR, concluded: "The possible association between long-term inhibition of thyroid hormone synthesis (goiter) and induction of thyroid follicular cell hyperplasia and neoplasia underscores the significance of these findings."[36,37]

Continuing this line of research with rats, the team found that dietary supplementation with the soy isoflavone genistein over a 20-week period from pregnancy through weaning resulted in a dose-dependent reduction in microsomal thyroid peroxidase (TPO). They also observed a reduction in TPO activity in rats fed a standard soy-feed diet (containing 60 mg/kg total isoflavones) compared to those fed a soy-free diet (containing 1 mg/kg total isoflavones). Even so, there were no differences in T3, T4, TSH, thyroid weights or histopathology between the two groups, suggesting that the rats were able to maintain normal thyroid activity—at least during the short term of the study.[38]

Another way goitrogens damage thyroid function is by increasing concentrations of thyroid binding globulin (TBG), a plasma protein involved in the inactivation and transport of T3 and T4.[39] This lowers free thyroxine concentrations and increases TSH secretions.

FORMULA FOR DISASTER

The first reports of thyroid damage suffered by human infants on soy formula appeared during the 1950s.[40-43] Most cases involved goiter, with no overt signs of hypothyroidism. Although iodine supplements helped, they did not entirely solve the problem. Researchers found that matters improved considerably if the processing of the soy formula included extraction with an organic solvent as well as heating.[44] Although no one at the time identified the principal goitrogens as the isoflavones, alcohol solvent extraction is, in fact, the only way to remove them. Heat, pressure and alkaline treatments used in ordinary soy processing will not remove the isoflavones.[45,46]

As a result of these studies, soy infant formula manufacturers changed their recipes, adding iodine and switching the main ingredient from soy flour to soy protein isolate, a product now known to have a lower isoflavone content.[47] Since these changes, there have been no reports of goiter in infants fed soy formula.[48] However, as discussed earlier, goiter is only one marker of thyroid health.

Infants with congenital hypothyroidism need 18 to 25 percent higher doses of thyroxine than expected replacement levels if bottle fed with soy formula. This increased requirement disappears if soy-based formula is discontinued.[49] Soy affects some infants so adversely that hypothyroidism persists despite medication.[50] Accordingly, the New Zealand Ministry of Health has advised that "clinicians closely monitor thyroxine levels in infants with hypothyroidism who were fed soy-based infant formula or high levels of other soy-containing infant foods."[51]

SUFFER THE LITTLE CHILDREN

Autoimmune thyroid disease is far more likely to occur in children who were fed soy formula. Researchers at North Shore University Hospital-Cornell University Medical College, Manhasset, New

York, made this discovery accidentally. They had set out to confirm something entirely different—a possible association of insulin-dependent diabetes with breast feeding. Instead, they found a high prevalence of antithryoid antibodies in patients with insulin-dependent diabetes who were fed soy-based formula during infancy.[52]

A follow-up study showed a significantly higher prevalence of feedings with soy formulas in patients with auto-immune thyroid disease as compared with their healthy siblings and healthy nonrelated control children. Pavel Fort, M.D., concluded: "Auto-immune thyroid alterations are among the most frequently encountered autoimmune conditions in children. The cause is generally considered to be multifactorial, involving a genetic predisposition to develop an autoimmune response which may be triggered by an environmental insult. Soy protein could be one of such environmental triggering factors."[53]

Evidence of other adverse effects from giving soy to children is mostly limited to anecdotal reports, but a *British Medical Journal* report warns that soy during childhood can lead to hypothyroidism and short stature.[54]

Does soy formula lead to later development of thyroid disease? Strong anecdotal evidence suggests that it does. Despite concerns raised by these reports and nearly 70 years of animal studies, no research group has attempted well-designed retrospective studies on the subject. On August 15, 2001, newspaper headlines announced publication of an article in the *Journal of the American Medical Association* asserting that soy infant formula had been proven safe.[55] Conspicuously missing in this study—funded in part by the infant formula industry—was a report on thyroid function. Instead, researchers focussed on evidence of endocrine disruption that would turn up "statistically insignificant." (For a full discussion of this study, see Chapter 28.) That many of the soy-fed subjects complained of lethargy and admitted the use of weight loss medications suggests—but does not prove—thyroid damage.

PICKLING ADULTS

The most powerful evidence of soy's adverse effects on the adult thyroid emerged from a study carried out at the Ishizuki Thyroid Clinic in Japan.[56] Dr. Yoshimochi Ishizuki of Aichi Medical University demonstrated that 30 grams of pickled soybeans per day, given to healthy adult men and women, induced thyroid disruptions in only 30 days. All the subjects consumed seaweed daily to ensure adequate iodine intake.

Compared to non-soy-eating controls, TSH levels increased significantly in a group of 20 adults fed soy for one month and in a second group of 17 fed for three months. Two individuals shot up from an optimum level of 1 uU/mL to a pronounced hypothyroid

MY SOY STORY: THYROID REMOVAL BIRTHDAY PRESENT

I will be turning 18 next week and will be celebrating my birthday by receiving nuclear radiation on my thyroid. This spring I was diagnosed with thyroid cancer, and thus had my thyroid removed. This occurrence boggled both my doctors and myself. I have pursued many leads on why a healthy 17-year-old could get this disorder. I just recently became aware of the alleged correlation between soy and thyroid function. I have been a vegetarian since before I began puberty. Soy products have constituted a large part of my diet in my attempt to provide my body with adequate protein. I also spent most of my life drinking soy sauce (I was a weird little kid). I would go through a few bottles a week. My mother did not breastfeed me, but used soy formula as an alternative. I hope that your study may result in more public attention of this issue to potentially prevent occurrences like the one which I had to suffer.

J.G., Boston, MA

state of 7uU/mL. Thyroxine levels decreased slightly. The second group experienced a significant increase in free thyroxine, indicating improved thyroid function, after they stopped eating the soy.

Goiter and hypothyroidism appeared in three members of the first group and eight of the second. Many of the three-monthers also suffered from symptoms associated with hypothyroidism: 53 percent from constipation, 53 percent from fatigue and 41 percent from lethargy. One case of subacute thyroiditis (inflammation of the thyroid) appeared in the first group. Although 9 of the 11 subjects saw a reduction in goiter size after they stopped eating the soy, goiter persisted in two subjects. These received thyroxine treatments and their goiters subsided in another two to six months.

Most notably, the subjects in this study started out healthy. During the course of the study, all had adequate iodine. Most importantly, the subjects did not eat very much soy—only 30 grams per day, with isoflavones of up to 23 mg total genistein and 10 mg of total daidzein.[57]

Even more frightening, the Ishizuki study shows that isoflavones exert harmful effects in healthy adults in amounts far below the levels of isoflavones administered to babies fed soy infant formula. This finding greatly concerned the United Kingdom's Committee on Toxicity of Chemicals in Food, Consumer Products and the Environment, which observed, "Even allowing for differences in absorption, the large differences in exposure would be expected to cause significant effects."[58] Likewise, the U.S. National Research Council has warned: "The concentration of soy phytoestrogens that inhibited thyroid hormone biosynthesis is within the range of exposure of infants maintained on soy formula. . . that concentration is six to eleven-fold higher than concentrations known to have hormonal effects in adults."[59]

Dr. Ishizuki's findings should also be sobering to another high-risk group—vegans, many of whom consume soy foods far in excess of the 30 grams used in the study. An earlier British study comparing the effects of vegan to omnivorous diets also found elevated

TSH levels and goitrogenic effects among the vegans, even after excluding the three persons with the highest TSH levels because they had taken kelp supplements.[60] Vegans with zinc and/or B_{12} deficiencies could be particularly vulnerable to thyroid damage. Zinc is required for adequate thyroid function and cobalt—central to the vitamin B_{12} molecule—is needed for synthesis of thyroxine.[61,62] Russian scientists found an inverse correlation between cobalt availability in food and drink and the incidence of goiter.[63]

Soy eaters are at risk for thyroid damage not only because of the goitrogens in soy but also because phytates contribute to zinc

MY SOY STORY: IF ONLY I HAD KNOWN

I am a healthy 48-year-old woman. An avid runner, I have followed a primarily vegetarian diet for over five years, and have always had excellent blood chemistry results at check-ups. Last year, however, I added something significant to my regular diet of fruits, vegetables, beans and grains: soy products. I followed the conventional wisdom that this would alleviate early menopausal symptoms, keep my heart healthy, etc. I ate tofu daily, consumed soy milk in abundance, snacked on soy nuts instead of regular snacks, and looked for soy isoflavones in my supplements. Results: I now am facing surgery for a goiter (enlarged thyroid) with multiple nodules. I have symptoms of thyroid damage. My skin, nails, hair are all suffering visibly. I have chest pain when I run. Worst of all my cholesterol has *risen* from 137 to 210 in the last six months. A nonsmoking, non-drinking vegetarian who eschews all dairy products simply cannot experience this kind of change in less than six months without some external factor. There is no thyroid disease in my family, and no other explanation other than the introduction of large amounts of soy into my diet. If only I had known.   L.T., Boulder, CO deficiency and an "anti-vitamin factor" results in greater needs of the body for vitamin B_{12}.[64]

OUT OF DATE, OUT OF MIND

The soy industry tends to dismiss these studies as either "out of date" (if they are old) or "poorly designed" (if recent).

In the Spring 2001 issue of *The Soy Connection*, Mark Messina, Ph.D., condemns the Ishizuki study because it "suffers from many design flaws" but fails to elucidate them. It is clear from his comments that Messina did not have a translation and relied on the abstract, or failed to read too carefully or he might have noticed that both men and women participated in the study at the Ishizuki Clinic, not just women.[65]

Apparently Messina thinks we can rely on abstracts alone for he praises a study by the authors "Bruce B, Spiller GA, Holloway L" entitled "Soy isoflavones do not have an antithyroid effect in post-menopausal women over 64 years of age." He lists the journal as *FASEB* and the year 2000, but includes no further information.[66] Neither Pub Med nor the Federation of Science and Experimental Biology (FASEB) website lists this article or any similar article by these or other authors. Dr. Northrup also admires this study—which she places in *Experimental Biology*.[67] When asked for a copy of this elusive study, Messina replied that it was "an abstract only" but that the full paper would be published in the *Journal of Medicinal Foods* in Fall 2003.[68]

The Journal of Medicinal Foods is owned by Mary Ann Liebert Inc., publisher of *Soya for Health* by Stephen Holt, M.D., and its editor-in-chief is Sheldon Saul Hendler, Ph.D., M.D., a member of the Scientific Advisory Council of Archer Daniels Midland.[69,70] Furthermore, the sponsor of this study was the same company, Archer Daniels Midland.[71]

Prior to publication, Leah Holloway, Ph.D., one of the three original authors and an expert on hormone therapies, was dropped without her knowledge[72] while Messina, a spokesperson for the soy industry, came on board. Neither of the two remaining authors has any apparent expertise in thyroid or other hormonal issues. Gene A. Spiller, Ph.D., of the Health Research and Studies Center in Los Altos, CA, has published extensively in the area of vegan nutrition. Bonnie Bruce, Ph.D., of the Division of Immunology and Rheumatology at Stanford University has been active with the Stanford Nutrition Action Program, an experimental trial aimed at reducing dietary fat intake among low-literacy, low-income adults. She has published articles on a variety of subjects, including low-fat vegan diets, lipid chemistry, bone density, obesity and bulimia.

Because the study was complete at the time Messina joined the team, his function was clearly that of putting an industry spin on the 70 years of research showing soy's adverse effects on the thyroid. Accordingly, he denigrates the work of four thyroid specialists from the renowned Ishizuki Clinic in Japan, relegates a major study by thyroid specialists Theodore Kay and Mieko Kimura of Kyoto University to a listing in the endnotes and skips over the pioneering findings of Daniel Sheehan, Ph.D., and Daniel Doerge, Ph.D, top toxicologists at the FDA's National Laboratory of Toxicological Research. To buttress his case, he even resorts to mention of unpublished favorable industry studies, referenced as "S. Potter, personal communication." Susan Potter, Ph.D., is Global Director for Health and Nutrition of the Solae Company, a joint venture of DuPont and Bunge which manufactures processed soy products.

In a letter to *Mothering* magazine, Messina states that this study "found no adverse effects of isoflavone (90 mg per day) supplements on thyroid function in postmenopausal women over a six-month period."[73] This statement omits both the title and the conclusion of the study, which holds that soy isoflavones do not affect thyroid function in individuals who are "iodine replete." The women in the study received the RDA of 150 ug per day of iodine in addition to iodine in their diet. The authors conclude that "It is important for all individuals regardless of their soy intake to consume adequate iodine" and recommend that those who consume large amounts of soy should make sure they consume "sufficient iodine."

UNSOLVED MYSTERY:
SOY, THE THYROID AND CHOLESTEROL

The soy industry urges men and women to take soy in order to lower their cholesterol. This happens in some cases but the results are not consistent. This is because soy lowers thyroid function, which in turn will raise cholesterol. When thyroxine levels drop, the liver no longer functions properly and produces excess cholesterol, fatty acids and triglycerides.

Curiously, T4 levels often go up after beginning feedings of soy protein. Although this effect is also not consistent, it has occurred often enough with hens, miniature pigs, hamsters, gerbils and rats fed soy or soy-corn diets—as compared to controls fed fish or casein-based diets—to lead to theories that soy protein lowers cholesterol because it induces an increase in plasma T4 concentrations.

This effect is not necessarily beneficial. As Richard L. Shames, M.D., and Karilee Halo Shames, R.N., Ph.D., authors of *Thyroid Power* put it, "An increase in T4, without a corresponding elevation of T3, not only results in weight gain but in impaired thyroid function generally."

SOURCES:
Staack R, Jeffrey E, Jimenez MD, Wang L, Potter SM. An extract of soy flour influences serum cholesterol and thyroid hormones in rats and hamsters. *J Nutr.* 1996; 126:3046-3053.

Forsythe WA. Soy protein, thyroid regulation and cholesterol metabolism. *J Nutr,* 1995, 125, 619S-623S.

Shames, Richard L. Shames, Karilee Halo. *Thyroid Power: Ten Steps to Total Health* (HarperResource, 2001).

This understates the fact that many parts of the world are iodine depleted and levels have also been decreasing in the American diet. The National Center for Health Statistics reports that median iodine intake decreased by more than 50 percent between the National Health and Nutrition Examination Surveys (NHANES) of 1970-1974 and 1988-1994. The Center also reports that several recent surveys indicate that the proportion of the U.S. population with low iodine levels is increasing.[74]

On the website www.veganhealth.org, Messina and his wife, Virginia Messina, M.P.H., R.D., issue the following warning to vegans: "It is possible that eating a diet with generous amounts of soyfoods could be a problem for people whose iodine intake is marginal. And that might just include some vegans, since the main sources of iodine in western diets are fish and milk." The Messinas conclude that

MY SOY STORY: TOTAL SOY KICK

I recently went through a thyroid scan, needle biopsy and a week of worry waiting to find out whether I had cancer of the thyroid. As it turns out, I have inflammation of the thyroid and have been taking 0.088 mcg of Synthroid. About a year and a half ago, I decided to make "healthy" changes in my life and started with a thorough medical exam at which time my thyroid was tested and I was told I had a normal thyroid. I also read a "makeover" book by Marilu Henner and one of her biggest points was that dairy was "evil" and soy was "king." I went on a total soy kick and over the last year have eaten tofu, edamame, soy meat substitute, soy cheese, soy butter, soy sour cream, soy cream cheese, soy yogurt and, the main culprit, Silk soy milk, especially the chocolate variety. Over the last three to six months, I have had 3-6 cups of soy milk a day. After reading your website about one week ago, I have thrown out *all* soy products and plan to let my endocrinologist know as I am now concerned about stopping the thyroid-depressing soy products and taking Synthroid. I want my doctor to be aware of the probable cause of my thyroid disease.   R.W., Portland, ME the "appropriate response to this is not to limit healthful soyfoods" but to "get enough iodine." They recommend iodized salt and "if this isn't a regular part of your diet, use an iodine supplement."[75]

Another of Messina's "well-designed" studies was completed at the University of Minnesota, St. Paul. Although he asserts that it shows the safety of an isoflavones-rich diet, the data actually show evidence of soy-induced endocrine disruption along the pituitary-hypothalamic-thyroid axis. However, the researchers dismissed these findings, stating that they were unable to fathom what they might mean. The researchers reported a decrease in T3 concentrations in premenopausal women receiving 128 mg isoflavones per day but concluded that because no effects were seen on total or free T4 or TSH, the results were "unlikely to be physiologically important."[76] In a second study by the same group, postmenopausal women on high-soy isoflavones diets (132 mg per day) showed higher thyroid binding globulin (TBG) levels while those on the lower isoflavones diet (65 mg per day) showed decreased TBG levels. These confusing results led the team to conclude that "while the changes are significant, they may not be physiologically relevant."[77]

Similarly, a human study partially funded by the Illinois Soybean Program, showed "small effects on thyroid hormone values that are unlikely to be clinically important."[78]

While none of these soy industry-endorsed studies contain data proving adverse effects on the thyroid, they do not establish safety either. On the contrary, they leave many unanswered questions. Further studies are needed, ones that might do well to enlist the services of thyroid specialists who comprehend the difference between "optimum" levels of TSH as opposed to "normal" or "average" levels and who would consider markers of thyroid function other than—or in addition to—those obtained by blood testing, a notoriously inaccurate marker of thyroid function. It would be interesting to see how the results might change if subjects had very healthy thyroids to begin with—as was the case with the subjects in the Ishizuki study—and not "average" thyroids that could already

MY SOY STORY: HEALTHIER TO SMOKE

I've just been diagnosed as having hyperthyroidism. This came out of nowhere and I can't believe it "just" happened. Several months ago, I quit smoking and having made that step, I decided to adopt a much healthier lifestyle. Part of this included becoming a vegetarian. I didn't worry about getting the right nutrients because I added soy to my diet. I started by replacing meat with soy products—Morningstar bacon 'burgers, hot dogs, etc. Then I read about the soy product Revival and began using it everyday for about a month, when I got what I thought at the time was the flu. The only symptoms I had were a very high temperature and a rapid heart rate. Well, the fever went down, but the heart rate never did. I thought I had a heart problem, but couldn't get a doctor to take me seriously. After all, I'm only 36 and in very good health. Or at least I was. The doctor finally ran some tests and found out that my thyroid had just "gone crazy." His words not mine. . . . I am so upset, what makes this really ironic is that if I would have just kept smoking I'd be healthier today.   B.F., Houston, TX

be considered subclinically hypothyroid.

Such considerations are important because moderately elevated TSH combined with a normal free thyroxine level indicates subclinical hypothyroidism, a condition in which increased TSH production compensates for reduced thyroid hormone secretion to maintain normal function. Mike Fitzpatrick, Ph.D., explains: "Subclinical hypothyroidism is a common condition that may eventually evolve toward overt hypothyroidism especially in persons with anti-thyroid antibodies. It is a condition of increasing importance, and its prevalence appears to be growing such that studies aimed at defining its evolution are warranted. Dietary factors may well play a major role in the development of this condition since high goitrogen intake can increase TSH secretion."[79]

Daniel R. Doerge, Ph.D., of the FDA's National Laboratory for Toxicological Research, adds, "The possibility that widely consumed soy products may cause harm in the human population via either or both estrogenic and goitrogenic activities is of concern. Rigorous, high-quality experimental and human research into soy toxicity is the best way to address these concerns."[80]

Claims of soy industry spokespersons to the contrary, such testing has yet to prove safety.

MY SOY STORY: NUTRITIONAL NIGHTMARE

Two years ago I was an energetic, happy-go-lucky, healthy person. Then I figured that I needed more protein and meat wasn't good for you, so I switched to soy: soy protein shakes, soy ice cream, soy milk, meal replacement bars, soy cereal, soy cookies, you name it . . . if it was soy, I ate it. I began to get run down, had severe leg cramps, muscle twitching, tinnitis, joint aches and stiffness, gastrointestinal problems, and worst of all, hair loss. I got colds with bronchitis one after another. I couldn't concentrate long enough to exercise and was terribly depressed. I felt like I was in a hole that I couldn't get out of. My doctor said that my thyroid and hormones fell into the "normal" range. She offered no explanation other than I was getting old and that's the way things are.

God bless all the people who are telling their stories. I never in my life thought that soy could be bad for people or that I would have reactions to it. I am going back to eating real, whole, natural foods like our elders ate. My "miracle food" turned into a nutritional nightmare.

P.F., Denver, CO

MY SOY STORY: THYROID STORM

I am fat and have high blood pressure so decided to go looking for lowfat and high-protein snack sources. I tried a Genisoy bar, liked it and went on a field trip with eight boxes. I consumed four to five bars a day (50-75 grams of soy protein total.) A few days after returning, I had my first attack of supraventricular tachycardia (severe heart arrhythmias). My wife was out of town, so while still able to, I called an ambulance. They took me in and my pulse was converted in the emergency room with IV calcium channel blocker. I was given an appropriate prescription for the drug, filled it, went home and tried to figure out what had hit me.

I woke up the next morning with another attack. Back to the hospital (wife driving now), ER conversion pulses, blood tests, chest X-ray, doctor's visit, elevated creatine and BUN, off to Tucson, AZ, to a cardiology hospital where a number of tests were made. Nothing wrong. Heart fine. No irregularities. Blood sugar, lungs, everything fine. Blood enzymes back to normal. They upped the medication and I went back home puzzled. I recollected tiredness for a few days before the first attack, a tightness or sense of swelling in the sides of my neck, and some poor sleeping and sweating several nights previously. After getting back home for the second time, once again I slept poorly, had rapid and anxious breathing and frequent light palpitations during the day. I am an herbalist, so I started doing 60 drops of Lycopus tincture. This stopped the palpitations, stopped the stressed breathing and allowed me to finally sleep on my left side again. Lycopus has thyroid-lowering properties. I have never consumed soy protein before and was shocked to learn that it causes thyroid damage and that I had almost died from "thyroid storms." Nothing else I had done prior to the attacks was different from the norm.   M.J., Denver, CO

28
SOY INFANT FORMULA
birth control for baby?

Parents who feed their infants soy formula are unwittingly giving them the hormonal equivalent of three to five birth control pills per day. The calculations are based on Swiss Federal Health Service figures and warnings; they represent a high dose of estrogen for anyone.[1] The amount is especially dangerous for infants whose very development requires the right hormones in the right place at the right time. Studies on rats, sheep, monkeys, and other animals—coupled with growing numbers of reports from pediatricians and parents—suggest that the estrogens in soy infant formula can irreversibly harm the baby's later sexual development and reproductive health.[2,3]

"Infants on soy formula have been identified as a high-risk group," writes Iain Robertson, Ph.D., senior toxicologist at Auckland University Medical School in New Zealand, "because the formula is the main source of nutrient, and because of their small size and developmental phase."[4] Bernard Zimmerli, Ph.D., of the Federal Office of Health, Berne, Switzerland, agrees: "The hormonal environment of the newborn child has profound effects on the individual development process."[5,6]

Robertson and Zimmerli do not speak alone. So many of the world's top pediatricians, endocrinologists and toxicologists have perceived a danger that the Weston A. Price Foundation in Washington, DC, and concerned citizens led by Valerie and Richard James in New Zealand have lobbied for a ban on the sale of soy infant formulas except by prescription.[7,8] Daniel Sheehan, Ph.D., formerly Senior Toxicologist at the U.S. Food and Drug Administration's National Center for Toxicological Research in Jefferson, Arkansas, states unequivocally that infants fed soy-based formulas have been placed at risk in a "large, uncontrolled and basically unmonitored human infant experiment."[9]

TIMING IS EVERYTHING

A crucial time for the programming of the human reproduction system is right after birth—the very time when many non-breastfed babies get bottle after bottle of soy formula. Normally during this period, the body surges with natural estrogens, testosterones and other hormones that Mother Nature intended to occupy receptor sites on cells where they serve to set off a series of biochemical reactions. The newborn's reproductive system is thus programmed to mature from infancy through puberty and into adulthood.[10-12]

For infants on soy formula, the programming may be interrupted. The phytoestrogens in soy formula—the isoflavones—bear a strong resemblance to the natural estrogens produced by the human body as well as to the synthetic estrogens found in contraceptive pills. Strictly speaking, soy estrogens are not hormones but "estrogen mimickers," but the bottom line is that the human body mistakes them for hormones.[13]

The result is that alien soy phytoestrogens can take over the receptor sites in cells and tissues intended for estrogen, progesterone, testosterone and other real hormones. Adults attempting to prevent hormonally driven breast and prostate cancers might possibly benefit from the pharmaceutical use of soy isoflavones acting as antagonists to endogenous estrogens. (The evidence is mixed.) Babies, however, can be irreversibly harmed if clogged receptor sites delay or stop normal, necessary development.[14]

Soy phytoestrogens can also obstruct the very production of estrogen and testosterone. By occupying—and inactivating—hormone receptor sites in the brain, they block messages normally transmitted by cell signal transduction pathways.[15-17]

Soy isoflavones also interfere by inhibiting the action of enzymes. The job of 17 β-hydroxysteroid oxidoreductase type 1 is to convert estrone into the body's principal form of estrogen, which is known as estradiol. This enzyme performs the same task of biosynthesis of testosterone from the androgen androstenedione. *In vitro* studies prove that soy isoflavones are potent inhibitors of 17 β-hydroxysteroid oxidoreductase and are able to inhibit the synthesis and metabolism of estradiol, testosterone and other steroid hormones.[18-20]

Isoflavones can also inhibit enzymes called protein tyrosine kinases, which add phosphate to intracellular proteins and are necessary for the action of insulin-like and epidermal growth factors. The soy isoflavone genistein, for example, blocks transforming growth factor, which in turn decreases the aromatization (that is, the transformation due to the action of the enzyme aromatase) of androgens to estrogens. Aromatase is an enzyme needed for many jobs related to fat accumulation, lipid metabolism, insulin resistance, vascular repair and bone mineralization.[21-26]

Some of soy's hormonal effects may be reversible in adults, following restoration of normal estrogen activity.[27-29] In newborns, the effects are more likely to be irreversible. Cliff Irvine, D.V.Sc., D.Sc., an endocrinologist at Lincoln University, New Zealand, explains:

"It has long been known that modification of the sex steroid milieu in neonatal rodents alters reproductive axis function and sexual behavior and leads to structural changes in specific areas of the brain. The effects of neonatal steroid treatment, although irreversible, are often not manifested until the reproductive system is activated at puberty. Moreover, there is only a limited window dur-

SOY ESTROGENS IN THE DIETS
OF ADULTS AND INFANTS

	Average Isoflavone Intake	Isoflavones per kg of body weight*
China (1990 survey)[108]	3 mg	0.05 mg
Japan (1996 survey)[109]	10 mg	0.17 mg
Japan (1998 survey)[110]	25 mg	0.42 mg
Japan (2000 survey)[111]	28 mg	0.47 mg
In iodine-replete men and women the amount causing thyroid suppression after 3 months [112]	35 mg	0.58 mg
In premenopausal women, causing hormonal changes after one month[113]	45 mg	0.75 mg
FDA recommended amount for adults to lower cholesterol[114,115]	25 mg	0.40 mg
In infants receiving soy formula[116]	38 mg	6.25 mg

*At 60 kg for adults, 6 kg for infants.

The average dose of isoflavones in soy formula is 38 mg isoflavones per day. On a body-weight basis, this intake of isoflavones is an order of magnitude higher than the amounts causing thryoid problems and endocrine disruption in adults. Would any parents, given these figures, take a risk by feeding their infants soy-based infant formula?

SOURCE: Table compiled by Sally Fallon, President of the Weston A Price Foundation.

ing development, the 'critical period,' when sex steroids can markedly influence neuronal structure and function.

"In humans, unlike rodents, this critical period was thought to occur before birth. However, recent theories on human sexual differentiation propose that there are several critical periods for development which occur not only prenatally but also during the early postnatal period. The timing of these critical periods seems to vary from tissue to tissue so that a temporary perturbation of the sex steroid environment may affect the development of only the one tissue that was passing through its critical period at that time. In extreme cases, this can lead to the development of sexual mosaics in which masculinized and feminized tissues coexist within the same body. Because the cerebral cortex develops late relative to other neural regions, the postnatal critical periods may be particularly important for cognitive development and other aspects of behavior that are mediated cortically."[30]

Most studies purporting to prove that infants on soy formula develop "normally" consider only height, weight and other obvious measurements of growth in infancy and early childhood. This does not prove safety or normal development. As Dave Woodhams, Ph.D., of the Soy Online Network in New Zealand, puts it, claims that soy babies have been "successfully raised" are mere speculation until "it has been determined that in all respects their histories are the same as those of people who were raised on breast milk or on alternative, non-soy formulas."[31]

SOY IMPEDES THE SEXUAL MATURATION OF BOYS

Male infants experience a testosterone surge during the first few months of life and produce androgens in amounts equal to those of adult men. So much testosterone at such a tender age is needed to program the boy for puberty, the time when his sex organs should develop and he should begin to express male characteristics such as facial and pubic hair and a deep voice. If receptor sites intended for the hormone testosterone are occupied by soy estrogens, however, appropriate development may never take place.[32-36]

Rats given the soy isoflavone genistein just after birth show significantly retarded spermatogenesis at puberty, smaller testicles, altered follicle stimulating hormone (FSH) levels, diminished fertility and altered mating behavior.[37] Soy estrogens given to newborn rats may also prevent proper development of the excurrent duct in the testes.[38] In mice, soy estrogens given to neonates have led to reduced expression in adulthood of estrogen receptor alpha and androgen receptors in the testes.[39]

In infant male monkeys, blocking the testosterone surge significantly delays puberty. Upon reaching puberty, such monkeys have lowers levels of plasma luteinizing hormone (LH) and testosterone concentrations, smaller testicles and lower sperm counts compared to normal controls.[40] Other problems seen include permanent impairment of the central nervous system pathway regulating gonadotropin-releasing hormone (GnRH) secretion, compromised sexual behavior and reduced bone density.[41,42] In all of these studies, researchers noticed no adverse effects whatsoever before puberty.[43]

Male marmoset monkeys given soy formula showed testosterone levels that were 53 to 70 percent lower than those of their dairy-formula fed twin brothers. This occurred even though the levels of isoflavones in the monkey diets were 40 to 87 percent lower than the levels reported in four-month-old human infants fed a 100 percent soy-based formula diet. Less clear is why the numbers of monkeys' Leydig cells (interstitial cells of the testis and chief source of androgens) increased by an average of 74 percent in soy formula-fed animals in that study although there were no consistent differences in Sertoli or germ cell numbers. A decrease in testosterone generally results in decreased Leydig cell numbers, so these results are confusing. What is clear is that significant endocrine disruption occurred and that long term effects need to be investigated. Richard Sharpe, M.D., Director of the Medical Research Centre for Reproductive Biology in Edinburgh, Scotland, pulled no punches when he concluded, "It is therefore considered likely that similar or larger effects to those shown here in marmosets may occur in human male infants fed with SFM [soy formula milk]."[44]

To date, most of the evidence damning either soy formula—or levels of phytoestrogens equivalent to those that would be found in soy formula—occurs only in animal studies. After all, investigators cannot ethically do sex steroid lowering experiments on humans. However, ample evidence exists of medical conditions in which a deficiency of male sex hormones in infancy have led to physical, mental and behavioral deficits at puberty. Such studies have shown that the androgens must be replaced at infancy—not later—for puberty to proceed normally.[45-47]

Now that sales of soy formula have been a growth industry for more than 30 years, it is probably not coincidental that pediatricians are reporting greater numbers of boys whose physical maturation is either delayed or does not occur at all. Breasts, underdeveloped gonads, cryptorchidism (undescended testicles) and steroid insufficiencies are increasingly common. Although an undescended testicle is a fairly easy matter to correct surgically, the condition increases a boy's risk of later developing testicular cancer. Unlike cases in the past, boys now diagnosed with delayed puberty are more likely

MY SOY STORY: A BIG DIFFERENCE

I have eleven-year-old fraternal twin boys. One of the boys (A) was fed soya milk formula due to lactose intolerance; he was approximately 3 months old at commencement. There is a marked difference in the boys' development and body shape. For example, his twin (B), breastfed and given regular formula only, is slim, wiry, active and highly articulate. A is overweight, sluggish and whilst tests show he is highly intelligent, he is underachieving. He also has excessively large breasts in relation to the size of the rest of his body.

C.S., London, UK

to be of normal weight or overweight and as tall as controls.[48-50]

Sperm counts are also falling. Between 1940 and 1990, sperm counts dropped from an average of 113 million sperm per milliliter of semen to 66 million. Since the 1970s, sperm counts have dropped about 2 percent per year and sperm quality has also declined.[51-53] "Our research suggests that the damage occurs during the first three months of development in the womb, during infancy and early childhood," says Dr. Sharpe. The cause? "The environmental chemicals in plastics and soy foods. Once taken into the human body, they both mimic the effects of the female hormone estrogen."[54]

Although some boys who experience delayed puberty normalize without apparent long-term, adverse effects on their sexual behavior or fertility, legitimate concerns remain.[55,56] The higher the level of estrogens at key developmental stages, the greater the interference with the production of androgens or androgen receptor sites and the greater the chance of emasculation.

Soy estrogens from infancy have also been linked to rising rates of ADD/ADHD and learning disabilities,[57-59] problems more often diagnosed in boys than girls. Childhood experts remain puzzled about the cause, but primate studies show that a deficiency of male hor-

MY SOY STORY: TEASED AT SCHOOL

My seven-year-old son was fed ISO formula for several months and grew in height and weight way off any of the normal charts. Despite making many enquiries about this, no doctor or hospital nutritionist has ever mentioned any possible link to thyroid problems. He is not a huge eater and is very active but is approximately 1.5 meters tall (4 foot, 11 inches) and weighs 55 kilograms (121 pounds) at age 7. Also, he has small genitals and is teased at school for both his weight and his "small willy."

D.G., Manchester, UK

mones will impair the development of spatial perception and visual discrimination. And human studies have shown diminished spatial ability in androgen-deficient men.[60] In monkeys, deficiency of male hormones impairs the development of spatial perception, which in humans is normally more acute in men than in women.[61] Future patterns of sexual orientation may also be influenced by the early hormonal environment.[62]

SOY ACCELERATES THE SEXUAL MATURATION OF GIRLS

Soy formula is bad news for girls as well. In female infants, natural estrogen levels approximately double during the first month of life, then decline and remain at low levels until puberty.[63-65] With increased estrogens in the environment and diet, an alarming number of girls are entering puberty much earlier than normal. One percent of all girls now show signs of puberty, such as breast development or pubic hair, before the age of three. By age eight, 14.7 percent of Caucasian girls and 48.3 percent of African-American girls had one or both of these characteristics.[66]

Environmental estrogens from plastics, pesticides and meats have been implicated, but some pediatric endocrinologists also believe that soy is contributing to the epidemic of a condition known as precocious puberty.[67] Precocious puberty is defined as puberty occurring in boys under the age of 9, white girls under the age of 7 and African American girls under the age of 6, and it involves premature activation of the hypothalamic-pituitary-gonadal axis. A variation known as precocious pseudopuberty involves the presence of sex steroids independent of pituitary gonadotropin release.

Early maturation in girls heralds reproductive problems later in life, including amenorrhea (failure to menstruate), anovulatory cycles (cycles in which no egg is released), impaired follicular development (follicles failing to mature and develop into healthy eggs), erratic hormonal surges and other problems associated with infertility. As the mammary glands depend on estrogen for their development and functioning, the presence of soy estrogens at a susceptible time might predispose girls to breast cancer, another condition that is on the rise and definitively linked to early puberty.

Although fewer researchers have looked at the sex steroid milieu in females than in males, enough animal studies exist to conclude that soy could compromise a girl's reproductive development. Soy protein isolate fed to female rats in various studies has accelerated puberty, increased uterine weight, decreased serum 17 β-estradiol

MY SOY STORY: OMINOUS CONCLUSIONS

My daughter was breastfed until I became ill when she was five months old. She was weaned very suddenly from me and suffered a serious body rash, which my doctor attributed to cow's milk formula. He suggested that I give her soy formula and informed me that it was a "healthier option" than cow's milk. This advice was given in August 1996, one month after the Ministry of Health warning about soy formula. I trusted my GP's expertise and I believed that a product could not possibly be on sale for consumption by infants, unless it had been tested and approved. I now fear that my trust was misplaced. My daughter consumed soy for just over 12 months. In her second year, she surged in growth beyond what our families or we would have expected according to our family sizes. Shortly after her fourth birthday, she began to experience a regular feminine discharge, which still persists today. The discharge has been repeatedly investigated, without conclusion, and she has seen a gynaecologist a number of times, something that strikes me as very odd at such a tender age. I recently learned about the potential dangers of soy formula and I have investigated matters as fully as I possibly can. My research has taken me around the world and my conclusions are very ominous.

P.W., Auckland, New Zealand

concentrations, caused premature anovulatory cycles and increased multioocyte follicles in their ovaries.[68-73] Mice injected with large doses of the soy isoflavones genistein soon after birth showed altered mammary gland development (possibly reducing their susceptibility to chemically induced tumor development as adults) as well as impaired ovarian follicular development and cycles (impairing fertility).[74-76]

To date, the most important study looking at effects on human female infants took place in Puerto Rico. Researchers investigating the possible cause of premature thelarche (breast development before the age of eight) evaluated a number of possible causative factors, including dietary and environmental estrogen exposure and maternal history of premature sexual development. No conclusive associations were found in subjects more than 2 years old at the onset of thelarche, but researchers found a significant association with

MY SOY STORY: KNOWLEDGE CONJURES RAGE

Personally, I am fortunate to have a friend who is very close to a scientist in England. Five years ago, he said, "No amount of soy is good for you, don't eat it." I don't, but 16 years ago, I fed it to my baby girl who had a problem with milk. She now has all the symptoms of a classic soy baby—menstruated at the age of 10, low thyroid, frequent intense migraines, learning disabilities and a skin disease that has been associated with thyroid called vitiligo. I believe that I harmed her by feeding her soy formula, and the fact that there wasn't even a whisper that I might be hurting her makes it worse. I recently picked up an old book (1950) on thyroid in the library which clearly stated that soy had negative impact on thyroids. That information was known 50 years ago, but it has been silenced by marketing payola. And knowledge of this conjures rage in me.   A. R., London, UK soy formula among the girls whose breasts developed before the age of 2. Two other—far less significant—associations were made: maternal cystic ovaries and eating chicken.[77] More recently, the high rates of premature breast development in Puerto Rico have been linked with phthalates, chemicals used in the manufacture of plastics, lubricants and solvents, that can mimic or alter activity of sex hormones in animals.[78] This data, too, fell short of proof, suggesting the need to consider multifactorial dietary and environmental causes.

Yet soy proponents have dismissed the very possibility that soy could be part of the problem, blaming "growth hormone factors" in meat products as the cause (though nothing in the study supports that conclusion) or by criticizing the methodology of the study, which depended upon interviews with subjects and accurate recall. The last is a common criticism of a retrospective study although the assumption that parents would accurately remember details as basic as the type of infant formula used and as alarming as the development of breasts in their toddlers is a reasonable one.

Researchers with ties to the soy industry tend to leave out the 1986 Puerto Rico study whenever they make claims for the safety of soy infant formula. For example, Karen Oeter Klein, M.D., of DuPont Hospital for Children wrote in *Nutrition Reviews* in 1998 that the medical

MY SOY STORY: NOT READY FOR PUBERTY

My daughter is 8 years old and she is beginning to develop breasts and hair under her arms. She was breastfed but ingested heavy amounts of soy products most of her life. We are no longer using soy, but her teeth have permanent staining and now the early development. Is there any doctor or person I can speak with about this? She is just not ready on so many levels for puberty and I am very concerned with the adverse effects of early onset puberty.

R.T., Kansas City, MO

literature provides "no evidence of endocrine effects . . . and no changes in timing of puberty." This statement is false. Had Dr. Klein found fault with the 1986 Puerto Rican study, then she had an obligation to describe her objections. Instead, she omitted the study altogether and noted the adverse effects of isoflavones on hormone levels, uterine weight and fertility in various animal species, concluding that "different species and different tissues are affected by isoflavones in markedly different ways. It is difficult to know which tissues, if any, are affected in infants, and the variation among species makes extrapolation to infants inappropriate."[79]

Dr. Klein may think "extrapolation" inappropriate; others might think that the lack of "extrapolation" constitutes treachery. Indeed, some tissues in every animal species studied to date have been adversely affected by soy—so adversely that Dr. Sharpe came to a more responsible conclusion: "I've seen numerous studies showing what soy does to female animals. Until I have a reassurance that it doesn't have this effect on humans, I will not give soy to my children."[80]

Furthermore, Dr. Klein appears to have redefined the endocrine system to exclude the thyroid gland, as she ignores extensive evidence of autoimmune and other thyroid damage (see Chapter 27). Finally, she fails to examine suppressant effects on the immune system (see Chapter 30) and ignores the fact of higher incidences of insulin dependent diabetes in soy-fed children.[81]

Dr. Klein's reluctance to extrapolate and her omission of the Puerto Rican study and all the thyroid studies may be due to the fact that DuPont, owner of Protein Technologies International, the leading manufacturer of soy protein isolate, supports the hospital where she works; that the Soy Infant Formula Council sponsored her review; and that the trustees of *Nutrition Reviews* include representatives from industry giants such as Monsanto, Cargill, Heinz and Kraft, among others.[82]

STROM ON THE HORIZON

Recently a team of researchers headed by Brian L. Strom, M.D., studied the use of soy formula and its long-term impact on reproductive health and announced only one adverse finding: longer, more painful menstrual periods among the women who'd been fed soy formula in infancy.[83] Dr. Strom's conclusion, that the results were "reassuring," made newspaper headlines all over the world. But the data in the body of the report was far from reassuring. Mary G. Enig, Ph.D., President of the Maryland Nutritionists Association; Naomi Baumslag, M.D., Clinical Professor of Pediatrics at Georgetown University and President of the Women's International Public Health Network; Lynn R. Goldman, M.D., M.P.H., Environmental Health Sciences, Johns Hopkins University; Retha Newbold, Ph.D., National Institute of Environmental Health Sciences, Research Triangle Park, NC; and other experts who analyzed the findings, noted numerous flaws in both the design and reporting of this study,[84,85] including:

+ Failure to include mention of statistically significant, higher incidences of allergies and asthma in the study's abstract— the only part read by most busy health professionals and media reporters.

+ Glossing over or omitting from the main body of the report gynecological problems such as higher rates of cervical cancer, polycystic ovarian syndrome, blocked fallopian tubes, pelvic inflammatory disease, hormonal disorders and multiple births.

+ Manipulation of statistics by not evaluating still births or failure to achieve pregnancy (higher in the soy-fed women) but evaluating miscarriages (slightly higher in the dairy-formula-fed group).

twenty-eight: soy infant formula

• Excluding thyroid function as a subject for study (although thyroid damage from soy formula has been the principal concern of critics for decades). Nonetheless, thyroid damage can be surmised by the fact that the soy-fed females grew up to report higher rates of sedentary activity and use of weight-loss medicines.

• Conducting the entire study by telephone interviews, asking subjective questions, and performing no medical examinations, laboratory tests or other objective testing. Breast development, for example, was gauged by asking participants at which age they first bought their bras.

MY SOY STORY: JUST WANTED TO DIE

My daughter was on soya milk formula from 4 weeks old to approximately 3 years old. The reason she was put on it was she couldn't tolerate my breast milk. At the age of 2, her whole body started to swell starting from her left arm and quickly spreading over her entire body. She was in hospital and swollen like this for 3 weeks despite being given steroids. They never did find out what caused it. She was tested for thyroid problems at 4 years old after an initial test showed a problem, but the second test came back clear. She has had lots of on-going problems, joint pains being the most frequent. She has had several broken bones, the worst was a spiral fracture of the femur caused simply by her jumping over my sewing machine cord. She developed breasts at a very early age and despite her tiny frame started her menstrual cycle at 11 years old. It was full on from the start, lasting up to 7 days and very heavy with terrible back pain. Sometimes she said she just wanted to die. Her GP is trying to find a contraceptive pill that will help.   E. S., Sydney, Australia

• Providing no information on the ages at which formula feeding ended, the dose length or the quantity of the soy isoflavones (all of which are basic requirements of valid toxicology studies).[86]

• Using the criteria "trade school, college and post college" as a measure of intelligence, thus rating a graduate of a beauty school at the same level as someone who received a doctorate degree. The researchers could only have obtained meaningful conclusions by breaking these out into separate categories.

• Following up infants who were given soy formula as infants for just 16 weeks (though serious damage can occur for at least the first nine months in boys and the first six months in girls) and failing to obtain any information about whether the subjects in the study took soy formula after the initial 16-week study period or ate soy foods during childhood.[86]

• Using a study group of 282 soy-fed persons that was too small for most of the negative findings to become "statistically significant."

The design and presentation of this study actually hide the adverse effects of soy, rather than reveal them. It was funded by the National Institutes of Health and the International Formula Council (a trade group that represents formula manufacturers) and carried out under the auspices of the Fomon Infant Nutrition Unit at the University of Iowa. The Fomon Infant Nutrition Unit receives support from the major formula manufacturers Ross Products Division of Abbott Laboratories, Nestlé and Mead Johnson Nutritionals. As Dr. Joseph Mercola commented in his weekly health ezine, "If you can believe a 'telephone interview' study funded by the baby-formula industry, then maybe you will believe this nonsense."[87]

twenty-eight: soy infant formula

SOY DANGERS ARE NOT EXAGGERATED

Most of the published data on the epidemic of emasculated boys, premature puberty, reproductive system abnormalities and infertility implicate environmental estrogens such as PCBs and DDE (a breakdown product of DDT), not soy phytoestrogens as the probable cause.[88]

GIRL INTERRUPTED: WHY AFRICAN-AMERICAN GIRLS GROW UP TOO SOON

Why are so many young girls entering puberty earlier than usual? And why are 48.3 percent of African-American girls—compared to 14.7 percent of Caucasian girls—developing breasts, pubic hair and even menstruating before the age of 8?[117] Although blacks now experience earlier puberties than whites, it is apparently a recent phenomenon and not a racial difference.[118,119]

Early puberty is generally blamed on exposure to the ever increasing numbers of xeno (foreign) estrogens in the modern environment. Estrogens—or estrogen mimickers—are widely found in plastics, pesticides and commercial animal products. Although it has been known for decades that soy estrogens trigger accelerated maturation in female animals of every species, few people, until recently, thought of putting soy foods on the estrogen danger list.[120,121]

Yet of all the estrogens to be found in the environment, soy is the likeliest explanation of why African-American girls reach puberty so quickly. Since its establishment in 1974, the federal government's WIC (Women, Infants and Children) program has provided free infant formula to teenage and other low-income mothers. Because of perceived lactose intolerance, African American babies are very likely to receive soy formula.

The media focus on the dangers of environmental chemicals but the "health" benefits of soy have also made it easy to overlook the role of soy estrogens. Unfortunately, a whole lot of people seem to think that soy formula has been around for centuries and so must be safe. As we discussed in Chapter 12, this is simply not true. Soy formula is neither natural nor traditional.

MY SOY STORY: SICKENED AND STUNNED

My nine-month-old daughter has been on soy formula since she was approximately three months old. In the past month, I noticed that her breasts were developing. At first, I thought it was because she is a chubby baby. Then I started noticing a clear mucus vaginal discharge occurring periodically. The second time I saw the discharge, I noticed a slight pink color in it. I called the pediatrician's office to see whether I should be concerned. They told me to just keep an eye on it. The discharge went away for approximately a week and finally, one morning when I changed her diaper I noticed that the diaper had a pinkish hue to it. I called the doctor and brought her in.

They examined her and found nothing. They suggested it might be a urinary tract infection or perhaps the diaper was just reacting to the acid in her urine, thus resulting in the pink color. They sent me home with a specimen bag to try to capture her urine. The bag did not work and I ultimately had to bring her in to be catheterized. The urine tested negative. I mentioned to the doctor that I did not think blood was in the urine. I thought it was just being washed out by the urine because I had seen some slight bloody discharge

ISOFLAVONES IN BREAST MILK

A popular argument in support of soy infant formula claims that Japanese women eat a lot of soy products and so must have high levels of soy phytoestrogens in their breast milk. Therefore, if problems could arise from soy phytoestrogens in infants, we would see it in Japanese children. When soy advocates came to this conclusion a decade ago, no one had actually measured the levels of soy isoflavones in breast milk. Since then, researchers have discovered that isoflavones are almost nonexistent in breast milk, even in vegetarian women who consume copious quantities of tofu, soymilk, soy protein shakes and other soyfoods. Cow's milk and goat's milk formulas are also almost entirely free of isoflavones.[89,90]

"Isoflavones were not detectable in human breast milk regardless of the mother's soy consumption," says Cliff Irvine, D.V.Sc., D.Sc., whose tests established a level of soy phytoestrogens in breast milk

the night before. He dismissed my claim.

Then the next evening she developed a fever so I brought her back again thinking it might be related to the bleeding. It turned out to be an ear infection. But during that visit, I asked if he thought the bleeding might be hormone related and I pointed out that her breasts seemed swollen. He looked and said it was normal for some babies. She was then put on antibiotics for her ear infection. Over the course of the next day or so the bleeding seemed to have gone away, but I noticed that her face was broken out and that she was developing brown "peach fuzz" in her pubic area. It was then completely clear to me that this was hormonal and I needed to take matters into my own hands to get her to a specialist. Today, my husband came across an article about the link of soy formula and premature puberty. I was sickened and stunned when I read it. I would never have linked the two.

H.S., Philadelphia, PA

at less than 0.01 mg per liter. In contrast, the total isoflavone concentrations in soy infant formula (properly diluted as per package instructions) were "at least 660 times higher than the maximum level possible in breastmilk." Irvine also reported that the hormones in oral contraceptive pills were transferred into breast milk in minuscule quantities, as were ovarian steroids used to induce lactation in cattle.[91]

Adrian Franke, Ph.D., of the Cancer Research Center of Hawaii in Honolulu found a maximum of 0.02 mg phytoestrogens per liter of breast milk, or about 1/1,000 of the concentration measured in soy infant formula.[92,93] In yet another study, Kenneth D. R. Setchell, Ph.D., of the Children's Hospital and Medical Center in Cincinnati, Ohio, arrived at similar figures and concluded, "The levels of phytoestrogens in soy formula are many times higher than in the breast milk of high soy consumers. Daily exposure of infants to isoflavones was four to eleven fold higher (on a body weight basis) than the dose that has hormonal effects in adults consuming soy foods. Circulating concentrations were 13,000 to 22,000 times higher than plasma estradiol concentrations in early life and sufficient to exert biological effects, whereas the contribution of isoflavones from breast milk and cow milk was negligible."[94]

MATERNAL HORMONES

Finally, soy advocates argue that the isoflavones in infant formula are not likely to be a problem because breastfed infants consume high levels of the maternal hormones estradiol, estriol and estrone—the principal forms of estrogen found naturally in the human body. This is true, but the estrogenic effect of the maternal hormones is far less—perhaps only one percent that of the phytoestrogens in soy formula. Although estradiol is 1,200 times stronger than the principal soy estrogen genistein, soy formula contains 130,000 times more isoflavones than human breast milk.[95,96] Furthermore, the level of estradiol in human milk declines soon after birth and nearly disappears after two to three weeks. The soy phytoestrogens in soy infant formula, however, remain at a consistently high level.

Woodhams concludes: "The human infant has adapted to the presence of maternal hormones in breast milk immediately after birth and evolved the means to metabolize them safely. It is only in the last few generations that infants have been challenged with the alien estrogen mimickers from soybeans."[97]

CAN INFANTS ABSORB ISOFLAVONES?

The answer is yes.

When Setchell quantified the phytoestrogens in breast milk, he also measured intake and excretion rates and concluded that he "had no doubt that soy phytoestrogens accumulated in the body."[98] Similarly P.S. Venkataraman found that babies fed from birth on soy formula partially absorb isoflavones in the stomach and small intestine; these isoflavones show up in hydrolyzed form in the blood, undergo further metabolization in the liver and then circulate to all organs and tissues of the body including the brain before excretion in the urine. Infants drinking soy formula excreted significantly more genistein in the urine than infants drinking cow's or mother's milk. This research shows that infants are very capable of hydrolyzing the soy isoflavones into active forms and absorbing them.[99]

At the Fourth International Symposium on the Role of Soy in the Prevention and Treatment of Chronic Disease in San Diego in November 2001, Setchell stated that infants cannot metabolize phytoestrogens into the more potent equol because they lack the gut flora. Yet in an earlier report Setchell stated: "Although the gut is sterile at birth, during the first week of life it rapidly develops a bacterial flora. Whether in early life the bacterial enzymes which in adults are responsible for the conversion of daidzein-glycoside in soya to equol are present, remains to be established. If so the infant may be subjected to concentrations of this weak estrogen which are well in excess of endogenous estrogen levels and if not it is probable that the precursor daidzein, itself a weak estrogen may be absorbed and excreted in the urine as the glucuronide conjugate, as shown in adults. Therefore, the potential effects of subjective infants as well as adults to relatively large amounts of dietary phytoestrogens remains to be evaluated."[100]

DARE WE "WAIT AND SEE?"

Until soy isoflavones are definitively linked to reproductive tract abnormalities, infertility and other health problems in humans, most health authorities recommend that we "wait and see." That could be a terrible mistake.

In the 1940s and 1950s, many western women took another estrogen, diethylstilbestrol (DES), early in their pregnancies in a misguided attempt to prevent miscarriage. That fact is relevant not only because DES bears a striking structural similarity to some plant estrogens—including soy isoflavones—but because it took more than 20 years before the full spectrum of harmful effects was observed. (The FDA did not ban DES until 1971.) Female offspring of women who took DES are prone to abnormalities of the vagina and cervix, reduced fertility and a high risk of developing a rare but lethal form of vaginal cancer called clear-cell adenocarcinoma. Male offspring show reduced fertility and a higher-than-normal incidence of genito-urinary tract abnormalities.[101]

DES is 100,000 times more potent than soy phytoestrogens. However, the large quantities of phytoestrogens in soy products are more than enough to compensate for their lower potency. When the effects of isoflavones in fetal and neonatal animals have been studied, they have paralleled those observed in human infants exposed to DES. While researchers need to be careful about extrapolating results from one species to another, it is prudent to heed warning signs.[102-104]

The soy industry has known about the DES connection for at least two decades. In 1985, Setchell wrote: "In spite of the controversy that surrounds the exogenous addition of estrogens such as diethylstilbestrol (DES) as a growth promoter in animals and its contamination in food, relatively little consideration appears to have been given to the contribution of naturally occurring plant estrogens in the diet. Indeed, while the potency of DES far exceeds that of either the endogenous estrogens or the phytoestrogens, the amounts consumed of the latter are significantly greater. The effects of plant estrogens in man should however be of some concern, particularly since it has been suggested that soya might be as beneficial a growth promoter as DES in animals. For example, the concentrations of phytoestrogens in soy, calculated to match 0.5 ppb of DES are well within the concentration range of commonly consumed soy products."[105]

In 1979, University of Wisconsin scientists warned that "likely human exposure to phytoestrogens when measured in DES equivalents is considerably higher than likely human exposure to DES in liver from cattle treated with DES as a growth stimulant."[106]

The soy-DES connection has, if anything, grown stronger with time. Recent studies indicate that genistein may be even more carcinogenic than DES, if exposure occurs during critical periods of differentiation—as is always the case with growing babies. Within one month, mice fed a modified soy protein diet had significantly higher incidences of vulvar carcinomas than mice fed control diet, leading Retha Newbold, Ph.D., of the National Laboratory of Toxicology, National Institute of Environmental Health Sciences, to conclude: "The use of soy–based infant formulas in the absence of medical necessity and the marketing of soy products designed to appeal to children should be closely monitored."[107]

BRITISH WARN AGAINST SOY FORMULA

In 2003 the British Dietetic Association issued a position statement warning against the possible dangers of soy infant formula. It advised dietitians to discourage the use of soy protein in children during the first six months of life "to avoid sensitization to soya protein and exposure to phytoestrogens while organ systems remain at their most vulnerable. This would include soy infant formula and soya products such as desserts, etc. When a soy-based formula is used parents should be informed of current findings relating to phytoestrogens and health on the clinical need for soy formula. Any parent choosing to refuse soya for their infant should be supported in their decision."

The BDA's decision followed a series of increasingly strong statements issued by the British government. In 1996, the Committee on Toxicity of Chemicals in Foods, Consumer Products and Environment (COT) completed a review of phytoestrogens in soy and concluded "that breast milk and cows' milk formulae are the preferred sources of nutrition for infants." The British Food Advisory Committee (FAC) then recommended that, "as a precautionary measure, infant formulae manufacturers should investigate ways to reduce the levels of phytoestrogens in soy-based formulae." In 1999, the Panel of Child and Maternal Nutrition (Committee on Medical Aspects of Food and Nutrition Policy, 1999-2000) endorsed this recommendation and noted that the clinical grounds for recommending a soy-based formula to parents were diminishing as more suitable hydrolysates based on cows' milk were becoming available."

SOURCES

British Dietetic Association. Paediatric group position statement on the use of soya protein for infants. *J Fam Health Care*, 2003, 13, 4, 93.

Committee on Toxicity (COT) Report on Phytoestrogens and Health. Chapter 16 International policy on soy-based infant formula. www.foodstandards.gov.uk/news/newsarchive/working_group

STRESSED OUT ON SOY

A recent study on the effects of soy isoflavones on rat behavior begins with the following statement: "Isoflavones form one of the main classes of phytoestrogens and have been found to exert both oestrogenic and anti-oestrogenic effects on the central nervous system. The effects have not been limited to reproductive behaviour, but include effects on learning and anxiety and actions on the hypothalamo-pituitary axis." Noting that most rat chow contains soy, the investigators compared the behavior of rats given isoflavones in their diets with those on an isoflavone-free diet. Rats fed isoflavones spent significantly less time in active social inter-action and had significantly elevated stress-induced corti-costerone concentrations. Their conclusion: "Major changes in behavioural measures of anxiety and in stress hormones can result from the soya isoflavone content of rat diet. These changes are as striking as those seen following drug admin-istration and could form an important source of variation between laboratories."

This study provides scientific support to numerous an-ecdotal reports of high levels of anxiety, extreme emotional behavior and difficulties with social contact in children fed soy as infants.

SOURCE: Hartley DC, Edwards JE et al. The soya isoflavone content of rat diet can increase anxiety and stress hormone release in the male rat. *Psychopharmacology* (Berl) 2003, 167, 1, 46-53.

MY SOY STORY: TEN SURGERIES

I'd like to add my two cents regarding the extreme health hazards of soy. My son was born with a third degree hypospadias which required ten—yes, ten surgeries to correct. He had the worst hypospadias a male can have, where his urethra's opening appeared at the base of his genitals. How did this utter nightmare occur? Well, I was foolishly a vegan and little did I know that the daily tofu and soymilk I was drinking for the past decade was highly estrogenating my already estrogenated body. Healthy women make enough estrogen as it is. The phytoestrogens disrupted my fetus's development. I have met other women who had sons with hypospadias and they ate soy daily all during pregnancy. Enough said.

S.D. Lincoln, NE

29
SOY AND THE
REPRODUCTIVE SYSTEM
breeding discontent

Herbalists, midwives and witches have long known that certain plants and herbs have a contraceptive effect.[1] Scientists first recognized the fact that plants contained such substances in 1926. Interest picked up in the mid-1940s when sheep were diagnosed with "clover disease." The cause was three phytoestrogens in clover: formononetin, biochanin A and genistein. Sheep can efficiently convert formononetin to equol, the highly estrogenic metabolite that also comes from the soy isoflavone daidzein. In female sheep, eating clover causes endometrial damage and cervical mucus changes associated with an inability to conceive. The problems are not unique to sheep; fertility problems from phytoestrogen exposure have also been reported in birds, cows, mice, cats and dogs as well as in humans.[2-14] Scientists have identified estrogenic activity in more than 300 plants,[15] but only one of these plants commonly appears in the food supply—soy.

FAST TRACK TO EXTINCTION

The best known case concerns the cheetahs at the Cincinnati Zoo. In the 1980s, Kenneth D. R. Setchell, Ph.D., discovered one reason the big cats were not reproducing. The female cheetahs were suffering from liver disease and reproductive failure caused by the high concentrations of genistein and daidzein found in the soy-protein portion of their feed. As Setchell put it, "Cheetahs have always been difficult to breed in captivity, but the additional insult of a diet rich in estrogens may well be one of the major factors in the decline of fertility in cheetahs kept in North American zoos."[16]

The soy estrogens in the cheetah feed not only disrupted hormonal activity along the hypothalamic-pituitary-gonadal axis, but damaged the endometrium, making normal implantation and nourishment of a newly fertilized egg difficult. In contrast, cheetahs fed whole carcasses of beef, chicken and other animals at the DeWildt Research Centre in South Africa showed no signs of liver damage and had no problems breeding.[17]

At both the Fourth and Fifth International Symposia on the Role of Soy in the Prevention and Treatment of Chronic Disease, Setchell and other industry faithfuls reassured attendees that this is a cheetah problem and not a human problem. Cheetahs are particularly susceptible to damage because they lack key liver enzymes needed to adequately deactivate estrogenic compounds. While this makes soy especially unsuitable for felines, Setchell's research provides ample evidence that soy estrogens are risky for animals of any species, including human animals. In the cheetah study, for example, he compares phytoestrogens with DES, a potent and dangerous estrogen with a chemical structure very similar to genistein, which has been withdrawn from agricultural use in the west. He writes: "Despite concerns over the deleterious effect of diethylstilbestrol and other anabolic agents contaminating meats consumed by humans, it is apparent that the contribution of naturally occurring plant estrogens to the diet is rarely considered. This is surprising particularly as the level of phytoestrogens in foods is substantially higher than estrogen levels in animal tissues. Interestingly, it has been claimed that soy may be as beneficial as diethylstilbestrol as a growth promoter in animals."[18]

CAT OUT OF THE BAG

Although the soy industry did its best to bury the cheetah study, researchers over the past 25 years have steadily turned up evidence of soy's probable role in today's epidemic of infertility, menstrual problems and other reproductive disorders. A team of researchers from the Karolinska Institute in Stockholm working with Setchell, for example, concluded a study in the *Journal of Endocrinology* with the words: "These findings have raised concerns about human exposures to phytoestrogens. The widespread use of soya beans as a protein food source makes it important to determine possible physiological effects of equol in man. The 'contraceptive' effect in animals suggests to us that it may be of interest to investigate the dietary habits and urinary excretion of equol in women with unexplained infertility or disorders of the menstrual cycle."[19]

Similarly, Setchell once proposed that women with menstrual cycle disorders and fertility problems consider their consumption of soy "in view of the various reproductive disorders in animals that have been associated with the ingestion of a variety of phytoestrogens."[20]

The soy industry has not publicized these recommendations. Instead, it has boldly promoted the adverse effects as beneficial—as the key to breast cancer prevention no less. An example of such positive spin applied to alarming study results appears in a 1994 article published in the *American Journal of Clinical Nutrition*.[21]

Aedin Cassidy completed an in-depth study of six women of childbearing age who were given 60 grams of textured vegetable protein (containing 45 mg total isoflavones) per day for 30 days. Compared to controls, the soy feeding resulted in "significant biological effects," including menstrual cycles lengthened by an average of two and a half days, a 33 percent reduction of mid-cycle levels of luteinizing hormone (LH) and a 53 percent reduction of follicle stimulating hormone (FSH). One woman saw her LH and FSH levels reduced to a mere 17 percent and 32 percent, respectively, of normal levels. LH and FSH are gonadotropins; they stimulate the gonads— in males the testes, and in females the ovaries. They are not necessary for life, but are essential for reproduction. Although none of the women in this short-term study stopped ovulating, the effects of the isoflavones continued for three months after they ceased eating the soy.

These findings clearly show that soyfood consumption can disrupt a woman's cycle and jeopardize her fertility. However, the study's authors chose to deemphasize this finding in favor of speculation

MY SOY STORY: GAINED 28 POUNDS, LOST PERIOD

I'm perimenopausal so I purchased a soy isoflavone supplement made by Sundown to help control my symptoms. I had read so much about how they would help ease my way through upcoming menopause. That was the biggest mistake of my life. I gained 28 pounds in three weeks time and felt the worse I have ever felt in my life. The caps actually stopped me from having any bleeding at all and it took me six months to have a period again. I was happy about the lack of bleeding, but this stuff stopped a lot of other things from working in my body. My thyroid for one. I experienced classic symptoms of a thyroid disorder and never had such symptoms until I took that stuff. I am not a person who was ever overweight and always had a normal thyroid. The supplements were on the shelves in the store to purchase so I thought they would be safe for me. Wrong, wrong, wrong! There ought to be a warning label on this stuff!

P.R. Columbus, OH

that the longer menstrual cycles experienced by the soy-fed women could result in lower lifetime levels of estrogen. This, in turn, was harnessed to the unproven theory that reduction in lifetime estrogen levels is the key to reducing breast cancer risk. They also suggested that soy isoflavones could be used prophylactically to prevent breast cancer in a manner similar to the liver-damaging drug Tamoxifen. The conclusion that made the 6 o'clock news—still widely cited by the media—is that soy reduces breast cancer risk.

SAME BUT DIFFERENT

A look at the original version of the Cassidy study provides a lesson in how the soy industry co-opts scientific research. The earlier study was Aedin Cassidy's 1991 Ph.D. dissertation from Cam-

STOPPING THE STORK

Might plants high in phytoestrogens such as soy, flax and alfalfa have value as contraceptive drugs? The World Health Organization once thought so. In the early 1970s, it funded a $5 million study through the University of Chicago and sent researchers out in the field in search of all-natural contraceptives. The idea was to find a safe and effective alternative to the high-dose birth control pills of that era. Researchers visited dozens of native cultures to discover which herbs and plants were being used to prevent pregnancy, examined hundreds of plants and analyzed their phytochemicals. Although they found many contraceptive plants—soy, flax and red clover among them—they ultimately abandoned the project. Not because "natural" methods didn't work, but because the side effects were similar to—and just as serious—as those of the birth control pill.

SOURCE: Farnsworth NR, Bingel AS et al. Potential value of plants as sources of new antifertility agents. II. *J Pharm Sci*, 1975, 64, 717-754.

bridge University in England. The later version, published in the *American Journal of Clinical Nutrition*, won her worldwide recognition, kudos from the soy industry and a job at Unilever.

Although the data is the same, Cassidy's dissertation includes a lengthy discussion of the ways that soy isoflavones inhibit the hypothalamic-pituitary-gonadal axis and contribute to reproductive disorders and infertility. She states clearly that her findings with human subjects were consistent with the "pathological changes" observed in animals, including the infertile sheep afflicted with clover disease, and links her own findings to earlier human studies showing increased incidences of menstrual irregularities among vegetarian women. Her summary directly addresses the issue of impaired fertility.

"The results of the present study provide evidence to show that the feeding of 60 g of soya protein per day to six premenopausal women over a single menstrual cycle resulted in significant biological effects. The plant oestrogens present in soya protein interfered with the mechanism responsible for ovulation . . ."[22]

Other researchers have also reported soy-induced perturbances in menstrual cycles[23] and some have directly stated that "isoflavones influence not only estrogen receptor-related functions but the entire hypothalamo-hypophysis-gonadal axis."[24]

THE HEAT IS ON

The industry also urges women to eat soy to reduce menopausal symptoms and to prevent osteoporosis. The evidence that soy could do either is inconsistent and contradictory, yet sales of soy foods and soy isoflavone supplements are booming because of the desire for a "safe and natural" alternative to hormone replacement therapy (HRT). Even the soy-industry faithful admit that more research is needed to assess the benefits. As Mindy Kurzer, Ph.D., of the University of Minnesota, St. Paul, put it, "the manufacturers are way ahead of the science."[25]

The British Committee on Toxicity summarized the research as

SOY: WORTHLESS FOR MENOPAUSE

Five recent studies have shown that soy is worthless in treating symptoms of menopause. A study carried out at Monash University, Clayton, Australia found that three months of soy supplements providing 188 mg of isoflavones daily did not improve menopausal complaints in 94 older women compared with those taking a placebo.[98]

Investigators at the Department of Food Science and Human Nutrition at Iowa State University examined changes in menopausal symptoms in response to 24 weeks of isoflavone-rich diets, comparing women receiving about 80 mg isoflavones per day with a group receiving 4 mg per day and a group receiving none. They found no treatment effect on frequency, duration or severity of hot flashes or night sweats. As in the Australian study, all groups reported a decline in overall symptoms, indicating either a placebo effect or simply an improvement in symptoms during the study.[99]

In a study carried out at the University of Milan patients were administered 72 mg per day of soy-derived isoflavones or placebo under double-blind conditions. Both groups recorded a 40 percent reduction in the number of hot flashes.[100] In a similar study carried out at the University of Pittsburgh, those women taking the placebo actually showed improvement! Hot flashes, night sweats and vaginal dryness improved from baseline in the placebo group but not in the soy group. In addition, insomnia was more frequent over the 6-month study in the soy group.[101]

And, finally, a study carried out in Helsinki University Central Hospital found no difference between phytoestrogens and a placebo for treating menopausal symptoms in breast cancer survivors.[105]

follows: "Studies examining the effect of soy-based products or isoflavones to relieve menopausal symptoms are inconclusive. Some studies have suggested that soy may be beneficial, especially if basal intake is low, or the vasomotor symptoms severe, but the data are equivocal, as positive results are often not statistically significant and strong placebo responses are observed."[26] Even soy spokesperson Mark Messina has admitted that soy foods did no better than wheat flour (the placebo) in a double blind study.[27] Although the benefits for symptoms of menopause remain unproven, the risks to the thyroid are well known (see Chapter 27).

MEAT ON BONES

Likewise, the soy industry has high hopes that soy will prove to be the panacea for osteoporosis. At the last two International Symposia on the Role of Soy in the Prevention and Treatment of Chronic Disease, entire sessions were devoted to the latest soy research on bones. On the whole, the results were disappointing, leading embarrassed researchers to explain that they haven't found a consistent bone-sparing effect because the dose must be either "suboptimal" or "excessive." In other words, they *know* soy works, if they could only find the perfect dose, the perfect formula, the right age to initiate preventive treatment.

POTENT DRUGS

Meanwhile, evidence is mounting that isoflavone supplements present a potential hazard to menopausal women. In 2004, Italian researchers called the supplements "potent drugs" after finding that they caused "significant increases in the occurrence of endometrial hyperplasia" (a thickening of the uterine lining) in menopausal women. Endometrial proliferation is a precursor of cancer, and was the first problem identified with synthetic estrogen replacement therapy (ERT). They concluded: "These findings call into question the long-term safety of phytoestrogens with respect to the endometrium."[28]

At Soyfoods 2001 in Phoenix, Arizona, Setchell repeatedly warned of the dangers of soy isoflavones: "There have been more than 10,000 publications in the last decade on the role isoflavones can play. These have significant biological benefit. This has driven the whole area of functional food. . . [and] and stimulated an industry that involves extracting and isolating these bioactive substances from soybeans and packaging them in various supplements and dietary drinks. This, I think, is one area where I have been relatively vocal in my concern because we know that there is a natural tendency to believe that if a small amount of something is good then if we take more it will be a lot better. With these compounds, let me stress there is a very real potential for deleterious effects. I'm absolutely appalled at some of the industries that are beginning to fortify and package foods and various beverages boasting isoflavone levels in excess of 90 mg and I've even seen 160 mg. It is so artificial and I'm not convinced there is any advantage. . ."[29]

Yet Revival Soy, the product offering the high 160 mg of isoflavones per serving claims that it came up with that dose based on the work of Setchell and others. At Soyfoods 2001, however, Setchell admitted having made a mistake back in 1984: "Now the other thing is if we must look at the usual dietary intake of Asia. Clinical work is driven by the idea that the isoflavone levels of Asians were extremely high and that low incidence of hormonal disease was due to high circulating levels of these compounds. If we look at a new cohort study in Japan, we see an average intake of 6-8 g per day. If you do rough calculations as I did, I would estimate that the approximate levels of isoflavones were 15-30 mg per day and not, as I must admit, I rather erroneously stated in 1984. We thought perhaps then that it was 150-200 mg. We were going on very little data at the time. . . ."[30]

SHOOTING BLANKS

Soy phytoestrogens also affect the fertility, the testosterone levels and probably the sex drive of men. Scientists first linked phytoestrogens with lowered sperm count and other reproductive problems in the 1940s when they diagnosed clover disease in sheep. Normal males became infertile, while castrated males—called wethers—had experienced teat enlargement and nipple discharge.[31,32] Sperm production of rodents, primates and humans is similar and known to be disrupted by estrogens that either interact directly with the testes or that affect plasma gonadotrophin or sex hormone concentrations. Compared to rodents, humans produce relatively low numbers of sperm, so even small effects may impair fertility.[33] As it happens, the changes in sperm quality and quantity over the past 60 years loom large.

In 1992 Danish researchers reported that sperm counts had dropped 50 percent worldwide between 1939 and 1990. The study was widely criticized, but a reanalysis confirmed the results. Other studies followed with reports that sperm counts have been going down at the rate of two percent per year since the 1970s. Sperm quality has also suffered.[34-40] The most probable cause is a combined assault by the environmental chemicals in pesticides and plastics

PLANT SURVIVAL MECHANISM

Like other antinutrients and toxins in soybeans, isoflavones seem to have evolved to ensure the plant's survival. In a dry year, desert annuals exhibit stunted growth but greatly increased levels of phytoestrogens. When eaten by California quail, these compounds inhibit their ability to reproduce and so prevent the birth of young who would starve because of insufficient food. In a wet year, the plants grow vigorously and contain few phytoestrogens. The quail then breed prolifically and feed their young through the winter on the abundant crop.

SOURCE: Leopold AS, Erwin M et al. Phytoestrogens: adverse effects on reproduction in California quail. *Science,* 1976, 9, 191, 4222, 98-100.

MY SOY STORY: LOW LIBIDO

I'm an over-50 natural bodybuilder who was always looking for a good source of protein. I reached a point where I had changed my protein intake to pure soy protein isolate, because it was inexpensive and at *first* made me feel good. I was also drinking soy milk and my wife and I were both eating a lot of fake soy foods.

In the spring of 1998, I spent three months away from home in Hawaii, running a gym and testing whether we wanted to move there. I was eating what we are told is the "perfect" diet: oatmeal, nuts, raisins, some fish and a lot of soy protein isolate. When I came home, I had reached a point where my energy levels were so low I would often spend a day or two doing nothing. My libido was also at an all-time low, and this was unusual and depressing. I didn't have a clue what was wrong, until my wife accidentally learned about the estrogens in soy foods.

We quit soy cold turkey! Today my old self is back—energy levels, libido and thought processes. This information is vital, and I have no problem walking up to perfect strangers in the supermarket and health food stores, and telling them to stay away from soy. In fact, I have one health food store owner very upset with me. Young mothers and fathers have even put soy milk back on the shelf and asked me about alternatives. L.W., Preston, AZ

along with the dietary phytoestrogens from soy.[41]

Although men produce sperm throughout their lives, serious damage is most likely to occur during the first trimester of pregnancy, and during infancy and early childhood. Adults who care about their sperm might also want to be cautious about soy consumption, however. Researchers at King's College in England who studied mouse sperm treated with the estrogens found in paint, beer and tofu found clear evidence that these natural and environmental estrogens all affected the sperm's ability to fertilize an egg. All three estrogens initially made the sperm friskier—a process known as capacitation—but then the sperm petered out before they could find an egg to penetrate.[42]

THE LOWDOWN ON TESTOSTERONE

Researchers have also reported lowered testosterone and higher estrogen levels in males who consume foods rich in soy estrogens.[43,44] Scientists have even induced "testosterone deprivation" in animals simply by feeding them isoflavone-rich diets.[45]

Just as soy industry spokesmen promote hormonal changes indicative of infertility as beneficial tools in the war against breast cancer, so they tout testosterone-lowering as protective against prostate cancer and atherosclerosis.[46,47] Although the possibility that soy foods or supplements could prevent these deadly conditions makes headlines, few men hear that the downside is demasculinization. This is not just a macho thing, for testosterone is an important hormone for growth, repair, red blood cell formation, sex drive and immune function.[48] Low levels of testosterone have also been linked to low thyroid function, another unwanted and common side effect of soy consumption.[49]

Recently scientists at the University of North Carolina at Chapel Hill completed a study for the National Cancer Institute in which the soy-eating men experienced "nipple discharge, breast enlargement and slight decreases in testosterone." The good news, according to lead researcher Steven H. Zeisel, M.D., was that nothing "serious" was found, even though they administered doses up to 30 times what one might get from "normal foods." To reassure men, he stated: "I don't think there are a lot of estrogenic worries. Your testicles will not shrink and you won't have massive breast enlargement."[50]

As Anthony Colpo commented in www.theomnivore.com, "Gee, it's such a relief to know that men won't experience 'massive'

PANDA PORN

Is she or isn't she? That's one of the most frequently asked questions at the National, Atlanta and San Diego Zoos. Pregnancies of pandas in captivity are rare, live births even rarer. Of the few pandas born alive, only 40 percent survive the first month and only a third make it into adulthood.

The challenge is great. Even in the wild, pandas are solitary creatures that can be finicky about finding a mate with the perfect smell. With the giant panda nearly extinct, zoo officials have tried everything imaginable to encourage the pandas to mate, including behavioral therapy to improve social skills. At the Chengdu Giant Panda Breeding and Research Base in China, encouragement includes showing X-rated "how to" videos of humping pandas. Even so, most zoos resort to artificial insemination.

Clearly, it's time to take a look at the panda diet. According to the *Washington Post*, Mei Xiang and Tian Tian, the couple at the National Zoo, are rewarded with treats, including apple slices and "vitamin-rich soy biscuits." Yet soy isoflavones have caused infertility, miscarriages, birth defects, decreased libido, anxiety, social isolation, aggression and other behavioral disorders in all animal species tested. Anecdotal evidence indicates that soy can even alter one's scent— and not for the better. Poor pandas!

SOURCES:
Fernandez, Manny. Hoping, but not necessarily expecting: zoo's panda staff on pregnancy watch. *Washington Post,* September 1, 2004, B3.

Walker, Camerson. Wong, Kathleen. Panda pornography inspires bashful bears. *This Week in Wild*, California Academy of Sciences, July 3, 2002.

What is captive breeding? and Do you know what pandas eat? www.marymount.k12/ny.us/maryet/Studentwebwork01/Thinkquest/Pandas/html.capt.

breast enlargement from copious soy consumption. See, nothing to worry about fellas; you won't end up looking like Anna-Nicole Smith up top, just a more modestly-proportioned Heather Locklear instead! As an added bonus, the testosterone reductions you experience won't be reflected by a visible decrease in the size of your family jewels, so even the tightest pants will fail to reveal your declining testosterone status! As for nipple discharge, c'mon what's a little lactation between friends?"[51]

SEX AND THE UNBORN BOY

Can soy phytoestrogens taken by the mother during pregnancy exert demasculinizing effects on the unborn baby boy? Human studies are sparse, but animal studies suggest this as a strong possibility.

From the outset, a fetus is genetically male or female. However, all mammalian fetuses develop into phenotypic females unless male hormones are produced. These change the phenotype of the fetus from female to male and play critical roles in masculinization. Testosterone is produced in the testes of the male fetus during the first trimester of pregnancy. Estrogens—including soy isoflavones—can interfere and suppress the unborn baby boy's testosterone production. The male fetus is extremely vulnerable to interference by estrogens during this time. Female genital development is largely independent of hormone interaction, but proper male genital development will occur only if male hormones are present.[52-55] This is why birth defects involving sex organs are over eight times more prevalent among males than females.[56]

Today more and more baby boys are born with genital anomalies caused by excess prenatal estrogen exposure. The stronger the interference by estrogens, the more severe the effects. Birth defects that are obviously recognizable at birth include genotypic males with female genitalia, hypospadias (a birth defect in which the opening of the penis is located on the underside of the shaft) and cryptorchidism (undescended testicles).[57]

When less extreme exposure to estrogens occurs, the consequences might not manifest until puberty or adulthood. As with the use of soy infant formula during the vulnerable neonatal period, these manifestations can include reduced sperm production and poor sperm quality. An estrogenized boy is also likely to have a smaller-than-average size penis. The reason is that testosterone must be present and bind to receptor cells in the penis both before and after birth for proper growth to occur during puberty. There are many receptors in the penis, so the amount of stunting will depend upon the levels of exposure and numbers of receptor sites that are blocked. In a worst case scenario, the penis fails to grow beyond its original size at infancy.[58,59] Estrogenized boys are also more likely to develop testicular cancer in early adulthood because of aberrant germ cells in the testes.[60]

Exposure to soy *in utero* may also put males at risk for later development of benign prostatic hypertrophy and prostate cancer. Prostate cells sensitized to estrogen during fetal development are more responsive to estrogens later in life and less responsive to the normal controlling mechanisms of prostatic growth.[61] Ironically, many spokesmen, including former junk bond salesman Michael Milken, are promoting soy as the all-natural way to prevent and reverse prostate disease and cancer.

SEX ON THE BRAIN

When male hormones needed to shape the reproductive system are scarce or absent, demasculinizing effects occur throughout the body. Environmental estrogens and phytoestrogens have been shown to alter the development of brain cells that control reproduction, sexual behavior and, possibly, sexual preference.[62,63]

Estrogenic disruption of embryonal programming is a likely reason that boys suffer from ADD/ADHD more often than girls.[64] Soy can also disrupt visual-spatial memory as shown in maze tests. Normally, males outperform female rats in this test, but those fed a phytoestrogen-rich soy diet lose their advantage. Females who stayed on the diet increased their visual-spatial memory and outperformed those switched to the soy-free diet. The opposite effect occured in males.[65]

During the past few years, researchers have coined the terms "Developmental Estrogenization Syndrome" and "Testicular Dysgenesis Syndrome" to describe the clusters of birth defects, the increased susceptibility to hormonal diseases and the altered behavioral patterns that occur in estrogenized boys.[66-68]

HYPOSPADIAS

Hypospadias is a disorder in which the meatus (the opening of the urethra) appears on the underside of the shaft of the penis. When this birth defect occurs, the opening can be anywhere from the tip to the scrotum or even the perineum, although it usually occurs an inch or so from the usual end site. In some cases, it appears so far back as to create doubt about the gender of the child. The condition can usually be repaired surgically so that it will not interfere with urination and sex.

Undescended testicles and inguinal hernia are the most common associated anomalies found in boys with hypospadias.[69,70]

Hypospadias is one of the most common congenital birth defects. It now occurs in one out of 125 live male births. Since the 1960s, seven European countries and the United States have published independent reports on increasing rates of hypospadias. Severe cases have seen the largest increase, so the phenomenon cannot be attributed to more sensitive reporting. This is not a worldwide trend, for hypospadias is rarely found in less affluent and less industrialized nations.[71-73]

Hypospadias results when hormonal disturbances result in incomplete virilization around the eighth week of gestation. Under normal conditions, fetal testosterone will be converted at that time to dihydrotestosterone (DHT) by the enzyme alpha reductase to initiate the simultaneous growth of the penis and the urethra. Agricultural and industrial chemicals can interfere with the masculinization of the external genitals and internal male gonads. However, not all endocrine disrupters are manmade. Naturally occurring phytoestrogens are present in foods, particularly soy foods and processed foods containing soy protein.[74-77]

Excess soyfoods in the pregnant mother's diet may contribute to the rising rates of hypospadias. In a longitudinal study of pregnancy and childhood, hypospadias was found in 51 out of 7,928 boys. Vegetarian mothers were five times more likely to give birth to a boy with hypospadias than a mother on an omnivorous diet. Lesser risk factors included taking iron supplements or catching the flu during the first trimester of pregnancy. There were no significant differences pertaining to maternal smoking, drinking, age or having twins. The researchers concluded: "It is important to note that there is biological evidence that vegetarians have a greater exposure to phytoestrogens and thus a causal link is biologically feasible. . . . As vegetarians have a greater exposure to phytoestrogens than do omnivores, these results support the possibility that phytoestrogens have a deleterious effect on the developing male reproductive system."[78] Soy is the likeliest culprit as no other commonly eaten food is high in phytoestrogens.[79]

Although this study falls far short of proving that soy in the diet is the culprit, the link is strong enough for several top urologists to call for further investigation.[80] A European Commission study of 3,000 babies is now underway to determine what might be causing the epidemic of hypospadias. The two main suspects are soy and pesticides. As Ieuan Hughes, M.D. of the Department of Pediatrics, Cambridge University, and chairman since 2002 of the British Committee on Toxicity of Chemicals in Food, Consumer Products and the Environment, puts it, "There is a clear association between child deformities and vegetarianism and this is a cause for concern."[81]

Another estrogenic substance linked to hypospadias is diethylstilbestrol (DES). Most laboratory studies have focused on its effects on the female offspring of mothers who took DES during pregnancy, but male rat pups exposed to DES on days 13 to 20 of gestation were born with hypospadias at all dose levels tested. Sons of DES daughters also have significantly increased risk of developing hypospadias, cryptorchidism and epidymal deformities compared to boys whose mothers were not exposed to DES prenatally.[82] As discussed in Chapter 28, DES is structurally similar to genistein and similar adverse effects have been reported in both animal and human studies.

BACK TO THE WOMB

Female genital development *in utero* is largely independent of hormone interaction. However, phytoestrogen exposure could program a girl for early breast development, precocious puberty and even estrogen-dependent diseases such as breast, ovarian or uterine cancers.[83-85]

The soy industry has responded with the suggestion that babies in the womb would only *benefit*. Coral A. Lamartiniere, Ph.D., of the University of Alabama, Birmingham, has proposed that the key to preventing breast cancer is giving shots of genistein to fetuses in the womb, thus preprograming girls so that they will have "reduced susceptibility to breast cancer" later in life.[86-89]

So far, Lamartiniere has experimented on rats, with results that have included "enhanced mammary gland maturation" and accelerated uterine weight gain—in other words, premature breast development and puberty. However, these early sprouting breasts have fewer terminal end buds and more lobules, changes that indicate greater differentiation and (possibly) decreased susceptibility to carcinogens. Because Lamartiniere found "no significant effect" on other reproductive markers, he reported that his breast-cancer prevention program did not "cause any significant toxicity." He concluded: "We hypothesize that the early genistein action promotes cell differentiation, resulting in a less active EGF signaling pathway in adulthood that, in turn, suppresses the development of mammary cancer. We speculate that breast cancer protection in Asian women consuming a traditional soy-containing diet is derived from early exposure to soybean products containing genistein. We believe that early events are essential for cancer-protection benefits."[90]

Lamartiniere's statement about "Asian women" is typical of the unreferenced claims made in the soy literature. Everyone, after all, "knows" that Asians practically mainline soy from the fetal period onward and that they have low rates of breast cancer because of it. Although the former statement is not true (see Chapter 3) and the latter statement is mostly speculation, most soy researchers introduce their claims of benefit with a statements like "Asian women and men who consume a traditional diet high in soy products . . . ." The fact that studies on soy and breast cancer have shown inconclusive and inconsistent results has greatly frustrated these researchers, many of whom stood up at the Fifth International Symposium on the Role of Soy in the Prevention and Reversal of Disease in Orlando, Florida in the fall of 2003 with the speculation that the problem is not soy itself but the fact that people aren't eating enough of it early enough. The solution offered by Lamartinere is to artificially "imprint" girls with the developmental "blueprint" of soy-eating Asian females. The proposed method? Administering shots of genistein at key developmental points from the fetal period to postpartum to prepuberty.

Other researchers see less cause for optimism—their work shows that perinatal genistein is an endocrine disrupter that contributes to or causes breast cancer.[91,92]

CROSSING THE PLACENTA

Many people question whether soy estrogens cross the placenta. The answer is yes.[93-95] The message published in the *Archives of Toxicology* is clear: "Since dietary phytoestrogens account for a significant proportion of human exposure to potential endocrine modulators and since the placenta does not represent a barrier to daidzein or related estrogenic isoflavones, the consequences of the exposures early in life should be examined and monitored carefully."

Claude Hughes,M.D., Ph.D., director of the Center for Women's Health at Cedars-Sinai Medical Center in Los Angeles agrees. He found that 30 percent of human fetuses are exposed to an anti-androgenic pesticide at concentrations of from one half to three times those of endogenous testosterone in males. However, 40 percent of human fetuses are exposed to estrogenic isoflavones at concentrations from 20 to 180 times that of estrogen produced by the mother.[96] His comment to the press? "If mom is eating something that can act like sex hormones, it is logical to wonder if that could change the baby's development."[97]

PULP FICTION

Soy oil and other vegetable oils contain plant estrogens known as phytosterols. The FDA allows the food industry to add plant-derived sterols to margarines, spreads, salad dressings, yogurts and orange juice and even make a health claim for their cholesterol-lowering benefits. However, the sterols in these foods do not normally come from soy but from wood pulp.

The most common sterols are beta-sitosterol, campesterol and stigmasterol. Drug companies used them in the 1960s to manufacture human sex hormones. Now these waste products are being singled out and sold for their supposed heart-protective benefits.

Like soy isoflavones—the phytoestrogens found in soy protein—sterols cause endocrine disruption throughout the body. They are structurally similar to the soy isoflavones genistein and daidzein as well as the synthetic estrogen diethylstilbestrol (DES). Accordingly, the Australia/New Zealand Food Authority (ANZFA)—though not our own FDA—requires that sterol-containing "functional foods" carry warning labels advising pregnant and lactating women, infants or children not to eat them.

By lowering cholesterol levels, sterols take away the

cholesterol the body needs to adequately synthesize hormones such as estrogen and testosterone. Sterols also resemble natural hormones closely enough to clog receptor sites needed by genuine hormones. This can result in birth defects, infertility, reproductive disorders, behavioral problems, greater risk of breast cancer and even atherosclerotic lesions. Fish swimming downstream in water polluted by the effluent from wood pulp plants have become "sex inverted," hermaphroditic and infertile. Sheep injected with sterols have shown ovarian and uterine damage.

Sterols can also cause a breakdown of the bone matrix, leading to a life-threatening condition called hypercalcemia, which is marked by a variety of physical and mental symptoms, including vomiting, diarrhea, abdominal pain, emotional instability, confusion, delirium, psychosis, stupor, muscle weakness, renal failure and cardiac arrythmias. Cytellin, a cholesterol-lowering drug made from sterols, was taken off the market because of some of those same side effects. Yet the food industry would like us to believe that sterols are natural and safe enough to add in highly unnatural amounts to processed food products.

SOURCE: James, Valerie. Toxins on your toast. www.westonaprice.org and www.soyonlineservice.co.nz/Phytosterols.htm. The article includes 23 references from medical, environmental and toxicology journals and official government documents.

MY SOY STORY: NO BASIS FOR SEED

I am a naturopath and a medical intuitive. I can virtually guarantee that men who have been eating quantities of soy will have a thyroid problem, no energy and very low libido. In a recent case a man declared quite proudly that he had been drinking soy milk for the previous seven years on a regular basis. He had come to see me because he and his wife had not been able to conceive. When intuitively checking out his reproductive area I found that there was no life there, no basis for any seed. The testes were as dead as a dodo.

J.C., Arlington, VA

MY SOY STORY: TWO MISCARRIAGES

I recently incorporated a protein shake into my diet, which contained soy protein isolate, soy lecithin and soybean oil. I thought I was being healthy. Almost immediately, my menses and ovulation started to change. I was ovulating a week to 10 days later than usual, but didn't think anything of it and became pregnant twice. I miscarried the first one 18 days post ovulation and the second at 20 days post ovulation. I have never had such irregularity in my cycles and have never before miscarried any pregnancy. I am not a vegetarian and eat wild game meat and vegetables from our organic garden so I knew I wasn't getting hormones from other foods. It had to be the soy.

L.M., Santa Rosa, CA

30

SOY AND CANCER
high hopes and hype

Soy protein and soy isoflavone supplements are being heavily promoted as "miracle cures" for cancer. With cancer rates at an all-time high and cancer the second leading cause of morbidity and mortality in the United States,[1] the idea that a simple food could save lives sounds like very good news indeed. Unfortunately, the truth is another soy story.

While a few studies suggest that soy protein—or its isoflavones—*might* help prevent cancer, far more studies show it to be ineffective or inconsistent. Some studies even show that soy can contribute to, promote or even cause cancer. Yet the soy industry persists in touting soy as the natural cancer answer.

In February 2004, the Solae Company submitted a petition to the FDA requesting permission for a cancer health claim for soy protein.[2] In a strategy reminiscent of Protein Technology International's establishment of the heart disease health claim in 1998 (see Chapter 13), Solae claimed that "there is scientific agreement among experts qualified by scientific training and experience to evaluate such claims regarding the relationship between soy protein products and a reduced risk of certain cancers." In fact, no such consensus exists, and numerous experts "qualified by scientific training and experience"— including scientists from the FDA's own National Laboratory for Toxicological Research—have warned of soy protein's carcinogenic potential and of the health dangers that ensue from excess soy-food consumption.[3]

The idea that scientists could even consider soy for a cancer health claim is ludicrous on the face of it. Soy isoflavones—the plant estrogens in soy most often credited with cancer prevention—are listed as "carcinogens" in many toxicology textbooks, including the American Chemical Society's 1976 *Chemical Carcinogens*. Over the

---

PRESTO CHANGO:
POISON TO PROFIT

Soy isoflavones are listed as "carcinogens" in the American Chemical Society's 1976 textbook *Chemical Carcinogens* as well as in other toxicology textbooks. Today they are credited with cancer prevention. How can this be? Patricia Murphy, Ph.D., of Iowa State University, explains: "It is true that isoflavones have been included as toxicants in publications prior to 1985. However, recently the health-protective effects of isoflavones and other constituents in soy have gained favor." Indeed, they have thanks to the work of industry-sponsored researchers such as Murphy herself, honored at the Fourth International Symposium on the Role of Soy in Preventing and Treating Chronic Disease in San Diego for her "outstanding contributions to increasing the understanding and awareness of the health effects of soyfoods and soybean constituents."

SOURCE: Murphy P. Rebuttal on isoflavones in soy-based infant formulas. *J Agri Food Chem*, 1998, 46, 3390-3399.

---

years, soy isoflavones have been proven to be mutagenic, clastogenic and teratogenic. In addition, the modern industrial soy processing techniques used to make soy protein isolate, textured vegetable protein and other modern soy products create toxic and carcinogenic residues (see Chapters 11 and 22-23). Finally, soybeans naturally contain goitrogens, allergens, protease inhibitors and other antinutrients and toxins that damage the digestive, immune and neuroendocrine systems, putting consumers at increased risk for many health problems, including cancer (see Chapters 16-20, 24-25 and 27).

Despite these well-known hazards, the soy industry makes the improbable claim that soybeans are the key to cancer prevention and reversal. After all, Asians eat a lot of soy and suffer less from cancer. Or so we are led to believe.

GEOGRAPHY LESSON

The death rate from breast cancer is four times lower and from prostate cancer eighteen times lower in China than in the United States.[4] Soy proponents often cite these and similarly favorable statistics on breast, prostate and colon cancers as good reasons to eat a lot of soy protein. But if decreased rates of breast and prostate colon cancer in Asia are to be attributed to soy consumption, then the same logic requires that soy take the blame for the higher rates of cancers of the esophagus, stomach, thyroid, pancreas and liver found in the countries of Asia.[5]

Not surprisingly, we hear only the good news. While soybeans in the diet *might* be a factor in either reduced or increased incidences of cancer in Asia, there is no direct evidence of cause and effect. Several dietary and lifestyle factors are undoubtedly involved. Epidemiological studies of prostate cancer, for example, have not only associated reduced cancer incidence with soy but also with rice, vegetables, fruits, nuts, grains, green tea, fish, other legumes and/or combinations of foods. None of the research supports crediting soy alone.[6-10] As Herman Adlercreutz, M.D., of the University of Helsinki, Finland, observed, "Whether these observed protective effects are caused by the presence of dietary phyto-oestrogens, or whether they are merely indicators of a healthy diet in general, has not been established."[11]

ESTROGEN AND ANTI-ESTROGENS

Those who look at the many laboratory studies on soy and cancer can only note that the results are contradictory—in some studies soy seems to prevent cancer, in some to cause it and in some to have no effect. Like most hormonally active agents, soy isoflavones can act as either estrogens or anti-estrogens, either stimulating or inhibiting cell growth. Although soy proponents often laud the ability of soy estrogens to act *against* human estrogens, soy estrogens are as likely to act *with* them. The former might decrease cancer, the latter increases the risk. Thus increasing soy food consumption for cancer prevention is unreliable, unpredictable and risky.

Kenneth D. R. Setchell, Ph.D., warned of the potential harm back in 1984 when he wrote: "Estrogens exert dose dependent dual effects upon tumour induction and growth. High doses inhibit tumour development and suppress growth while physiological doses stimulate growth of human tumour cells."[12] This warning has proven true in a number of recent studies.

In 1997 researchers from the University of Minnesota at St. Paul found that phytoestrogens inhibited breast cancer cells at high concentrations but stimulated growth at low concentrations. They concluded: "The current focus on the role of phytoestrogens in cancer prevention must take into account biphasic effects observed in this study, showing inhibition of DNA synthesis at high concentrations but induction at concentrations close to probable levels in human diets."[13]

In 2001, the British Columbia Cancer Agency in Vancouver reported that genistein and daidzein at high concentrations inhibited tumor growth and enhanced the effect of Tamoxifen *in vitro* (in laboratory cell lines or test tubes). However, at dietary levels soy stimulated existing breast tumor growth and antagonized the effect of

Tamoxifen both *in vivo* (in living organisms) and *in vitro*. Accordingly, the agency warned that "women with current or past cancer should be aware of the risks of potential tumor growth when taking soy products."[14]

Likewise, Craig Dees, Ph.D., of the Oak Ridge National Laboratory in Tennessee came to the conclusion that "dietary estrogens at low concentrations do not act as anti-estrogens, but act like DDT and estradiol to stimulate breast cancer cells to enter the cell cycle."[15]

These findings suggest that high concentrations of soy isoflavones might prove useful as a potent drug, but do not portend well for those who eat soy foods to prevent or treat cancer.

GOOD NEWS, BAD NEWS

"Soy prevents stomach cancer and heart disease" was the proclamation heard 'round the world in 2000 when Japanese researchers provided "modest support for the preventive role of soy." Modest isn't much, but then, every little bit helps in the fight against cancer and heart disease.

Indeed, the study does provide "modest support." What the conclusion omits is the fact that soy might possibly provide some protection from stomach cancer—but only if you happen to be male; and that soy might possibly provide some protection from heart disease—but only if you are female! Conspicuously missing from the researchers' well-publicized conclusion was the fact that they found "significant positive correlations" between higher rates of colorectal cancer mortality and soy product intake. In other words the soy that will save you from stomach cancer could kill you with colon cancer! Call it a "killer cure!"

SOURCE: Nagata C. Ecological study of the association between soy product intake and mortality from cancer and heart disease in Japan. *International Epidemiological Association*, 2000. 29, 832-836.

BREAST CANCER

Women eating soy to prevent breast cancer risk developing the very disease they are trying to prevent. Although some *in vitro* studies show that isoflavones inhibit the proliferation of breast cancer cells,[16-18] there are plenty of contradictory findings. *In vitro* studies dating back to the 1970s show that soy causes the proliferation of breast cancer cells.[19-21]

In animal models, soy protein and miso have reduced the incidence and size of radiation-induced and chemically-induced breast tumors in rats.[22-24] But other studies have shown no effect.[25-27] Both soy protein isolate and whey have protected rats from chemically-induced breast tumors, but whey-fed rats enjoy protection in the first generation while soy-fed rats enjoy protection in the following generations.[28] Solae recently cited this study as evidence of soy's protective effect but failed to mention that the rats fed soy protein experienced a "one-day advance in vaginal opening."[29] This is evidence of premature sexual maturation and suggests that high soy intake in the human diet could put young girls at risk for precocious puberty, itself a well-known risk factor for breast cancer (see Chapter 28).

Warning bells also sounded with a series of rodent studies led by William Helferich, M.D., at the University of Illinois at Urbana-Champaign.[30-34] The researchers tested soy protein isolate-based feeds—containing increasingly high concentrations of the soy isoflavone genistein—and discovered that the more isoflavones the mice ate, the higher the incidence of breast cell proliferation and cancer growth. The researchers also found that tumors regressed when the mice were switched back to an isoflavone-free diet. Dietary genistein notably stimulated the growth of mammary tumors in a low-estrogen hormonal environment similar to that found in menopausal women. Dietary genistein also negated the effects of the drug Tamoxifen, suggesting that women undergoing cancer treatment should avoid soy foods.

In the most recent of the studies, Dr. Helferich announced that soy products (such as NovaSoy) that contain isoflavones in purified forms provoked far greater tumor growth than minimally processed products such as soy flour. The takeaway from all five studies? Dr. Helferich is clear: "Our preclinical laboratory animal data suggest that caution is warranted regarding the use of soy supplements high in isoflavones for women with breast cancer, particularly if they are menopausal."[35]

In humans, results have been equally sobering. Phytoestrogens in the diet have proved to be estrogenic stimuli[36] or caused the proliferation of breast cells.[37] Researchers at the University of California at San Francisco who hoped to find that soy foods had a protective effect against premenopausal breast cancer found instead that six months' consumption of soy protein containing the isoflavones genistein and daidzein had a "stimulatory effect on the premenopausal female breast, characterized by increased secretion of breast fluid, the appearance of hyperplastic epithelial cells and elevated levels of plasma estradiol."[38] Breast cancer risk is higher for women with abnormal cells in their breast fluid.[39]

Soy protein has caused the proliferation of breast cancer cells in laboratory, animal and human studies, linking soy consumption to increased breast-cancer risk, especially for those already afflicted with the disease. The latter group includes not only women who have already been diagnosed with breast cancer, but those in the early stages prior to diagnosis. Postmenopausal women may be at even greater risk. Barry Golden, Ph.D., of Tufts University warns that high soy consumption might increase the estrogenic activity in cells by as much as 25 to 30 percent in women who have gone through menopause and so have low levels of natural estrogen. Golden believes that premenopausal women are less at risk because their own estrogens "overpower" the plant estrogens from soy, but he warns that soy might pose "an added potential risk" for women who either have breast cancer or are at risk for the disease.[40]

Proponents of soy foods often claim that soy foods provide protection against the growing numbers of carcinogens in the environment. But a study of 34,759 women in Hiroshima and Nagasaki,

Japan, found no significant association between breast cancer risk and consumption of soy foods.[41] In their petition, the Solae Company dismisses this study as irrelevant because it was carried out in cities where women were exposed to high levels of ionizing radiation after the atomic bomb,[42] but the fact that women consuming high levels of soy protein did not enjoy special protection is very significant.

Meanwhile, Dutch researchers from the University Medical Center in Utrecht reported on 15,555 women aged 49 to 70 years who were studied from 1993-1997. The news was not good for the soy industry. After analyzing data on isoflavone and lignan intake, and adjusting for known breast cancer risk factors and other variables, the team found no significant trends between breast cancer risk and dietary phytoestrogens.[43,44] This spurred Regina G. Ziegler, Ph.D., a nutritional epidemiologist at the National Cancer Institute in Bethesda, MD, to speak out against the soyfood fad. Summarizing the soy and breast cancer research to date, she warned that it was "complicated, inconsistent and inconclusive" and concluded that when patients ask whether they should eat more soy foods, "I think we have to be cautious."[45-46]

PROSTATE CANCER

Despite the endorsement of junk bond dealer and prostate cancer survivor Michael Milken, soy does not emerge as the best option for prevention or treatment of prostate cancer. While it is true that a few laboratory and human studies have suggested that soy protein—or its estrogens—might reduce the incidence of prostate cancer, far more studies show no effect. And many studies link soy consumption to *increased* prostate cancer risk.

Epidemiological studies indeed show lower rates of prostate cancer in Asia but provide little or no proof that soy consumption should take the credit. A 1979 Japanese study of 122,261 men over the age of 40 revealed that green and yellow vegetables appeared protective and that soy miso—a food category that would have included cheap, fast-fermented misos that became popular after World War II—significantly increased the risk.[47] Over the years researchers have concluded that anything and everything—from dietary choices such as green tea, rice, nuts and fish to lifestyle factors such as monogamy, fidelity and poverty—could be responsible for lower rates of prostate cancer.[48-53]

Most of the studies suggesting that soy could protect men from prostate cancer are *in vitro* studies using genistein and other isoflavones [54-59] or animal studies using genistein injections of high level isoflavone concentrates.[60-62] The results of these studies cannot be interpreted to mean that men should eat more soy. Rather they suggest that researchers might develop useful and profitable drugs derived from soy.

Animal studies using soy foods with isoflavones are at best inconclusive. Soy flour inhibited the development of transplanted prostate tumors in rats.[63] But rye bran beat soy protein in a mouse study.[64] Both soy protein isolate (SPI) and conjugated linoleic acid (CLA), a substance found in butter, have been associated with reduced risk of prostate cancer, but researchers found that neither of them, singly or in combination, inhibited prostate cancer growth. Moreover, at the highest concentrations of SPI, there was a significant increase in tumor size. The researchers concluded, "These results, in an established rat model, suggest caution in using isoflavone-rich SPI in human studies involving advanced hormone-refractory prostate cancer until further investigation of these effects are completed."[65]

One study presented to the FDA as proof that soy reduces prostate cancer incidence concludes with a most revealing statement: "Dietary soymeal found in most natural ingredient diets may promote PC (prostate cancer) tumorigenesis but only in L-W rats." Researchers use L-W (Lobund-Wistar) rats because they were bred to exhibit a unique model of spontaneous prostate cancer that "shares many of its characteristics with the natural history of PC in man, including (a) inherent predisposition, high production of testosterone and aging risk factors, (b) endogenous tumorigenic mechanisms, and (c) early state testosterone-dependent and late stage testosterone-independent tumors."[66,67]

In the human animal, soy either failed to improve PSA or actually increased levels in middle-aged and elderly men.[68-70] PSA (prostate specific antigen) is a marker of prostate tumor growth. However, a few human studies suggest that if soy, in fact, can reduce rates of prostate cancer it does so only for those who produce equol.[71-72] Equol is a metabolite of the soy isoflavone daidzein that some people produce in the intestines (see Chapter 26). If so, only some males can benefit from soy protein consumption. Furthermore, green tea drinking might be needed to improve the capacity for equol production.[73]

Soy proponents rarely tell men that the reason why soy might protect them against prostate cancer is because it has a feminizing effect. Levels of soy that might be useful in prostate cancer prevention or treatment will significantly decrease testosterone and androgen and increase estrogen.[74-77] Doctors believe that prostate cancer depends on exposure to male reproductive hormones and thus recommend soy because its estrogens perturb natural hormone concentrations and ratios. While this theory might lead to valid pharmaceutical applications in cancer treatment, it seems inadvisable as a preventative treatment for the entire male population.

Men who have been urged to consume soy to prevent or reverse prostate cancer might also consider the warnings of Daniel Doerge, Ph.D., and Hebron C. Chang, Ph.D., of the FDA's National Laboratory for Toxicological Research, who discovered that "genistein interferes with estrogen receptors in rat prostate glands" and warned that this finding might "have implications for reproductive toxicity and carcinogenesis."[78]

Brain damage is yet another possibility. Soy isoflavones decreased both brain and prostate weights of rats and also altered the structure of the sexually dimorphic brain region.[79] The sexual dimorphic nucleus is located in the diencephalons at the base of the hypothalamus and is sensitive to estrogen and testosterone in gender-specific ways, that is, differently for males and females.

Finally, researchers who tested a low-fat, high-soy diet on prostate cancer patients found an insignificant decline in PSA levels, a modest effect on time to progression (TTP, another prostate cancer marker) and an undesirable increase in IGF-1 serum levels.[80] IGF-1 stands for Insulin-like Growth Factor. Circulating IGF-1 concentrations increase the risk of prostate, bladder, colorectal and breast cancer and have been implicated in heart disease, Type 2 diabetes and osteoporosis. Research indicates that soy increases IGF-1 levels only in men.[81]

GASTROINTESTINAL CANCERS

The soy industry tells us that soy has a long track record in the prevention and treatment of gastrointestinal cancers.[82] Yet the most notable study to come along in recent years reveals that soy protein is associated with a lowered risk of stomach cancer but a higher risk of death from colorectal cancer.[83]

Most epidemiological studies, whether carried out in Asia or elsewhere, show little or no association. The most promising foods for cancer protection appear to be green and yellow vegetables and those from the allium family, such as garlic and onions. Tomatoes, snap beans, tea, eggplant, celery, fish, poultry, milk and various other foods have variously been found protective. Soy does not stand alone as a potential dietary savior.

These studies provide excellent support for the FDA's promotion of fruits and vegetables as a way to prevent cancer, but fail to support the Solae Company's petition for a health claim for soy protein. The foods most often linked to cancers of the stomach and colon are pickled, smoked and fried foods, processed meats, vegetable cooking oils, high-salt dishes and fermented beans, particularly soy miso. Noodles, bread and other starchy carbohydrates, alcohol, smoking, "speed eating" and binge eating have also been implicated.[84-93]

The fact that miso and other fermented soybean products are

linked to gastrointestinal cancers [94-96] is not surprising given the fact that many people in Japan and Korea do not eat the old-fashioned, slow-fermented products but modern commercial versions manufactured using hydrolyzation and other fast-fermenting processes that leave toxic residues and carcinogens. These products may also contain additives such as caramel, sugar and MSG. The studies do not distinguish between the various processing methods for miso.

Animal studies also send conflicting messages. While a few studies suggest that dietary genistein can protect against chemically induced pre-cancerous lesions,[97,98] others show no protection.[99,100] Still other studies suggest that soy can *cause* pre-cancerous lesions. Certainly soybeans have the potential to induce epithelial cell damage and proliferation, markers of colon cancer risk.[101-103] Finally, soy is highly unlikely to be protective against colon cancer because it is seriously low in the amino acid methionine (see Chapter 13). Methionine has been shown to prevent colon cancer.[104,105]

A few *in vitro* studies suggest that high levels of genistein can interfere with cell cycle processes to inhibit the growth of human colon cancer cells.[106-108] Once again, these findings do not mean that we should all eat more soybeans but rather indicate that isoflavones might have promise as a pharmaceutical drug. Indeed, in one case study, a 66-year-old man who took 160 mg of phytoestrogens daily for one week before a radical prostatectomy showed benefit from cancer cell death and tumor regression.[109] This short-term course of genistein drug therapy gave him soy's benefits without much risk.

OTHER CANCERS

So little proof exists that soy protein prevents or reverses other forms of cancer that the Solae Company did not even attempt to claim benefits against lung, thyroid, pancreatic, ovarian, bladder or other cancers when it petitioned the FDA for a qualified health claim.[110]

In fact, many studies show adverse effects. Recently, findings from the Singapore Chinese Health Study sent shock waves through the industry: soy was associated with a two- to three-fold increase in bladder cancer risk. A follow-up study strengthened the connection. No other food in the diet was associated with the increase, just soy.[111,112]

Soy can almost certainly be blamed for at least some of the increase in thyroid cancers in that soy isoflavones induce both goiters and thyroid tumors (see Chapter 27). As for the rising rate of pancreatic cancer, scientists have known for half a century that trypsin inhibitors in soy protein put stress on the pancreas, contributing to and possibly causing pancreatic cancer (see Chapter 16).

Recently, four alarming studies linked soy estrogens to infant leukemia.[113-116]

The immune system—which plays a critical role in cancer prevention and effective treatment—has also proved vulnerable to the soy assault. [117,118]

Finally, soy isoflavones are clastogenic and mutagenic. This means that they cause chromosomal breaks and genetic aberrations, the precursors to cancer.[119-125]

IRRESPONSIBLE

Cancer is not a single disease but a group of different diseases that develop over the course of many years in a multistage process involving both initiation and promotion. Biochemical individuality, diet, lifestyle, environmental and other factors all play roles in any individual's vulnerability to the disease. Consequently, as Mike Fitzpatrick, Ph.D., put it, "There can be no blanket approach to cancer prevention and an agent that may reduce the risk of cancer in one person may increase the risk of cancer in another. It is completely irresponsible for the soy industry or isoflavone supplement manufacturers to promote (or even suggest) that their products are cancer preventing without any reference to individual case history, any real idea of what constitutes a safe dose, or any mention of the fact that soy may increase the risk of cancer. Those soy food or isoflavone manufacturers that proclaim the anti-cancer properties of their products are guilty of giving false hope to millions; but worse, they may be placing consumers at greater risk of contracting the same horrendous diseases they are trying to avoid."[126]

HEALTH CLAIM MUDDLE

In February 2004 the Solae Company, a manufacturer of processed soy products, filed a petition with FDA for a soy protein and cancer health claim. Approval of the claim would result in additional billions of dollars in profits to the industry and the harm of countless American citizens. Although the FDA was expected to make its ruling in November 2004, the agency extended the deadline by 90 days in order to consider a soy industry rebuttal of the 50-page protest filed by the Weston A. Price Foundation.

Solae actually has conceded that its original qualified health claim was not warranted and proposed new, more ambiguous language including "New scientific research suggests, but does not prove, that soy protein may reduce the risk of certain cancers" and "Soy protein may reduce the risk of certain cancers. The scientific evidence is promising but not conclusive."

Clearly Solae hopes that an unproven claim—boldly stated—will have the desired effect of encouraging Americans to eat more of its soy protein products. In its petition to the FDA, Solae estimated that winning the health claim would double soy protein sales with the average consumer increasing his or her soy consumption to 4.49 grams per day. Solae noted that the soy protein/heart disease health claim of 1998 doubled the average consumption of soy protein from 0.78 to 2.23 grams per day. These are average figures; many people consume amounts well in excess of the average. Many people who would not otherwise choose soy would consciously add more soy foods carrying a cancer health claim to their diets.

The cancer health claim would run on packages with no consumer warning. It would promote an indiscriminate increase in consumption of soy protein for men, women and children with no admission of the fact that a substance that might possibly be helpful in one stage of the life cycle could be harmful in another. And consumers would receive no warning about the fact that the isoflavones in soy protein exert their influence throughout the body in many different ways and have shown the potential to contribute to and even cause cancer.

Finally, people would not be warned that increased levels of soy estrogens in the diet have a cumulative or exponential effect when combined with other environmental estrogens. Toxicologists at the Centre for Toxicology, the School of Pharmacology at the University of London, have stated that "estrogenic agents are able to act together to produce significant effects when combined at concentrations below levels that would be toxic separately."

If Solae's petition is defeated—as it ought to be—consumers will still lack a warning label. But it would be good news indeed if the FDA would choose not to purposely mislead Americans with the false claim that soy prevents cancer.[127-131]

A CANCER

The story of soy sheds light on the dirty little secrets of the modern food processing industry, the power of public relations, the corruption of scientific inquiry and the collusion of FDA and other government agencies that are mandated to protect us.

In the first half of the 20th century, John Harvey Kellogg, Henry Ford and others envisioned a grand future for soy. By the 1960s, vegetarians, hippies, environmentalists and other idealists joined the cry, recommending soy foods as the solution to world hunger, the path to good health, the key to healthy aging and the way to preserve our environment.

Sadly, big business and big government have usurped their impossible dream. Old-fashioned whole soy foods that contribute to health if eaten in moderation have given way to ersatz products that lead inevitably to malnutrition and disease. Gigantic corporate farms and billion dollar soybean-crushing and food processing plants have driven out small farmers and cottage industries. The result worldwide is an epidemic of disease in humans and other life forms mirrored by a malignant increase in pollution and overall damage to the planet—a kind of cancer on the body of Mother Earth.

What will the coming years bring? More false claims for soy protein—and new claims for soy oil—as the healer of everything from cancer to ingrown toenails? Or a genuine, consumer-driven, grassroots movement demanding honesty, integrity, common sense and "real food?" The challenge and choice is ours.

END NOTES

Chapter One: Soy in the East

1. Liu, KeSun. *Soybeans: Chemistry, Technology and Utilization* (Gaithersburg, MD, Aspen) xvii.
2. Katz, Solomon H. Food and biocultural evolution: a model for the investigation of modern nutritional problems. In *Nutritional Anthropology*, Francis E. Johnston ed. (NY, Alan R. Liss, 1987) 50.
3. Katz.
4. Liu, 1, 9-10.
5. Liu, 218.
6. Shurtleff, William, Aoyagi, Akiko. *The Book of Miso: Food for Mankind* (New York, NY, Ballantine, 1976) 488.
7. Katz.
8. Shurtleff, William. Aoyagi, Akiko. *The Book of Miso: Savory Soy Seasoning* (Berkeley, CA, Ten Speed Press, 2001) 215-216.
9. Shurtleff, Aoyagi. *The Book of Miso: Food for Mankind*, 488.
10. Shurtleff, Aoyagi. 507-511.
11. Shurtleff, William. Aoyagi, Akiko. *The Book of Tofu* (NY, Ballantine, 1979) 72.
12. Shurtleff, William. Aoyagi, Akiko. *The Book of Tempeh* (Berkeley, CA, Ten Speed Press, 2001) 145.
13. Shurtleff, Aoyagi. *The Book of Miso: Food for Mankind*, 490.
14. Shurtleff, Aoyagi. 494.
15. Shurtleff, Aoyagi. *The Book of Miso: Food for Mankind, 493.*
16. Shurtleff, Aoyagi. *The Book of Miso: Savory Soy Seasoning*, 218.
17. Shurtleff, Aoyagi. 220-221.
18. Shurtleff, Aoyagi. *The Book of Miso: Food for Mankind*, 503-505.
19. Shurtleff, Aoyagi. *The Book of Tofu*, 115.
20. Shurtleff, Aoyagi, 61, 113.
21. Liu, 166.
22. Fallon, Sally. Enig. Mary G. Tragedy and Hype: The Third International Soy Symposium. *Nexus*, April-May 2000, 21.
23. Shurtleff, Aoyagi. 113-114.
24. Fallon, Sally. Enig, Mary. Human Diet Series: China. *Price-Pottenger Nutrition Foundation Health Journal*, Fall 1997.
25. Simoons, Frederick J. *Food in China: A Cultural and Historical Inquiry.* (Boca Raton, FL, CRC Press, 1991) 87.
26. Liu, 166
27. Shurtleff, Aoyagi. 114-115.
28. Shurtleff, Aoyagi. *The Book of Tempeh*, 145-148.
29. Shurtleff, Aoygai. *The Book of Tofu*, 63, 73-75.
30. Shurtleff, William and Aoyagi, Akiko. History of Soybean Crushing: Soy Oil and Soybean Meal. In *History of Soybeans and Soyfoods: Past, Present and Future* (Lafayette, CA. Soyfoods Center), unpublished manuscript, 27.
31. Shurtleff, Aoyagi, 27-28.
32. Shurtleff, Aoyagi. 27.
33. Robbins, John. Letter to Peggy O'Mara, Editor, *Mothering* magazine, April 30, 2004.
34. Willcox, Bradley. Willcox, D. Craig, Suzuki, Makoto. *The Okinawa Program: How the World's Longest-Lived People Achieve Everlasting Health – And How You Can Too* (Clarkson-Potter, 2001).
35. Willcox, Bradley. Willcox, D. Craig, Suzuki, Makoto. *The Okinawa Diet Plan: Get Leaner, Live Longer and Never Feel Hungry* (Clarkson-Potter, 2003).
36. Suzuki M, Willcox BJ, Willcox CD. Implications from and for food cultures for cardiovascular disease and longevity. *Asia Pac J Clin Nutr*, 2001, 10, 2, 165-171.
37. Taira, Kazuhiko. In Franklyn, Deborah. Take a Lesson from the People of Okinawa, *Health*, September 1996, 57-63.
38. Akisaka M, Suzuki M. Okinawa Longevity Study. Molecular Genetic Analysis of HLSA Genes in the Very Old. *Nippon Ronen Igakkai Zasshi*, 1998, 35, 4, 294-298.

end notes - 2, 3

Chapter 2: Soy Goes West

1. Kahn EJ Jr. Staffs of life V: The future of the planet. *The New Yorker*, 1985. 56, 61, 65.
2. Dies, Edward J. *Soybeans: Gold from the Soil* (NY, Macmillan, 1942). Summarized by William Shurtleff in *USDA-ARS National Center for Agricultural Utilization Research, Peoria Illinois* (Lafayette, CA, Soyfoods Center). Entry #155
3. Shurtleff, William. Aoyagi, Akiko. *The Book of Tofu* (NY Ballantine, 1979). 63-66.
4. Shurtleff, William. Aoyagi, Akiko. *The Book of Miso: Savory Soy Seasoning* (Berkeley, CA, Ten Speed, 2001). 231-234.
5. Swingle Walter T. Our agricultural debt to Asia. Arthur E. Christy, ed. *The Asian Legacy and American Life* (NY John Day, 1945) Summarized by William Shurtleff in *USDA-ARS National Center for Agricultural Utilization Research, Peoria Illinois* (Lafayette, CA, Soyfoods Center). Entry #167.
6. Shurtleff, William. *USDA-ARS National Center for Agricultural Utilization Research, Peoria Illinois* (Lafayette, CA, Soyfoods Center). Entries # 121-133,136
7. Shurtleff, William. Aoyagi, Akiko. *Bibliography and Sourcebook on Seventh-Day Adventists, 1866-1992* (Lafayette, CA, Soyfoods Center). Numerous entries.
8. Horvath AA. Soya flour as a national food. *Scientific Monthly*, 1930, 33, 251-260. Quoted in Messina, Mark. Messina, Virginia. Setchell, Kenneth DR. *The Simple Soybean and Your Health* (Jersey City Park, NY, Avery, 1994) 38.
9. Shurtleff, William. *USDA-ARS National Center for Agricultural Utilization Research, Peoria.* Entries # 71, 111, 117.
10. Lewis, David L. *The Public Image of Henry Ford: An American Folk Hero and His Company* (Detroit, Wayne State University Press, 1987) 282-283.
11. Lewis, 284.
12. Bryan, Ford R. Robert Allen Boyer (1909-1989), Unpublished manuscript. Summarized by Shurtleff and Aoyagi in *Bibliography and Sourcebook on Seventh Day Adventists.* Entry #1573.
13. Lewis, 285.
14. Erickson, David R. *Practical Handbook of Soybean Processing and Utilization* (Champaign, IL. AOCS Press, 1995) 392.
15. Kahn, 68.
16. Lewis, 285.
17. Lewis, 291
18. Shurtleff, William. The history of soybean margarine. In *History of Soybeans and Soyfoods: Past, Present and Future* (Lafayette, CA. Soyfoods Center, 1983) 15.
19. Horvath AA. Soya flour as a national food. *Scientific Monthly*, 1931, 33, 252-260. Summarized by William Shurtleff and available through Soyfoods Center, Lafayette, CA.
20. Soya Flour, *Food Manufacture* (London), 1929, 4, 35-36. Reprinted in *Publications on Berczeller's Soy Flour*, Volume III, 1930. L. Berczeller, ed. Summarized by William Shurtleff in Entry #2 of a SoyaScan data base search of Mussolini (Lafayette, CA. Soyfoods Center).
21. Oldfield, Josiah. Eating for victory. *B Med J*, 1940, I (4145), 994-995. Summarized by William Shurtleff in Entry #4 of a SoyaScan data base search of Mussolini (Lafayette, CA. Soyfoods Center).
22. Food and the war. The soybean has come to have a prominent place in the military dietetics of Germany. *Good Health* (Battle Creek, MI) 1940, 75, 9, 125. Summarized by William Shurtleff as Entry #5 of a SoyaScan data base search of Mussolini.
23. Horvath AA. The soy bean as human food. *Industrial and Engineering Chemistry*, News Edition, May 10, 1931, 9, 9, 136. Summarized by William Shurtleff in *USDA-ARS National Center for Agricultural Utilization Research, Peoria Illinois* (Lafayette, CA, Soyfoods Center). Entry #106.
24. Peterson, Franklynn. The bean that's making meat obsolete. *Popular Mechanics*, October 1974, 142, 84-87.
25. Shurtleff, William. Soyfoods in Cuba. http://www.thesoydailyclub/com/Food/soyfoodsinccuba05272004.asp.
26. Shurtleff, Aoyagi. *Book of Tofu*, 66.
27. Kahn, 75.
28. Shurtleff, William. USDA-ARS National Center for Agricultural Utilization Research, Peoria, IL. (Lafayette, CA. Soyfoods Center), Entries #66-69.
29. Papanikolaw, Jim. Soybean oil demand can grow with new industrial uses. *Chemical Market Reporter*, 1999, 256, 15, 9.
30. Insta-Pro extruder provides a money saving solution. *Soya Bluebook* Update, April-June 1996.
31. Author's telephone interview with Nabil Said, November 5, 2002.
32. Rampton, Sheldon. Stauber, John. *Mad Cow U.S.A.* (Monroe, ME, Common Courage Press, 2004).61-72.

Chapter 3: The Ploy of Soy

1. Kilman, Scott. Cooper, Helene. Crop Blight: Monsanto falls flat trying to sell Europe on bioengineered food. Its soybeans are safe, say trade officials, but public doesn't want to hear about it. *Wall Street Journal*, May 11, 1999. A1, A10.
2. Lagnado, Lucette. Group sows seeds of revolt against genetically altered foods in U.S. *Wall Street Journal*, October 12, 1999. B1.
3. Hart, Kathleen. *Eating in the Dark* (NY Pantheon, 2002).
4. Lambrecht, Bill. *Dinner at the New Gene Café: How Genetic Engineering Is Changing What We Eat, How We Live, and the Global Politics of Food.* (Thomas Dunne Books, 2001).

5. Fallon, Sally. Enig, Mary G. A reply to Mr. Peary's defense of soybeans. *Health Freedom News*, February 1996.
6. Rohter, Larry. Relentless foe of the Amazon jungle: soybeans. *New York Times,* September 17, 2003.
7. Golbitz, Peter. Soyfoods consumption in the United States and worldwide, a statistical analysis. www.soyatech.com.
8. Organisation for Economic Co-operation and Development. *Food Consumption Statistics.* (Paris, OECD Publications, 1991).
9. Chen J. Campbell TC et al. *Diet, Lifestyle and Mortality in China: A Study of the Characteristics of 65 Counties* (Oxford University Press, Cornell University Press, China People's Medical Publishing House, 1990).
10. Messina, Mark. Letter to Peggy O'Mara, Editor, *Mothering* magazine, May 5, 2004.
11. Japanese soyfoods: Will western foods change eastern tastes? www.soyatech.com. Posted 10/8/2002.
12. DuPont begins third soy protein joint venture in China. SinoCast China Business NEWS VIA NewsEdge Corporation. www.soyatech.com. Posted 10/21/2002.
13. Prospectus 2004 Soyfoods: US Soyfoods Market Report. www.soyatech.com.
14. Golbitz, Peter. Demand, availability drive new growth in soyfoods market. *The Soy Connection,* Spring 2002.
15. Golbitz, Peter. Soyfood sales up 21% in 2000, will grow 15-25% in 2001, says new report. Posted 10/16/2001. www.soyatech.com
16. Coleman, Richard J. Vegetable protein – a delayed birth? *J Amer Oil Chem Soc*, 1975, 52, 238A. Quoted by Fallon, Sally. Enig, Mary G. Tragedy and Hype – The Third International Soy Symposium. *Nexus*, April-May 2000. 18. www.westonaprice.org
17. Gilbert, Linda, President of HealthFocus, the publisher of *Soyfoods Shoppers 2001: Who They Are, Why They Buy.* Quoted in Golbitz, Peter. Study focuses on who consumes soy. www.soyatech.com.
18. Fass, Philip. Mount, Mary Jane. Increasing consumer awareness of soy. *Soyfoods 2001: New Technology Innovations and Effective Marketing Tactics,* January 17-19, 2001. Hyatt Regency, Phoenix, AZ.
19. April 2003 SoySource, United Soybean Board. www.thesoydailyclub.com.
20. Osborn & Barr Communications Press Release. Soybean Checkoff Program yields additional research money to examine soy health benefits. www.unitedsoybean.org/news/20030930.htm.
21. Wansink, Brian. Hasler, Clare et al. How consumers interpret two-sided health claims. www.soyfoodsillinois.uiuc.edu.
22. Sansoni, Brian. Quoted in Henkel, John. Soy: Health claims for soy protein, questions about other components. *FDA Consumer Magazine,* May-June 2000.

Chapter 4: Green Peas, Yellow Beans and Black Eyes

1. Liu, KeShun. *Soybeans: Chemistry, Technology*, Utilization (Gaithersburg, MD, Aspen, 1999). 1-24.
2. Liu, 20.
3. Liu, 10, 20-22.
4. Health drives Cargill "ramp up" for soybean oil. www.novisgroup.com. 8/23/04.
5. World soybean: production and area harvested 1999-2005, Soya Blue Book. www.soyatech.com.
6. Woerfel, John B. Harvest, storage, handling and trading of soybeans. In *Practical Handbook of Soybean Processing and Utilization.* David R. Erickson, ed. (Champaign, IL, AOCS Press, 1995). 39-55.
7. Genetically modified crops in the United States. Pew Initiatives on Food and Technology Fact Sheet. http://pewagbiotech.org.
8. Kilman, Scott. Cooper, Helene. Crop blight: Monsanto falls flat trying to sell Europe on bioengineered foods – its soybeans are safe, say trade officials, but public doesn't want to hear it – mad cow and Englishmen. *Wall Street Journal,* May 11, 1999. A1, A10.
9. Monsanto genetically engineered soya has elevated hormone levels: public health threat. International scientists appeal to governments world wide. Press Release. Third Meeting of the Open-ended Ad hoc Working Group on Biosafety of the UN-Convention on Biological Diversity. Montreal, October 13, 1997.
10. Kawata, Masaharu. Monsanto's dangerous logic as seen in the application documents submitted to the Health Ministry of Japan. Third World Biosafety Information Service, July 28, 2003. www.organicconsumers.org.
11. Hart, Kathleen. *Eating in the Dark: America's Experiment with Genetically Engineered Foods* (NY Pantheon, 2002).
12. Liu, KeShun. *Soybeans: Chemistry, Technology and Utilization* (Gathersberg, MD Aspen, 1999). 203-205.
13. Shurtleff, William. SoyaScan Notes. Chronology of soy sprouts worldwide. In *USDA-ARS National Center for Agricultural Utilization Research, Peoria, IL. Bibliography and Sourcebook* (Soyfoods Center Lafayette, CA) Entry #207.
14. Shurtleff.
15. Shurtleff.
16. Shurtleff , William. On the Etymology of "green vegetable soybeans," "edamame," "vegetable-type soybeans," and "food-grade soybeans": a chronology of terminology. Summarized in *USDA-ARS National Center for Agricultural Utilization Research, Peoria, IL. Bibliography and Sourcebook* (Lafayette, CA, Soyfoods Center) Entry #206.
17. Shurtleff, William. Chronology of green vegetable soybeans and edamame (including maodou) worldwide. Special Exhibit Museum of Soy. www.thesoydailyclub.com.
18. Liu, 209-210.
19. Shurtleff.
20. Shurtleff.
21. Shurtleff.
22. Morse, WJ. Letter (July 20, 1929) read before the tenth annual field meeting of the American Soybean Ssociation, Guelph, Ontario, Canada. Quoted in Shurtleff, William. *USDA-ARS National Center for Agricultural Utilization Research, Peoria, IL. Bibliography and Sourcebook* (Lafayette, CA, Soyfoods Center) Entry #83.

end notes - 5

23. Liu, 17-21.
24. Liu. 208-209.
25. Horvath AA. The soybean as human food. *Chinese Economic Journal*, 1, 1, 24-32. Summarized in Shurtleff, William. *USDA-ARS National Center for Agricultural Utilization Research, Peoria, IL. Bibliography and Sourcebook* (Lafayette, CA, Soyfoods Center), Entry #71.
26. Liu, 208-209.

Chapter 5: The Good Old Soys – Soybeans with Culture

1. Shurtleff, William and Aoyagi, Akiko. *The Book of Miso: Savory Soy Seasoning* (Ten Speed Press, Second Edition, 2001), 20-44.
2. Shurtleff, Aoyagi. 28-29.
3. Shurtleff, William. Aoyagi, Akiko. *The Book of Miso: Food for Mankind* (NY, Ballentine, 1976), 43-45.
4. Fallon, Sally. Enig, Mary. *Nourishing Traditions* (Washington, DC, New Trends, Second Edition, 1999). 89-91.
5. Mihagi Y, Shinjo S et al. Trypsin inhibitor activity in commercial soybean products in Japan. *J Nutr Sci Vitaminol*, 1997, 43, 5, 575-580.
6. Shurtleff, William, Aoyagi, Akiko. *The Book of Tempeh* (Berkeley, CA, Ten Speed Press, Second Edition, 2001) 34-35.
7. Visser A, Thomas A. Review: Soya protein products—their processing, functionality and application aspects. *Food Rev Int*, 1987, 3, 1&2, 1-32.
8. Anderson RL, Wolfe WJ. Composition changes in trypsin inhibitors, phytic acid, saponins and isoflavones related to soybean processing. *J Nutr*, 1995, 125, 581S-588S.
9. Calloway DH, Hickey CA, Murphy EL, Reduction of intestinal gas-forming properties of legumes by traditional and experimental food processing methods. *J Food Sci*, 1971, 36, 251-255.
10. Liu, Keshun. *Soybeans: Chemistry, Technology and Utilization* (Gaithersburg, MD, Aspen, 1999), 278.
11. Shurtleff, Aoyagi. *Book of Miso: Savory Soy Seasoning*, 22.
12. Shurtleff, Aoyagi. *Book of Tempeh*, 33.
13. Keuth S, Bispin B. Formation of vitamins by pure cultures of tempe moulds and bacteria during the tempe solid substrate fermentation. *J Appl Bacteriol*, 1993, 75, 5, 427-434.
14. Katsuyama H, Ideguchi S et al. Usual dietary intake of fermented soybeans (natto) is associated with bone mineral density in premenopausal women. *J Nutr Sci Vitaminol* (Tokyo), 2002, 48, 3, 207-215.
15. Matsuo M, Nakamura N et al. Antioxidative mechanism and apoptosis induction by 3-hydroxyanthranilic acid, an antioxidant in Indonesian food tempeh, in the human hepatoma-derived call line, HuH-7. *J Nutr Sci Viaminol*, 1997, 43, 2, 249-259.
16. Chen LH, Packett LV, Yun I. Tissue antioxidant effect of ocean hake fish and fermented soybean (tempeh) as protein source in rats. *J Nutr*, 1972, 102, 2, 181-185.
17. Specker BL, Miller D et al. Increased urinary methylmalonic acid excretion in breast-fed infants of vegetarian mothers and identification of an acceptable dietary source of vitamin B-12. *Am J Clin Nutr*, 1988, 47, 1, 89-92.
18. Ensminger AH et al. *Encyclopedia of Foods and Nutrition*, (Boca Raton, FL, CRC Press, 1994) 1284.
19. Shurtleff, Aoyagi, *Book of Tempeh*, 33-34.
20. Keuth S, Bisping B formation of vitamins by pure cultures of tempe moulds and bacteria during the tempe solid substrate fermentation. *J Appl Bacteriiol*, 1993, 75, 5, 427-434.
21. Keuth S, Bisping B Vitamin B12 production by Citrobacter freudii or Klebsiella pneumoniae during tempeh fermentation and proof of enterotoxin absence by PCR. *Appl Environ Microbiol*, 1994, 50, 5, 1495-1499.
22. Vinh LT, Dworsechak E. Phytate content of some foods from plant origin from Vietnam and Hungary. *Nahrung*, 1985, 29, 2, 161-166.
23. Golbitz, Peter. *Tofu and Soyfoods Cookery* (Book Publishing Company, 1998) 22.
24. Liu. 270, 278.
25. Kristofikova L, Rosenberg M et al. Selection of Rhizopus strains for L (+) lactic acid and gamma-linolenic acid production. *Folia Microbiol (Praha)*, 1991, 35, 5, 451-451-455. Medline abstract.
26. Enig, Mary G, *Know Your Fats*, (Silver Spring, Bethesda Press, 2000).
27. Horrobin, David F. The regulation of prostaglandin biosynthesis by manipulation of essential fatty acid metabolism. *Reviews in Pure and Applied Pharmacological Sciences*, Vol 4, pp 339-383, Freund Publishing House, 1983
28. Lappe, Frances Moore. *Diet for a Small Planet* (NY Ballentine, 1982).
29. Protein Quality (NPU) of Various Foods, Figure 2.3 in Shurtleff, Aoyagi, *Book of Tempeh*, 31.
30. Shurtleff, Aoyagi. *Book of Tempeh*, 32.
31. Shurtleff, Aoyagi. *Book of Miso: Savory Soy Seasoning*, 21, 253.
32. Setchell, Kenneth DR. Safety and toxicity of soyfoods and their constituent isoflavones. Presentation at *Soyfoods 2002: New Technology Innovations and Effective Marketing Tactics*, January 17-19, 2001, Hyatt Regency, Phoenix, AZ. Educational Audio Cassettes.
33. Nakamura Y, Tsuji S , Tonogai Y. Determination of the levels of isoflavonoids in soybeans and soy-derived foods and estimation of isoflavonoids in the Japanese daily intake. *JAOAC Int*, 2000, 83, 3, 635-650.
34. Fallon, Sally. Enig, Mary G. Tragedy and Hype: The Third International Soy Symposium, *Nexus*, 2000, 7, 3.
35. Shurtleff, Aoyagi. *Book of Tempeh*, 35.
36. Masuda S, Hara-Kudo Y, Kumaga S. Reduction of Escherichia coli 0157: H7 populations in soy sauce, a fermented seasoning. *J Food Prot*, 61, 6, 657-661.
37. Matsushima K, Yashiro K et al. Absence of aflatoxin biosynthesis in koji mold (aspergillus sojae). *Appl Microbiol Biotechnol*, 2001, 55, 6, 771-776.

38. Wei RD, Chang SC, Lee SS. High pressure liquid chromatographic determination of aflatoxins in soy sauce and fermented soybean paste. *J Assoc Off Anal Chemi*, 1980, 63, 6, 1269-1274.
39. Sripathomaswat N, Thasnakorn P. Survey of aflatoxin-producing fungi in certain fermented foods and beverages in Thailand. *Mycopathologia*, 1981, 73, 2, 83-88.
40. Vietnam finds aflatoxin contamination in soy, peanut products. *Vietnam News Briefs* via NewsEdge Corporation 1/15/02 www.soyatech.com.
41. Shurtleff, Aoyagi. *Book of Miso:Savory Soy Seasoning*, 25-26.
42. Shurtleff, Aoyagi.
43. Ohara M, Lu H et al. Radioprotective effects of miso (fermented soybean paste) against radiation in B6C3F1 mice: increased small intestinal crypt survival, crypt lengths and prolongation of average time to death. *Hiroshima J Med Sci*, 2001, 50, 4, 83-86.
44. Shurtleff, Aoyagi, 26.
45. Fallon, Sally, Enig, Mary. Food in China – Variety and Monotony www.westonaprice.org.
46. Shurtleff, Aoyagi. *Book of Miso: Savory Soy Seasoning*, 98.
47. Shurtleff, Aoyagi. 48.
48. Shurtleff, Aoyagi. 48.
49. Shurtleff, Aoyagi. 50.
50. Liu, 218-237.
51. Shurtleff, Aoyagi, 39·
52. Shurtleff, Aoyagi, 261.
53. Dorsett PH, Morse WJ. Miso in Japan. 1930 document from Agricultural Explorations in Japan Summarized by William Shurtleff and Akiko Aoyagi in *USDA-ARS National Center for Agricultural Utilization Research, Peoria, IL. Bibliography and Sourcebook* (Lafayette, CA, Soyfoods Center. Entry #97.
54. Shurtleff, Aoyagi, 30, 43-44.
55. Sugiyama, Shin-ichi. Fermented soy bean products, IFINR.2-1990, 19-24.
56. Shurtleff, Aoyagi. *Book of Miso: Food for Mankind*, 521-530.
57. Shurtleff, Aoyagi. *Book of Miso: Savory Soy Seasoning*, 30, 32, 43-44.
58. Shurtleff, Aoyagi.
59. Shurtleff, Aoyagi, *Book of Tofu*, 71-72.
60. Katsuyama H, Ideguchi S et al. Usual dietary intake of fermented soybeans (natto) is associated with bone mineral density in premenopausal women. *J Nutr Sci Vitaminol* (Tokyo), 2002, 48, 3, 207-215.
61. Liu, 260-273.
62. Shurtleff, Aoyagi, *Book of Tempeh*, 8-16, 37-40.
63. Shurtleff, Aoyagi
64. Shurtleff, Aoyagi.
65. *Bon Appetit*, March 2003 reported on www.thesoydailyclub.com.
66. Shurtleff, Aoyagi, *Book of Miso: Savory Soy Seasoning*, 49, 222-223.
67. Liu, 237-250.
68. Liu, 239.
69. Shurtleff, Aoyagi, *Book of Miso: Savory Soy Seasoning*, 50.
70. Morse WH. Letter read to the 1929 convention of the American Soybean Association, July 20, 1929. Summarized by William Shurtleff in *USDA-ARS National Center for Agricultural Utilization Research, Peoria Illinois. Bibliography and Sourcebook* (Lafayette, CA, Soyfoods Center. Entry #83.
71. Shurtleff, Aoyagi. *Book of Miso: Food for Mankind*, 522-524.
72. Shurtleff, Aoyagi.
73. Liu, 250-260.
74. Sugiyama.
75. Liu, 248-251.
76. Liu, 250.
77. Elliott, Valerie. Cancer link prompts soy sauce recall, *Times of London*, June 21, 2001. www.mercola.com.
78. More soy sauce products fail tests. *New Zealand Herald*, September 21, 2001.
79. Soy Sauce Products – Consultation Paper – Proposal for the permanent regulation of 'soy sauces.' *News and Issues*, New Zealand Ministry of Health. www.moh.govt.nz.
80. Li X, Hiramoto K et al. Identification of 2,5-dimethyl-4-hydroxy-3(2H)-furanone (DMHF) and 4-hydroxy-2(or5)-ethyl-5(or2)-methyl-3(2h)-furanone (HEMF) with DNA breaking activity in soy sauce. *Food Chem Toxicol*, 1998, 36, 4, 305-3224.
81. Colin JC. The naturally occurring furanones: formation and function from pheromone to food. *Biol Rev Camb Philos Soc*, 1999, 74, 3, 259-276. Medline abstract.
82. Jung YJ, Youn JY, et al. Salsolinol, a naturally occurring tetrahydroisoquinoline alkaloid, induces DNA damage and chromosomal aberrations in cultured Chinese hamster lung fibroblast cells. *Mutat Res*, 2001, 474, 1-2, 35-33.
83. Kim YK, Koh E, et al. Determination of ethyl carbamate in some fermented Korean foods and beverages. *Food Addit Contam*, 200, 17, 6, 469-475.
84. Fujie K, Nishi J et al. Acute cytogenetic effects of tyramine, MTCAs, NACl and soy sauce on rat bone marrow cells in vivo. *Mutat Res*, 1990, 240, 4, 281-288.
85. Higashimoto M, Matano K, Ohnishi Y. Augmenting effect of a nonmutagenic fraction in soy sauce on mutagenicity of 3-diazotyramine produced in the nitrite-treated sauce. *Jpn J Cancer Res*, 1988, 79, 12, 1284-1292.
86. Nagahara A, Ohshita K, Nasuno S. Relation of nitrite concentration to mutagen formation in soy sauce. *Food Chem Toxicol*, 1986, 24, 1, 13-15.

87. Nagao M, Wakabayashi K et al. Nitrosatable precursors of mutagens in vegetables and soy sauce. *Princess Takamatsu Symp*, 1985, 16, 77-86.
88. Ochiai M, Wakabayashi K et al. Tyramine is a major mutagen precursor in soy sauce, being convertible to a mutagen nitrite. *Gann*, 1984, 75, 1, 1-2.
89. Wakabayashi K, Nagao M et al. Appearance of direct-acting mutagenicity of various foodstuffs produced in Japan and Southeast Asia on nitrite treatment. *Mutat Res*, 1985, 158, 3, 119-24.
90. Wakabayashi K, Nagao M, Sugimura T. Mutagens and carcinogens produced by the reaction of environmental aromatic compounds with nitrite. *Cancer Surv*, 1989, 8, 2, 385-399.
91. Kimura S, Okazaki K et al. Mutagenicity of nitrite-treated soy sauce in Chinese hamster V79 cells. *Tokushima J Exp Med*, 1990, 37, 1-2, 31-34.
92. Shulman KI, Walker SE. Refining the MAOI diet: tyramine content of pizzas and soy products. *J Clin Psychiatry*, 1999, 60, 3, 191-193.
93. Walker SE, Shulman KI et al. Tyramine content of previously restricted foods in monoamine oxidase inhibitor diets. *J Clin Pschopharmacol*, 1996, 16, 5, 383-388.
94. Iron-fortified soy sauce to help Chinese combat anemia. Xinhua via NewsEdge Corporation, Beijing, September 24, 2002. www.soyatech.com.

Chapter 6: Not Milk and UnCheese – The Udder Alternatives

1. Soymilk: opportunity for the dairy industry? Posted 12/26/2001. www.soyatech.com.
2. Shurtleff, William, Chronology of soymilk worldwide: Part I, 220AD to 1949, Special Exhibit, Museum of Soy, 2001, www.soydailyclub.com.
3. Guy RA. The diets of nursing mothers and young children in Peiping. *Chinese Med J*, 1936, 50, 434-442.
4. Guy RA, Yeh KS. Roasted soybean in infant feeding. *Chinese Med J*, 1938, 54, 2, 101-110.
5. Guy RA, Yeh KS. Soybean "milk" as a food for young infants. *Chinese Med J*, 1938, 54, 1, 1-30.
6. Shurtleff.
7. Miller HW, Wen CJ. Experimental nutrition studies of soymilk in human nutrition, *Chinese Medl J*, 1936, 50, 4, 450-459.
8. Moore, Raymond S. *China Doctor: The Life Story of Harry Willis Miller* (Harper, 1961). Summarized by William Shurtleff, Akiko Aoyagi in Bibliography and Sourcebook on the Seventh Day Adventists, 1866-1992. (Lafayette, CA, Soyfoods Center). Entry #444.
9. Miller, Harry W. Why Japan needs soy milk. *Soybean Digest*, April 1959, 16-17. Summarized by Shurtleff, Aoyagi in *Bibliography and Sourcebook on Seventh Day Adventists, 1866-1992*, Entry #419.
10. Wilson, Lester A. Soy Foods. In *Practical Handbook of Soybean Processing and Utilization*. David R. Erickson, ed. (Champaign, IL, AOCS Press, 1995), 432.
11. Kahn EJ Jr. Staffs of Life Part V: The future of the planet. *The New Yorker*, March 11, 1985, 65.
12. Shurtleff.
13. Shurtleff.
14. Wallace GM. Studies on the processing and properties of soymilk. *J Sci Food Agric*, 1971, 22, 526-535.
15. Japanese food maker to use new technology to create whole bean soyfoods. JIJI via NewsEdge Corporation. www.soyatechn.com. Posted 4/27/04.
16. Liu, KeShun. *Soybeans: Chemistry, Technology and Utilization* (Gaithersburg, MD, Aspen, 1999) 151-153.
17. Golbitz, Peter. Traditional soyfoods: processing and products, *J Nutr*, 1995, 125, 570S-572S.
18. Liu, 147.
19. Golbitz.
20. www.adltechnology.com
21. Study by Arthur D. Little & Soyatech shows soymilk falls short of taste standards. Business Wire via NewsEdge Corporation. Posted 8/21/01. www.soyatech.com.
22. Producers struggle to make soymilk palatable. *Boston Globe* via NewsEdge Corporation, August25. www.soyatech.com.
23. Benchmarking soymilk flavor: US. market 2001: new soymilk flavor study shows wide range in quality. Soyatech Press Release. Posted 6/18/01. www.soyatech.com
24. Liu, 161-162.
25. Huang AS, Hsieh OAL, Chang SS. Characterization of the nonvolatile minor constituents responsible for the objectionable taste of defatted soybean flour. *J Food Sci*, 47, 19.
26. Shurtleff, Aoyagi. Product name: Madison Soy Milk. In *Bibliography and Sourcebook on Seventh Day Adventists, 1866-1992*. (Lafayette, CA, Soyfoods Center). Entry # 102.
27. Fallon, Sally. Enig, Mary G. *Nourishing Traditions*. (Washington, DC, New Trends, 1999) Second Edition, 39.
28. Song, Sora. Beyond Brown Cow: Specialty yogurts are multiplying. But do they taste any better? *Time*, March 31, 2003, 191.
29. Thickener used in soymilk may cause health problems, study says. Environmental News Network, Sun Valley ID, via. NewsEdge Corporation. Posted 10/22/01. www.soyatech.com.
30. Words used by Amazon readers who reviewed vegan recipe books. www.amazon.com.
31. Hurley, Jayne. Liebman, Bonnie. The udder alternative: the soy dairy case, *Nutrition Action Newsletter*, Nov 2002, 14.
32. Hurley, Liebman.
33. Kraft develops method for preparing cheese with high levels of soy protein. *Food Ingredient News*, October 2002. www.soyatech.com.

34. Golbitz,, Peter. Traditional soyfoods: processing and products. *J Nutr,* 1004, 125, 570S-572S.
35. Shurtleff, Aoyagi. 367, 374.
36. Liu, 198-200.
37. Wilson, Lester A. Soy Foods. In *Practical Handbook of Soybean Processing and Utilization.* David R. Erickson, ed. (AOCS Press, 1995), 446-447.
38. Edible soy protein film may replace plastic wrap. Delta Farm Press via NewsEdge Corporation. Posted 2/25/2002 on www.soyatech.com
39. Madison, Deborah. *This Can't Be Tofu: 75 Recipes to Cook Something You Never Thought You Would — And Love Every Bite!* (NY Bantam Doubleday, 2000).
40. Liu, 184-191.
41. Shurtleff, Aoyagi, 110
42. Shurtleff, Aoyagi, 311-320
43. Liu, 168-169.
44. Shurtleff, Aoyagi, 137-138.
45. Liu, 197.
46. Haumann, Barbara Fitch. Food technology soy protein foods gain store space, INFORM, 1997, 8, 6, 588-592.
47. *Faces of Asia: A Tale of Tofu,* National Geographic Channel.
48. Shurtleff, Aoyagi. *Book of Tofu* 358-366.
49. Liu, 284-289.
50. Shurtleff, Aoyagi. 87-100.
51. Liu, 205-207.
52. Shurtleff, Aoyagi. *Book of Tempeh,* 114.
53. Liu 205-207.
54. New soymilk flavor study shows wide range in quality. Posted 6/18/2001.www.soyatech.com.
55. Soyatech president Peter Golbitz receives 2004 Soyfoods Industry Leadership Award. Posted 12/3/2004. www.soyatech.com.

Chapter 7: All American Soy – First Generation Soybean Products

1. Liu, KeShun. *Soybeans: Chemistry, Technology and Utilization* (Gaithersburg, MD, Aspen 1999) 207-208, 401.
2. Visser A, Thomas A. Review: Soya protein products: their processing, functionality, and application aspects. *Food Rev Int,* 1987, 3, 1&2, 6.
3. Hoover, WJ. Use of soy proteins in bakery products. *J Oil Chem Soc,* 1975, 52, 267A-269A.
4. Shurtleff, William, Aoyagi, Akiko. The History of Soybean Crushing: Soy Oil and Soybean Meal. From *The History of Soybeans and Soyfoods: Past, Present and Future.* Unpublished manuscript. (Lafayette, CA, Soyfoods Center) 27.
5. Piper, Charles V, Morse, William J. Soybean flour. In Piper and Morse, *The Soybean* (McGraw Hill, 1923). Summarized by William Shurtleff in *Bibliography and Sourcebook: USDA-ARS National Center for Agricultural Utilization Research,* Entry #61.
6. Klein BP, Perry AK, Adair N. Incorporating soy proteins into baked products for use in clinical studies. *J Nutr,* 125, 666S-674S.
7. Liu.
8. Rackis JJ. Biologically active components. In *Soybeans: Chemistry and Technology, Volume 1, Proteins,* Allan K. Smith and Sidney J Circle, eds. (Westport, CT, Avi, 1972)., 158-162.
9. Eldridge AC. Organic solvent treatment of soybeans and soybean fractions. In Smith and Circle, 150.
10. Lusas EW, Riaz MN. Soy protein products: processing and use. *J. Nutr,* 1995, 125, 573S-580S.
11. Klein, Perry, Adair.
12. Lusas.
13. Rackis JJ. Flatulence caused by soya and its control through processing. *J Am Oil Chem Soc,* 1981, 58, 503.
14. Rackis JJ. Flavor and flatulence factors in soy protein products. *J Agric Food Chem,* 1970, 18, 977.
15. Calloway DH, Hickey CA, Murphy EI. Reduction of intestinal gas-forming properties of legumes by traditional and experimental food processing methods. *J Food Sci,* 1971, 36, 251.
16. Suarez FL et al. Gas production in humans ingesting a soybean-flour derived from beans naturally low in oligosaccharides. *Am J Clin Nutr,* 1999, 69, 1, 135-139.
17. Crowley PR. Practical feeding programs using soy protein as base, *J Am Oil Chem Soc,* 1975, 52, 277A-279A.
18. Klein, Perry, Adair.
19. Klein, Perry, Adair.
20. Gunn RA, Taylor PR, Gangaros EJ. Gastrointestinal illness associated with consumption of a soybean protein extender. *J Food Sci,* 1980, 43, 525-527.
21. Moroz LA, Yang WH. Kunitz soybean trypsin inhibitor. *New Eng J Med,* 1980, 302, 1126-1128.
22. Hoover.
23. Liu.
24. Visser, Thomas.
25. Lusas.
26. Visser, Thomas.
27. Klein, Perry, Adair.
28. Liu.

29. Liu, 207-208.
30. Dorsett PH, Morse WJ. 1928-1932 Agricultural Explorations in Japan. Chosen (Korea), Northwestern China, Taiwan (Formosa0, Singapore, Java, Sumatra and Ceylon. USDA Bureau of Plant Industry, Foreign Plant Introduction and Forage Crop Investigations (Washington DC). Unpublished Log. Summarized by William Shurtleff in *Bibliography and Sourcebook: USDA-ARS.* Entry #93.

Chapter 8: All American Soy – Second Generation Soy Products

1. Schultz, Stacey. Pass the tofu tacos. *US News and World Report,* November 22, 1999, 77-78.
2. Barry, Dave. Big fat coverup. *Miami Herald,* November 3, 1996, 5.
3. Cargill billing new soy protein isolate as "inconspicuously good." Soy Protein Solutions Press Release, September 17, 2002. www.soyatech.com.
4. Visser A, Thomas A. Review: Soya protein products – their processing, functionality and application aspects. *Food Rev Inter,* 1987, 3, 1&2, 20.
5. Liu, KeShun. *Soybeans: Chemistry, Technology and Utilization* (Gaithersburg, MD, Aspen, 1999) 401.
6. Terrell RN, Staniec WP. Comparative functionality of soy proteins used in commercial meat food products. *J Am Oil Chem Soc,* 1975, 52, 263A-282A.
7. Martin, RE. Legal problems faced by soy proteins on state and national levels. *Soybean Digest,* November 1969. 19, 51.
8. Rakosky, Joseph. Soy protein in foods: their use and regulations in the US. *J Am Oil Chem Soc,* 1975, 52, 272A-274A.
9. Berkowitz DB, Webert DW. Determination of soy in meat. *J Assoc Off Anal Chem,* 1987, 70, 1, 85-90.
10. Wansink B, Park S-B et al. How soy labeling influences preference and taste. Illinois Center for Soy Foods, Research abstracts. www.soyfoodsillinois.uiuc.edu/abstracts.html.
11. Wolf, Walter J. Report of the Working Group respecting vegetable protein production and utilization for human use. Joint FAO/WHO Food Standards Programme Codex Committee on Vegetable Proteins, Fifth session, Ottawa, Canada, February 6-10, 1989.
12. Liu, 426.
13. Liu, 425.
14. Visser, 20, 21.
15. Lusas EW, Rhee, KC. Soy protein processing and utilization. In *Practical Handbook of Soybean Processing and Utilization.* David R. Erickson, ed. (AOCS Press, 1995) 154-155.
16. Boismenue, Clyde. The market for soy protein isolates, concentrates, textured soy protein products and soy flour in America today Interview with William Shurtleff. SoyaScan Notes. November 12, 1990. Summarized by William Shurtleff and Akiko Aoyagi in *Bibliography and Sourcebook on Seventh Day Adventists, 1866-1992* (Lafayette, CA Soyfoods Center) Entry # 1495.
17. Martin.
18. Making it cheaper to eat protein. *Business Week,* May 12, 1973 184, 186. Summarized by William Shurtleff and Akiko Aoyagi in *Bibliography and Sourcebook on Seventh Day Adventists, 1866-1992* (Lafayette, CA, Soyfoods Center) Entry # 671.
19. Liu, 425-436.
20. Visser, 20-21.
21. Berk, Zeki. Technology of production of edible flours and protein products from soybeans. *FAO Bulletin,* Food and Agriculture Organization of the United Nations, Rome, 1992, 24.
22. Lusas EW, Riaz MN. Soy protein products: processing and use. *J Nutr,* 1995, 125,573S-580S.
23. Fischer RW. The use of soy in food products, *Soybean Digest,* May 1967. Summarized by Shurtleff and Aoyagi in *Bibliography and Sourcebook on Seventh Day Adventists, 1866-1992* (Lafayette, CA, Soyfoods Center) Entry #551.
24. Lusas EW, Rhee KC. Soy protein processing and utilization. In *Practical Handbook of Soybean Processing and Utilization* (AOCS Press, 1995) 149-151.
25. Klein BP, Perry AK, Adair N. Incorporating soy proteins into baked products for us in clinical studies. *J Nutr,* 1995, 125, 666S-674S.
26. Rackis JJ. Biological and physiological factors in soybeans. *J Am Chem Soc,* 1974, 51, 161A-169A.
27. Visser. 7, 20.
28. SCOGS-101. Evaluation of the health aspects of soy protein isolates as food ingredients, 1979. Prepared for Bureau of Foods, Food and Drug Administration by the Life Sciences Research Office, FASEB.
29. Rackis.
30. Liener IE. Implications of antinutritional components in soybean foods. *Crit Rev Food Sci Nutr,* 1994, 34, 1, 50-51.
31. Food Labeling: Health Claims, Soy Protein and Coronary Heart Disease. Federal Register, October 26, 1999.64, 206, Food and Drug Administration. 8-9.
32. SCOGS 101
33. Friedman M. Lysinoalanine in food and in antimicrobial proteins. *Adv Exp Med Biol,* 1999, 459, 145-159.
34. Lusas EW, Rhee, KC. Soy protein processing and utilization. In *Practical Handbook of Soybean Processing and Utilization* (AOCS Press, 1995) 140.
35. Berk, 83-85, 94.
36. Visser, 7-8.

37. Liu, 386-390.
38. Lusas, Rhee, 137-147.
39. Klatt, Craig. Best-selling Worthington and Loma Linda food products in Northern California (interview) SoyaScan Notes, July 18, 1990. Summarized by Shurtleff and Aoyagi in *Bibliography and Sourcebook on Seventh Day Adventists, 1866-1992*, Entry #1526.
40. Liu, 329-399, 429-430.
41. Berk, 4.
42. Visser, 23.

Chapter 9: Soy Oil and Margarine – Fat of the Land

1. Visser A, Thomas A. Review: Soya protein products – their processing, functionality, and application aspects. *Food Rev Int*, 1987, 3, 1 &2, 1-32.
2. Eldridge, AC. Organic Solvent treatment of soybeans and soybean fractions. In *Soybeans: Chemistry and Technology, Volume 1, Proteins*. Allan K. Smith and Sidney J. Circle, eds. (Avi, 1972) 150.
3. Berk, Z. Technology of production of edible flours and protein products from soybeans. Food and Agriculture Organization of the United Nations, Rome, 1992, 12, 22.
4. Liu, KeShun. *Soybeans: Chemistry, Technology and Utilization* (Gaithersburg, MD,Aspen, 1999) 57.
5. Sipos, Andre. Szuhaj, Bernard F. Chapter 11, Soybean Oil. In YH Hui, ed. *Bailey's Industrial Oil and Fat Products*, (NY Wiley-Interscience, Fifth Edition, 1995) Volume 2, 527-528.
6. Shurtleff, William and Aoyagi, Akiko. *The History of Soy Oil Hydrogenation and of Research on the Safety of Hydrogenated Soy Oils*, Unpublished manuscript, (Lafayette, CA, Soyfoods Center), 21.
7. Shurtleff, William and Aoyagi, Akiko. *The History of Soybean Crushing: Soy Oil and Soybean Meal*, Unpublished manuscript (Lafayette, CA, Soyfoods Center), 21-22, 26, 38, 42-43, 49.
8. Johnson LA, Myers DJ. Industrial uses for soybeans. In *Practical Handbook of Soybean Processing and Utilization*. David R. Erickson, ed. (Champaign, IL, AOCS Press, 1995)
9. Shurtleff, Aoyagi, 28-37.
10. Shurtleff, Aoyagi, 21-24, 38-41.
11. Fallon S, Enig MG. Food in China – Variety and Monotony. www.westonaprice.org.
12. Shurtleff, Aoyagi, *The History of Soybean Crushing*, 24.
13. Shurtleff, Aoyagi, 22-24.
14. Shurtleff, Aoyagi, 133-134.
15. Shurtleff, Aoyagi. 136.
16. Enig, Mary. *Know Your Fats* (Silver Spring, Bethesda Press, 2000) 258-259.
17. Shurtleff, William and Aoyagi, Akiko. *The History of Soy Oil Margarine*, Unpublished manuscript. (Lafayette, CA, Soyfoods Center) 3-5, 35-41.
18. Moustafa, Ahmad. Consumer and industrial margarines. In Erickson, David R, ed. *Practical Handbook of Soybean Processing Utilization* (Champaign, IL, AOCS Press, 1995) 339-362.
19. Enig. 194, 269.
20. Erickson, 363-379.
21. Shurtleff, William, Aoyagi, Akiko. *The History of Soy Oil Shortening*. Unpublished manuscript (Lafayette, CA, Soyfoods Center) 3-8.
22. Forristal, Linda Joyce. The rise and fall of Crisco. *Wise Traditions*, 2001, 2, 2, 56-57. www.westonaprice.org.
23. Shurtleff, Aoyag. *The History of Soy Margarine*, 44-45.
24. Basiron, Yusof. Palm oil. In Hui YH, ed. 336.
25. Achaya, KT. Concerns over vegetable oils. NFI (Nutritional Foundation of India) Publications, July 1984. www.nutritionfoundationofindia.org.
26. Shurleff, Aoyagi. *The History of Soy Oil Hydrogenation*, 3.
27. Enig, Mary G. Fallon, Sally. The Oiling of America. www.westonaprice.org.
28. Shurtleff, Aoyagi. *The History of Soybean Hydrogenation*, 13-22.
29. Shurtleff, Aoyagi. *The History of Soybean Crushing*, 71.
30. Morse, WJ. Letter to C.V. Piper, Bureau of Plant Industry, USDA, Washington, DC, January 14, 1921. Summarized by William Shurtleff in USDA-ARTS National Center for Agricultural Utilization Research, Peoria, IL. (Lafayette, CA, Soyfoods Center). Entry #37.
31. Shurtleff and Aoyagi. *The History of Soy Oil Margarine*. 15.
32. Shurtleff, Aoyagi.
33. Shurtleff, Aoyagi, 17.
34. Shurtleff, Aoyagi, 28.
35. Shurtleff, Aoyagi, 31.
36. Shurtleff, Aoyagi. *The History of Soybean Crushing*, 95.
37. Enig, Fallon. 4
38. Shurtleff, Aoyagi. *The History of Soybean Margarine*, 23.
39. Frazer, Alastair. Nutritional and dietetic aspects. In JH van Stuyvenberg, ed. *Margarine: An Economic, Social and Scientific History, 1869-1969* (Toronto University Press, 1969). 158-162.
40. Shurtleff, Aoyagi, *The History of Soybean Crushing*, 118.
41. Enig, Mary G, Fallon, Sally. The skinny on fats. www.westonaprice.org.
42. Erickson DR. Erickson MD. Hydrogenation and base stock formulation procedures. In David R. Erickson, ed. *Practical Handbook of Soybean Processing and Utilization*, 218-238.

43. Anderson, Dan. A primer on oils processing technology. Chapter 1 in YH Hui,, ed. *Bailey's Industrial Oil and Fat Products*, Volume 4, 35-39.
44. Sipos, Szuhaj.
45. Enig, 19.
46. Mercola, Joseph. *Trans* fat much worse for you than saturated fat. July 21, 2001. www.mercola.com.
47. Enig, 20, 259.
48. Erickson, 277-296.
49. Gorman, Jessica. *Trans* Fats: New studies add to these fats' image problem. *Science News*, 2001, 160, 301.
50. Shurtleff, Aoyagi, *The History of Soybean Crushing*, 137.
51. Enig, Fallon. Oiling of America.
52. Mercola, Joseph. The case of the phantom fat: the dangers of *trans* fat. January 16, 2000. www.mercola.com.
53. Japanese scientists develop cholesterol-lowering agent from edible oil byproduct. Nikkei English News Service via NewsEdge Corporation, 12/21/2001. www.soyatech.com.
54. Doctor calls plant sterol spreads "significant development." Unilever PR Newswire via NewsEdge Corporation, Posted 9/11/01. www.soyatech.com.

Chapter 10: Soy Lecithin – Sludge to Profit

1. Smith, Allan K and Circle, Sidney J. *Soybeans: Chemistry and Technology, Vol 1, Proteins* (Westport CT, Avi, 1972) 79.
2. Berk, Zeki. Technology of production of edible flours and protein products from soybeans. *FAO Agricultural Services Bulletin*, Food and Agriculture Organization of the United Nations, 97, 14.
3. Nash AM, Eldridge AC, Wolf WJ. Fractionation and characterization of alcohol extractions associated with soybean proteins: nonprotein components. *J Agr Food Chem*, 1967, 15, 1, 106-108.
4. Shurtleff, William and Aoyagi, Akiko. What is lecithin? Chapters 1-6 from History of Soy Lecithin. In *Soyfoods: Past, Present and Future*. Unpublished manuscript, (Lafayette, CA, Soyfoods Center, 1981).
5. Wood and Allison, Effects of consumption of choline and lecithin on neurological and cardiovascular systems, Life Sciences Research Office, Federation of American Societies for Experimental Biology (FASEB), 1981.
6. Liu, KeShun. *Soybeans: Chemistry, Technology, Utilization* (Gaithersburg, MD, Aspen, 1999) 32.
7. Shurtleff.
8. Shurtleff.
9. Berk.
10. Shurtleff.
11. Gu X, Beardslee T et al. Identification of IgE-binding proteins in soy lecithin. *Int Arch Allergy Immunol*, 2001, 126, 3, 218-225.
12. Mortimer EZ. Anaphylaxis following ingestion of soybean. *Pediatr*, 1961, 58, 90-92.
13. Moroz LA, Yang WH. Kunitz soybean trypsin-inhibitor: a specific allergen in food anaphylaxis *NEJM*, 1980, 302, 1126-1128.
14. Shurtleff.
15. Davis, Adelle. *Let's Get Well* (NY, Signet/New American Library, 1965).
16. Clark, Linda. *Secrets of Health and Beauty* (NY, Jove, 1969).
17. Crenshaw, Mary Ann. *The Natural Way to Super Beauty* (NY, Dell, 1974).
18. Shurtleff.
19. Lecithin demand poised to gain on choline health claims. Chemical Business NewsBase, *Chemical Market Reporter* via NewsEdge Corporation. Posted 10/8/2201. www.soyatech.com.
20. FDA clears health claim for choline. National Press Club, Washington, DC.PR Newswire via NewsEdge Corporation. Posted 9/10/2201 www.soyatech.com.
21. Soy products high in choline win labeling right. *News Observer*, Raleigh, NC via NewsEdge Corporation. Posted 9/12/2201 www.soyatech.com.
22. Amenta F, Parnetti L et al. Treatment of cognitive dysfunction associated with Alzheimer's disease with cholinergic precursors. Ineffective treatments or inappropriate approaches? *Mech Ageing Dev*, 2001, 122, 16, 2025-2040.
23. Ceda GP, Ceresini G et al. Alpha-Glycerylphosphyorylcholine administration increases the GH responses to gHR of young and elderly subjects. *Horm Metab Res*, 1992, 24, 3, 119-121.
24. Parnetti L et al. Choline alphoscerate in cognitive decline and in acute cerebrovascular disease: an analysis of published clinical data. *Mec Ageing Dev*, 2001, 122, 16, 2041-2055.
25. Atkins, Robert. *Dr. Atkins' Vita-Nutrient Solution* (NY Simon and Schuster, 1998). 78-80.
26. Zeisel SH, Gettner S, Youssef M. Formation of aliphatic amine precursors of N-nitrosodimethylamine after oral administration of choline and choline analogues in the rat. *Food Chem Toxicol*, 1989, 27, 1, 31-34.
27. Fiume Z. Final report on the safety assessment of lecithin and hydrogenated lecithin. *Int J Toxicol*, 2001, 20, Suppl 1, 21-45.
28. Gelbmann CM, Muller WE. Chronic treatment with phosphatidylserine restores muscarinic cholinergic receptor deficits in the aged mouse brain. *Neurobiol Aging*, 1992, 3, 1, 45-50.
29. Crook TH, Tinklenberg J et al. Effects of phyosphatidylserine in age-associated memory impairment. *Neurology*, 1991, 41, 5, 644-699.
30. Crook T, Petrie W et al. Effects of phosphatidylserine in Alzheimer's disease. *Psychopharmacol Bull*, 1992, 28, 1, 61-66.

31. Monteleone P, Beinat L et al. Effects of phosphatidylserine on the neuroendocrine respone to physical stress in humans. *Neuroendocrinology*, 1990, 52, 3, 243-248.
32. Sakai M, Yamatoya H, Kudo S. Pharmacological effects of phosphatidylserine enzymatically synthesized from soybean lecithin on brain function in rodents. *J. Nutr Sci Vitaminol* (Tokyo), 1996, 42, 1, 47-54.
33. Enig, Mary. *Know Your Fats* (Silver Spring, MD, Bethesda Press, 2000), 60-61.
34. Blokland A, Honig W, et al. Cognition-enhancing properties of subchronic phosphatidylserine (PS) treatment in middle-aged rats: comparison of bovine cortex PS with egg PS and soybean PS. *Nutr*, 1999, 15, 10, 778-783.
35. Schreiber S, Kampf-Sherf O et al. An open trial of plant-source derived phosphatydilserine for treatment of age-related cognitive decline. *Isr J Psychiatry Relat Sci*, 2000, 37, 4, 302-307.
36. Sakai, Yamatoya, Kudo.
37. Blaylock, Russell. Not just another scare: toxin additives in your food and drink. www.aspartamekills.com/blayart1.htm.
38. Ripening agent made from soy granted EPA approval. Nutra-Park Inc., Madison, WI. Business wire via NewsEdge Corporation. Posted 4/4/2002. www.soyatech.com.

Chapter 11: Not Trusting the Process

1. Two such sites are: http://chetday.com and www.vegan-straight-edge.org.uk/soyfood.htm.
2. Archer, Michael C. Hazards of nitrate, nitrite and N-nitroso compounds in human nutrition. In John Hatchcock, ed. *Nutritional Toxicology,* Volume 1, (NY, Academic Press, 1982) 328-381.
3. Wasserman Aaron E. Wolff, Ivan A. Nitrites and nitrosamines in our environment: an update. In Robert L. Ory, ed. *Antinutrients and Natural Toxicants in Foods* (Westport, CT, Food and Nutrition Press, 1981).
4. Evaluation of the health aspects of soy protein isolates as food ingredients. Prepared by Life Sciences Research Office, Federation of American Societies for Experimental Biology for the Bureau of Foods, Food and Drug Administration, 1979. Contract # FDA 223-75-2004.
5. Archer, 366.
6. Atkins, Robert. *Dr. Atkins Vita-Nutrient Solution* (NY, Simon and Shuster, 1998), 234-235.
7. Rackis JJ, Gumbmann MR, Liener IE. The USDA trypsin inhibitor study: I. Background, objectives and procedural details. *Qual Plant Foods Hum Nutr*, 1985, 35, 225.
8. Fazio T, Havery DC. Volatile n'nitrosamines in direct flame-dried processed foods. *IARC Sci Publ* , 1982, 41, 277-286
9. Nagahara A, Ohshita K, Nasuno S. Relation of nitrite concentration to mutagen formation in soy sauce. *Food Chem Toxicol*, 1986, 24, 1, 13-15.
10. Nagao M, Wakabayashi K et al. Nitrosatable precursors of mutagens in vegetables and soy sauce. *Princess Takamatsu Symp*, 1985, 16, 77-86.
11. Ochiai M, Wakabayashi K et al. Tyramine is a major mutagen precursor in soy sauce, being convertible to a mutagen nitrite. *Gann*, 1984, 75, 1, 1-2.
12. Wakabayashi K, Nagao M et al. Appearance of direct-acting mutagenicity of various foodstuffs produced in Japan and Southeast Asia on nitrite treatment. *Mutat Res*, 1985, 158, 3, 119-24.
13. Wakabayashi K, Nagao M, Sugimura T. Mutagens and carcinogens produced by the reactionof environmental aromatic compounds with nitrite. *Cancer Surv*, 1989, 8, 2, 385-399.
14. Kimura S, Okazaki K et al. Mutagenicity of nitrite-treated soy sauce in Chinese hamster V79 cells. *Tokushima J Exp Med*, 1990, 37, 1-2, 31-34.
15. Fitzpatrick, Mike Response to a submission by Protein Technologies International (PTI), n.d.
16. Evaluation.
17. Friedman M. Lysinoalanine in food and in antimicrobial proteins. *Adv Exp Med Biol*, 1999, 459, 145-159.
18. Evaluation.
19. Liener IE Implications of Antinutritional components in soybean foods. *Crit Rev Food Sci Nutr*, 1994, 34, 1, 31-67.
20. Yannai, Shmuel Toxic factors induced by processing. In IE Liener, ed. *Toxic Constituents in Plant Food Stuff* (NY Academic, Second Edition, 1980), 408-409.
21. Sternberg M, Kim CY, Schwende FJ. Lysinoalanine: presence in foods and food ingredients. *Science*, 1975, 190, 992-994.
22. Kraft develops process to deflavor soy-based foods, ingredients. European Patents via NewsEdge Corporation. Posted 6/20/2002. www.soyatech.com.
23. Yannai.
24. Liener.
25. Yannai.
26. Liener.
27. Friedman.
28. Sarwar G, L'Abbe MR, et al. Influence of feeding alkaline/heat processed proteins on growth and protein and mineral status of rats. *Adv Exp Med Biol*, 1999, 459, 161-177.
29. Sarwar, L'Abbe.
30. Eck, Paul C and Wilson, Larry. *Toxic Metal in Human Health and Disease* (Phoenix, AZ, Eck Institute of Applied Nutrition and Bioenergetics) 1989.
31. Sarwar.
32. Blaylock, Russell. *Excitotoxins: The Taste that Kills* (NM Health Press, 1996).

33. Blaylock, Russell. Not just another scare: toxin additives in your food and drink. www.aspartamekills.com/ blayart1.htm.
34. Park CH, Choi SH et al. Glutamate and aspartate impair memory retention and damage hypothalamic neurons in adult mice. *Toxicol Lett*, 2000, 115, 2, 117-125.
35. Sugimura T, Wakabayashi K et al. Heterocyclic amines produced in cooked food: unavoidable xenobiotics. *Princess Takamatsu Symp*, 1990, 21, 279-288.
36. Nagao M. A new approach to risk estimation of food-borne carcinogens – heterocyclic amines – based on molecular information. *Mutat Res*, 1999, 431, 1, 3-12.
37. Ohgaki H, Takayama S, Sugimura T. Carcinogenicities of heterocyclic amines in cooked foods. *Mutat Res*, 1991, 259, 3-4, 399-410.
38. Felton JS, Malfatti MA et al. Health risks of heterocyclic amines. *Mutat Res*, 1997, 376, 1-2, 37-41.
39. Adamson RH, Thorgeirsson UP. Carcinogens in foods: heterocyclic amines and cancer and heart disease. *Adv Ex Med Biol*, 1995, 369, 211-220.
40. Higashimoto M, Yamamoto T et al. Mutagenicity of 1-methyl-1,2,3,4-terahydro-beta-carboline-3-carboxylic acid treated with nitrite in the presence of alcohols. *Mutat Res*, 1996, 367, 1, 43-49.
41. Wakabayashi K. Nagao M. Recently identified nitrite-reactive compounds in food: occurrence and biological properties of the nitrosated products. *IARC Sci Publ*, 1987, 84, 287-291.
42. Higashimoto M, Yamato H et al. Inhibitory effects of citrus fruits on the mutagenicity of 1-methyl 1,2,3,4-tetrahydro-beta-carboline-3-carboxylic acid treated with nitrite in the presence of ethanol. *Mutat Res*, 1998, 4155, 3, 219-226.
43. Diem S. Herderich M. Reaction of tryptophan with carbohydrates: identification and quantitative determination of novel beta-carboline alkaloids in food. *J Agric Food Chem*, 2001, 49, 5, 2486-2492.
44. Torreilles J, Guerin MC, Previero A. Smple compounds with high pharmacologic potential: beta-carbolines. Origins, syntheses, biological properties. *Biochimie*, 1985, 67, 9, 929-947. Med Line abstract. Article in French.
45. Lan CM, Chen BH. Effects of soy sauce and sugar on the formation of heterocyclic amines in marinated foods. *Food Chem Toxicol*, 2002, 40, 7, 989-1000.
46. Sugimura T, Wakabayashi K et al. Heterocyclic amines produced in cooked food: unavoidable xenobiotics. *Princess Takamatsu Symp*, 1990, 21, 279-288.
47. Tsuda M, Nagao M, et al. Nitrite converts 2-amino-alpha-carboline, an indirect mutagen, into 2-hydroxy-alpha-carboline, a non-mutagen, and 2-hydroxy-3-nitroso-alpha-carboline, a direct mutagen. *Mutat Res*, 1981, 83, 1, 61-68.
48. Hashizume T, Santo H et al. Mutagenic activities of tryptophan metabolites before and after nitrite treatment. *Food Chem Toxicol*, 1991, 29, 12, 839-844.
49. Wakabayashi K, Nagao M et al. Food-derived mutagens and carcinogens. *Cancer Res*, 1992, 52, 7 Suppl, 2092s-2098S.
50. Hiramoto K, Sekiguchi K et al. DNA breaking activity and mutagenicity of soy sauce: characterization of the active components and identification of 4-hydroxy-5-methyl-3(2H)-furanone. *Mutat Res*, 1996, 359, 2, 119-132.
51. Li X, Hiramoto K et al. Identification of 2,5-dimethyl-4-hydroxy-3(2H)-furanone (DMHF) and 4-hydroxy-2 (or 5-ethyl-5(or2)methyl-3(2H)-furanone (HEMF) with DNA breaking activity in soy sauce. *Food Chem Toxicol*, 1998, 36, 4, 305-314.
52. Slaughter C. The naturally occurring furanones: formation and function from pheromone to food. *Biol Rev Camb Philos Soc*, 1999, 74, 3, 259-276.
53. Aaslyng MD, Martens M. Chemical and Sensory characteristics of hydrolyzed vegetable protein, a savory flavoring. *J Agric Food Chem*, 1998, 16, 46, 2, 481-489.
54. Li X, Hiramoto K et al. Identification of 2,5-dimethyl-4-hydroxy-3(2H)-furanone (DMHF) and 4-hydroxy-2(or5)-etyl-5(or2)-methyl-3(2h)-furanone (HEMF) with DNA breaking activity in soy sauce. *Food Chem Toxicol*, 1998, 36, 4, 305-3224.
55. Colin JC. The naturally occurring furanones: formation and function from pheromone to food. *Biol Rev Camb Philos Soc*, 1999, 74, 3, 259-276. Medline abstract.
56. Soy Sauce Products – Consultation Paper – Proposal for the permanent regulation of "soy sauces." *News and Issues*, New Zealand Ministry of Health. www.moh.govt.nz.
57 Soy Sauce Products – Consultation Paper – Proposal for the permanent regulation of "soy sauces." *News and Issues*, New Zealand Ministry of Health. www.moh.govt.nz.
58. Elliott, Valerie. Cancer link prompts soy sauce recall. *Times of London*, June 21, 2001. www.mercola.com.
59. More soy sauce products fail tests. *New Zealand Herald*, September 21, 2001.
60. Chung WC, Hui KY, Cheng SC. Sensitive method for the determination of 1,3-dichloropropano-2,3-chloropropane-1,2-diol in soy sauce by capillary gas chromatography with mass spectrometric detection. *J Chromatogr A*, 2002, 952, 1-2, 185-192.
61. Crews C, LeBrun G, Brereton PA. Determination of 1,3-dichloropropanol in soy sauces by automated headspace gas chromatography-mass spectrometry. *Food Addit Contam*, 2002, 19, 4, 343-349.
62. Shurtleff, William and Aoyagi, Akiko. The History of Soybean Crushing, Soy Oil and Soybean Meal. From *History of Soybeans and Soyfoods: Past, Present and Future*, Unpublished manuscript (Lafayette, CA, Soyfoods Center, 1981) Section 26, p. 101.
63. Liu, KeShun. *Soybeans: Chemistry, Technology and Utilization*. (Gaithersburg, MD, Aspen, 1999) 304.
64. Eldridge AC. Organic solvent treatment of soybeans and soybean fractions. In Smith, Allan K and Circle, Sidney J. *Soybeans: Chemistry and Technology* (Westport, CT, Avi, 1972) p. 153.
65. Shurtleff, Aoyagi, 132.
66. Boatright WL, Crum AD. Non-polar-volatile lipids from soy protein isolates and hexane-defatted flakes. *JAOCS*, 1997, 74, 461-467.

Chapter 12: Formula for Disaster

1. Messina, Mark. Statement made at Fifth International Symposium on the Role of Soy in the Prevention and Treatment of Chronic Disease, September 21-24, 2003. Disney Contemporary Resort, Orlando, FL.
2. Shurtleff, William. Letter to *Mothering* magazine, February 25, 2004.
3. Ruhrah, J. The soy bean in infant feeding: a preliminary report. *Arch Ped*, 1909, 26, 496-501.
4. Ruhrah J. The soybean as an article of diet for infants *JAMA*, 1910, 54, 1664.
5. Ruhrah J. The soybean and condensed milk in infant feeding. *Am J Med Sci*, 1915, 140, 502.
6. Sinclair, JF. The soybean in infant feeding. *JAMA*, 1916, 66, 841.
7. Tso E. The development of an infant fed eight months on a soybean milk diet. *Chinese J Physiol*, 1928, 2, 1, 33-40.
8. Tso E, Yee M, Chen T. The nitrogen, calcium and phosphorous metabolism in infants fed on soybean "milk." *Chinese J Physiol*, 1928, 2, 409.
9. Chang KC, Tso E. A soluble soybean milk powder and its adaptation to infant feeding. *Chinese J Physiol*, 1931, 5, 199.
10. Guy RA. The diets of nursing mothers and young children in Peiping. *Chinese Med J*, 1936, 50, 434-442.
11. Guy RA. Roasted soybean in infant feeding. *Chinese Med J*, 1938, 54, 2, 10'-110.
12. Guy RA, Yeh KS. Soybean "milk" as a food for young infants. *Chinese Med J*, 1938, 54, 1, 1-50.
13. Guy. Diets of nursing mothers. 440-441.
14. Chou CY. Studies on the use of soybean food in infant feeding in China and the development of Formula 5410, 1983. Unpublished manuscript in the library of Bernard Zimmerli at the Federal Office of Health, Berne, Switzerland.
15. Miller, Harry W. Articles from *Soybean Digest*. Quoted in Shurtleff, William, Aoyagi Akiko. *Bibliography and Sourcebook on Seventh Day Adventists*, 1866-1992. (Lafayette, CA, Soyfoods Center) Entries #342,501,506.
16. Fitzpatrick, Mike. Quoted in *Soy Information Network Newsletter*, March 5, 1996. 6-7.
17. Ruhrah.
18. American Academy of Pediatrics, Committee on Nutrition. Soy protein-based formulas: recommendations for use in infant feeding (RE9806). *Ped*, 1998, 101, 1, 148-153.
19. Rittinger FR, Dembo LH. Soy bean (vegetable) milk in infant feeding: preliminary report. *Am J Dis Children*, 1932, 44, 1221-1238.
20. Rittinger FR, Dembo LH, Torrey GG. Soy bean (vegetable) milk in infant feeding: Results of three and one-half years' study on the growth and development of 205 infants. *J Ped*, 1934, 6, 517-532.
21. Horvath AA. Quoted in Shurtleff, William. *USDA-ARS National Center for Agricultural Utilization Research, Peoria, Illinois*.(Lafayette, CA. Soyfoods Center.) Entry # 117.
22. Horvath AA. *Am J Digest Dis*, 1938, 5, 177. Quoted in MacKay H. Flour with dried milk: a cheap and efficient substitute for breast milk. *Arc Dis Childhood*, 1939?, vol. ?, 1-9.
23. MacKay H. Flour with dried milk: a cheap and efficient substitute for breast milk. *Arc Dis Childhood*, 1939?, vol. ?, 1-25.
24. Hill LW, Stuart HC. A soybean food preparation for feeding infants with milk idiosyncrasy. *JAMA*, 1929, 93, 985.
25. Blackfan KD. Wollbach SB. *J Ped*, 1933, 3, 679.
26. Horvath.
27. MacKay, 1-9.
28. Rittinger, Dembo, 1224.
29. Rittinger, Dembo, Torrey. 520.
30. Stearns, Genevieve. Soy bean flour in infant feeding: A study of the relation of the comparative intakes of nitrogen, calcium and phosphorous on the exretion and retention of these elements by infants. *Am J Dis Childhood*, 1933, 46, 7-16.
31. Melick, Weldon. Self-supporting college. *Reader's Digest*, May 1938, 105-108. Summarized in Shurtleff, Aoyagi. Seventh Day Adventists, Entry #218.
32. MacKay, 9.
33. Eastham EJ. Soy protein allergy. In Hamburger, Robert N., ed. *Food Intolerance in Infancy. Allergology, Immunology and Gastroenterology* (NY Raven, 1989). 224.
34. Cornfield D, Cooke RE. Vitamin deficiency: unusual manifestation in a 5-1/2 month old baby. Case report. *Ped*, 1952, 20, 33-35.
35. Goldman HI, Desposito F. Hypoprothrombinemic bleeding in young infants: association with diarrhea antibiotics and milk substitutes. *Am J Dis Child*, 1966, 111, 430-432.
36. American Academy of Pediatrics.
37. Eastham, 224.
38. Jung AL, Car SL. A soy protein formula and a milk-based formula. A comparative evaluation in milk-tolerant infants showed no significant nutritional differences. *Clin Ped*, 1977, 16, 11, 982-985.
39. SCOGS-101. Evaluation of the health aspects of soy protein isolates as food ingredients, 1979. Prepared for the Bureau of Foods, Food and Drug Administration by the Life Sciences Research Office, FASEB.
40. Eastham, 223.
41. Eastham. 225.
42. Bates RD, Barreet WW et al. Milk and soy formulas: a comparative growth study. *Ann Allergy*, 1968, 26, 577.
43. Fomon SJ, Ziegler EE et al. Methionine fortification of a soy protein formula fed to infants. *Am J Clin Nutr*, 1979, 32, 2460-71.
44. American Academy of Pediatrics.

45. Fleischer DS, DiGeorge AM et al. Hypoproteinemia and edema in infants with cystic fibrosis of the pancreas. *J Ped*, 1964, 64, 341-348.
46. American Academy of Pediatrics.
47. Peace RW, Sarwar G et al. Trypsin inhibitor levels in soy-based infant formulas and commercial soy protein isolates and concentrates. *Food Res Int*, 1992, 25, 137-141.
48. American Academy of Pediatrics
49. American Academy of Pediatrics
50. Steichen JJ, Tsang RC. Bone mineralization and growth in term infants fed soy-based or cow milk-based formula. *J Ped*, 1987, 110, 687-692.
51. Eastham, 224.
52. Köhler L, Meeuwisse G, Mortensson W. Food intake and growth of infants between six and twenty six weeks of age on breast milk, cow's milk formula, or soy formula. *Acta Pædiatr Scand*, 1984, 73, 40-48.
53. Hillman LS, Chow W et al. Effects of soy formulas on mineral metabolism in term infants. *Am J Dis Child*, 1987, 141, 527-530.
54. Mimouni F, Campaigne B et al. Bone mineralization in the first year of life in infants fed human milk, cow-milk formula or soy based formula. *J Ped*, 1993, 122, 348-354.
55. Venkataraman PS, Luhar H, Heylan MJ. Bone mineral metabolism in full-term infants fed human milk, cow milk-based and soy-based formulas. *Am J Dis Child*, 1992, 146, 1302-1305.
56. American Academy of Pediatrics
57. Glasgow JF, Elmes Me. Exacerbation of acrodermatitis enteropathica by soya-bean milk feeding. *Lancet*, 1975, ii, 769.
58. Hertrampf E, Cayazzo M et al. Bioavailability of iron in soy-based formula and its effect on iron nutriture ininfancy. *Ped*, 1986, 78, 640-645.
59. Linshaw MA, Harrison HL et al. Hypochloraemic alkalosis in infants associated with soy protein formula. *J Ped*, 1980, 96, 635-640.
60. Fomon SJ, Ziegler EE et al. Sweetness of diet and food consumption by infants. *Proc Soc Exper Biol Med*, 1983, 173, 190-193.
61. Young JB, Landsberg L. Stimulation of the sympathetic nervous system during sucrose feeding. *Nature*, 1977, 269, 615-617.
62. American Academy of Pediatrics.
63. Fallon, Sally. Enig, Mary. Soy infant formula – better than breastmilk? www.westonaprice.org.
64. Fallon, Sally. Enig, Mary. *Nourishing Traditions* (Washington, DC. New Trends, 2nd Edition, 1999). 599.
65. Kellogg JH. Method of making acidophilus milk (from soymilk). US Patent 1,982,994. December 4. 2 p, Appliation filed 14 June 1933. Summarized by Shurtleff and Aoyagi in *Bibliography and Sourcebook on Seventh-Day Adventists 1866-1992*. (Lafayette, CA, Soyfoods Center). Entry #131
66. Thrapp, Dan L. Thousands owe lives to doctor's soybean "milk." Noted surgeon nutritionist, now 86, devised formula as missionary in 1925. *Los Angeles Times*, July 31, 1965, 19. Summarized by Shurtleff and Aoyagi, Entry # 506.
67. Loma Linda Soyalac Infant Powder. Shurtleff and Aoyagi, Entry # 357
68. Meyer, Herman Frederic. *Infant Foods and Feeding Practice* (Springfield, IL Charles Thomas, 1960).
69. Royal College of Australian Physicians. Paediatric Policy: Soy Infant Formula. www.racp.edu.au.
70. Eastham, 230.
71. Eastham.
72. Shurtleff, Aoyagi. Entry # 1509.
73. Moss, Malcolm H. Hypoprothrombinemic bleeding in a young infant. Association with a soy protein formula. *Amer J Dis Child*, 1969, 117, 540-543.
74. Eastham, 224.
75. RA, Wolf A. Infantile beriberi associated with Wernicke's encephalopathy. *Ped*, 1958, 21, 409-413.
76. Siegel-Itzkovich, Judy. Police in Israel launch investigation into deaths of babies given formula milk. *BMJ*, 2003, 327, 1128.
77. Plaut M and Yated Ne-eman Staff. Remedia soy infant formula scandal. *Dei'Ah veDibur*, November 12, 2003. http://chareidi.shemayisrael.com.
78. American Academy of Pediatrics.
79. Fitzpatrick, Mike. Dibb, Sue. Soya Infant formula: The Health Concerns. A Food Commission Briefing Paper. October 1998.
80. Woodhams, Dave. Nutritional deficiencies of soy protein based infant formulas. *Soy Information Network Newsletter*, March 5, 1995. 1-15.

Chapter 13: Soy Protein – The Inside Scoop

1. Jackson AA. Amino acids: essential and non-essential. *Lancet*, 1983, I, 1034-1037.
2. Jackson AA. Critique of protein-energy interactions in vivo: urea kinetics. In Protein-Energy Interactions: Proceedings of an I/D/E/C/G Workshop held in Waterville Valley, NH, USA, October 21-25, 1991 NS Scimshaw. B. Schurch, eds. (Lausanne, Switzerland, Nestle Foundation).
3. Persaud C, et al. The excretion of 5-oxoproline in urine as an index of glycine status during normal pregnancy. *Br J. Obstet. Gynaecol*, 1989, 96, 440-444.
4. Irwin, MI, Hegsted DM. A conspectus of research on amino requirements of man. *J Nutr*, 1971, 101, 387-429.
5. Fallon, Sally. Enig, Mary. *Nourishing Traditions* (Washington, DC, New Trends, Second Edition, 1999).

end notes - 13

6. United States Department of Agriculture. Composition of Foods: Legumes and Legume Products. (USDA, Washington, DC, 1986) 8-16.
7. FAO/WHO/UNU, 1985. Energy and protein requirements. Report of a Joint FAO/WHO/UNU Expert Consultation, WHO Tech. Rep. Ser. No 724, Geneva.
8. Wolf WJ. *Soybean Proteins in Human Nutrition*, 770.
9. www.brinkone.com/soy/html.
10. Sarwar G, Peace RW, Botting HG. Effect of amino acid supplementation on protein quality of soy-based infant formulas fed to rats. *Plant Foods Hum Nutr*1993, 43, 3, 259-266.
11. US Food and Drug Administration. Federal Register, 21, CFR, Part 101. Part III. Food labeling. Washington, DC, 1991.
12. Sarvar.
13. Sarvar.
14. Sarvar.
15. Friedman et al, Protein alkali reactions: chemistry, toxicology, and nutritional consequences. In *Nutritional and Toxicological Aspects of Food Safety*. M. Friedman,ed. (NY Plenum Press, 1984). 367-412.
16. Sarvar.
17. Wilcke, Harold L, Hopkins, Daniel T and Waggle, Doyle H. *Soy Protein and Human Nutrition* (NY, Academic Press, 1979).
18. Wilcke, 346.
19. Torun, Benjamin. Nutritional quality of soybean protein isolates: studies in children of preschool age. In *Soy Protein and Human Nutrition*, 106.
20. Fallon, Sally. Enig, Mary G. A reply to Mr. Peary's defense of soybeans. *Health Freedom News*, February 1996.
21. Bressani R et al. A critical summary of a short-term nitrogen balance index to measure protein quality in adult human subjects. In Wilcke, 313-323.
22. Kies, C. Comparison of human and animal studies in Nebraska. In Wilcke, 326-327.
23. Torun.
24. Register UD, Inano M et al. Nitrogen-balance studies in human subjects on various diets, *Am J Clin Nutr*, 1967, 20, 7, 753-759.
25. Beer WH et al. A long-term metabolic study to assess the nutritional value and immunological tolerance to two soy-protein concentrates in adult humans. *Am J Clin Nutr*, 1989, 50, 997-1007.
26. Young VR. Soy protein in relation to human protein and amino acid nutrition, *J Amer Diet Assoc*, 1991, 91, 7, 828-835.
27. Friedman M, Brandon DL. Nutritional and health benefits of soy proteins. *J. Agric Foods Chem*, 2001, 49, 3, 1069-1086.
28. Snyderman SE et al. Unessential: nitrogen: a limiting factor for human growth. *J Nutr*, 1962, 57-114.
29. McCully, Kilmer. *The Heart Revulution: The Extraordinary Discovery that Finally Laid The Cholesterol Myth to Rest* (Perennial, 2000).
30. McCully, Kilmer. *The Homocysteine Revolution* (McGraw Hill, 1999).
31. McCully,Kilmer. Email to author, August 25, 2004.
32. MannGV, Andrus SB et al. Experimental atherosclerosis in cebus monkeys.. *J Exp Med*, 953, 98, 195-218.
33. Mann GV, McNally A,, Prudhomme C. Experimental atherosclerosis. Effects of sulfur compounds on hypercholesterolemia and growth in cysteine deficient monkeys. *Am J.Clin Nutr*, 1960, 8, 491-498.
34. Stolzenberg-Solomon RZ, Miller ER, et al. Association of dietary protein intake and coffee consumption with serum homocysteine concentrations in an older population. *Am J Clin Nutr*, 1999, 69, 467-475.
35. Gaull GE, Sturman Ja, Raiha NCR. Development of mammalian sulfur metabolism: absence of cystathionase in human fetal tissues. *Pediatr Res*, 1972, 6, 538-547.
36. Gotoh N et al. Inhibition of glutathione synthesis increases the toxicity of oxidized low-density lipoprotein in human monocytes and macrophages. *Biochem J*, 1993, 296, Pt 1, 151-154.
37. Gaull GE and Wright CE. Protein and growth modulators. In SJ Fomon and WC Heird, eds *Energy and Protein Needs during Infancy*. (NY Academic Press, 1986). 870-897.
38. Gaull GE et al. Milk protein quantity and quality in low-birth weight infants III. Effects on sulfur amino acids in plasma and urine. *J Pediatr*, 1977, 90, 348-355.
39. Gaull, Wright.
40. Atkins, Robert. *Dr Atkin's Vita-Nutrient Solution* (NY Simon & Shuster, 1998) 176-178.
41. Atkins, 184-187.
42. Sarvar, Ghulam. The Protein Digestibility-Corrected Amino acid score method overestimates quality of proteins containing anti-nutritional factors and of poorly digestible proteins supplemented with limiting amino acids in rats. *J Nutr*, 1997, 127, 5, 758-764.
43. Sarvar.
44. Kawamura and Hayashi, Lysinoalanine-degrading enzymes of various animal kidneys. *Agric Biol Chem*, 1987, 51, 2289-2290.
45. Atkins, 171-172.
46. Rath, Matthias. Pauling, Linus. A unified theory of human cardiovascular disease, leading the way to the abolition of this disease as a cause for human mortality. www.mercola.com.
47. Marz, Russell B. *Medical Nutrition from Marz,* (Portland, OR, Omni Press, Second Edition 1999) 83.
48. Atkins, 192.
49. Atkins.
50. Eggum BO, Hansen I, Larsen T. Protein quality and digestible energy of selected foods determined in balance trials with rats. *Plant Foods Hum Nutr*, 1989, 39, 13-21.

51. Sarvar G, Peace RW. Comparisons between true digestibility of total nitrogen and limiting amino acids in vegetable proteins. *J Nutr*, 1986, 116, 1172-1184.
52. Emmert JL, Baker DH. Protein quality assessment of soy products. *Nutr Res*, 1995, 15, 1647-1656.
53. Brandon DL, Bates AH and Friedman M. Elisa Analysis of soybean trypsin inhibitors in processed foods. In M. Friedman, ed. *Nutritional and Toxicological Consequences of Food Processing.* (NY, Plenum, 1991) 331.
54. Rackis JJ. The USDA trypsin inhibitor study. I. Background, objectives, and procedural details. *Qual Plant Foods Hum Nutr*, 1985, 215.
55. Yannai Shmuel. Toxic factors induced by processing. In Irvin E. Liener, ed. *Toxic Constituents in Plant Foodstuffs* (NY Academic Press, 1980).408-410.
56. Sarwar G, L'Abbe MR et al. Influence of feeding alkaline/heat processed proteins on growth and protein and mineral status of rats. *Adv Exp Med Biol*, 1999, 4459, 161-177.
57. SCOGS 101. Evaluation of the health aspects of soy protein isolates as food ingredients. Life Sciences Research Office, Food and Drug Administration, Washington DC. FDA/BF-80/3.
58. Steinke FH. Measuring protein quality of foods In Wilcke, 307-308.
59. Nordlee JA et al. Identification of a Brazil nut allergin in transgenic soybeans. *NEJM*, 1996, 334,688-692.
60. Messina, Mark. Messina, Virginia. Setchell, Kenneth DR. *The Simple Soybean and your Health* (Garden City Park, NY, Avery, 1994) 25.
61. Breslau, NA et al. Relationship of animal protein-rich diet to kidney stone formation and calcium metabolism. *J Clin Endocrinol Metabol*, 1988, 66, 140-146.
62. Messina, Messina, Setchell, 116-117.
63. Mindell, Earl. *Earl Mindell's Soy Miracle* (NY Fireside, 1995) 77.
64. Whiting SJ, Draper HH. Effect of chronic acid load as sulfate or sulfur amino acids on bone metabolism in adult rats. *J Nutr*, 1981, 111, 1721-1726.
65. Spencer H, Kramer L, Osis D. Do protein and phosphorous cause calcium loss? *J Nutr*, 1988, 118, 657-660.
66. Liener IE, Kakade ML. Protease inhibitors. In Irvin E. Liener, ed. *Toxic Constituents in Plant Foodstuffs*, (NY Academic Press, Second Edition, 1980). 7-71.
67. Food and Drug Administration. Food Labeling: Health Claims: Soy Protein and Coronary Heart Disease. 21 CFR Part 101. Docket #98PO683.
68. Weber, Jennifer. The impact of the FDA health claim on the soyfoods market and where do we go from here? *Soyfoods 2001*, January 17-19, 2001. Phoenix, AZ. Educational Audio Cassettes.
69. The phrase is used repeatedly on the FDA website's www.usfda.gov The website also includes the FDA's Mission Statement: "The FDA is responsible for protecting the public health by assuring the safety, efficacy, and security of human and veterinary drugs, biological products, medical devices, our nation's food supply, cosmetics, and products that emit radiation. The FDA is also responsible for advancing the public health by helping to spread innovations that make medicines and foods more effective, safer, and more affordable, and helping the public get the accurate, science-based information they need to use medicines and foods to improve their health."
70. Proposed Health Claim for Soy Protein-Containing Products and a Reduced Risk of Heart Disease. Petition submitted by Marshall McMarcus, Director of Regulatory and Trade Affairs, Protein Technologies International, May 4, 1998.
71. Fallon, Sally. Enig, Mary G. Tragedy and Hype: The Third International Soy Symposium. *Nexus*, 2000, 7, 3.
72. James, Valerie. Letter to Documents Management Branch (H.F.A. 305), Food and Drug Administration quoting Section 403. James reminds the FDA that it is "not authorized to regulate on anything other than the petition to the agency. That is, it cannot 'substitute' a variation on the claim and make a proposed (or actual) ruling on this substituted purpose." September 16, 1999.
73. James.
74. Sheehan, Daniel M. Doerge, Daniel R. Letter to Dockets Management Branch (HFA305) February 18, 1999.
75. Fitzpatrick, Michael. Response to a submission by Protein Technologies International (PTI), n.d.
76. IEH Assessment on Phytoestrogens in the Human Diet. Final Report to the Ministry of Agriculture, Fisheries and Food, United Kingdom, November 1997, 11
77. Dibb, Sue. Co-Director The Food Commission UK. Letter to Dockets Management Branch (HFA-305) on Docket No 98P-0683 Food Labelling: Health Claims; Soy Protein and Coronary Heart Disease, January 25, 1999.
78. Liener IE. Letter to Dockets Management Branch, Food and Drug Administration, December 31, 1998.
79. Anderson JW, Johnstone BM, Cook-Newell ME. Meta-analysis of the effects of soy protein intake on serum lipids. *NEJM*, 1995, 333, 276-282.
80. Fitzpatrick M. Soy formulas and the effects of isoflavones on the thyroid. *NZ Med J*, 2000, 113, 1103, 24-26.
81. Ishizuki Y, Hirooka, Maruta Y, Tigashi K. The effects on the thyroid gland of soybeans administered experimentally in healthy subjects. *Nippon Naibundi Gakkai Zasshi*, 1991, 67, 622-629. Translation by Japan Communication Service, Wellington. Courtesy Valerie and Richard James.

Chapter 14: Soy Fat – Shortening Life

1. Enig, Mary G. *Know Your Fats: The Complete Primer for Understanding the Nutrition of Fats, Oils and Cholesterol* (Silver Spring, MD, Bethesda Press, 2000).
2. Fallon, Sally. Enig, Mary G. *Nourishing Traditions*, (New Trends, Second Edition,1999). 4-20.
3. Schmidt, Michael. *Smart Fats: How Dietary Fats and Oils Affect Mental Physical and Emotional Intelligence* (Berkeley, CA, Frog Ltd, 1997).
4. Enig, 104.
5. Fallon, Enig. 10.

6. Enig, 196, 259, 268.
7. Chrysam, Michael M. Margarines and spreads. In YH Hui, ed. *Bailey's Industrial Oil and Fat Products*, Volume 3, Edible Oil and Fat Products: Products and Application Technology (NY,Wiley, 1996). 77.
8. Ashbridge, David D. Soybeans vs other vegetable oils as a source of edible oil products. Huth PJ. Nutritional aspects of soybean oil and soy proteins. In David R. Erickson, ed. *Practical Handbook of Soybean Processing and Utilization* (Champaign, IL, AOCS Press, 1995) 4, 460.
9. Commodity Economics Division, Economic Research Service, US Department of Agriculture, OCS-41, July 1994. Summarized in Erickson, 463.
10. Enig.
11. Messina, Mark. Messina, Virginia. Setchell, Kenneth DR. *The Simple Soybean and Your Health* (Garden City Park, NY, Avery, 1994) 31.
12. Holt, Stephen. *The Soy Revolution* (NY, Evans, 1998) 25.
13. Solomon, Neil. *Soy Smart Health* (Pleasant Grove, UT, Woodland, 2000).
14. Golbitz, Peter. *Tofu and Soyfoods Cookery* (Summertown, TN, Book Publishing Co 1998) 23.
15. Enig, 123.
16. Visser A, Thomas A. Review: soya protein products – their processing, functionality and application aspects. *Food Rev Int*, 1987, 3, 1&2, 1-32.
17. Berk, Z. Technology of production of edible flours and protein products from soybeans. *FAO Bulletin,* Food and Agricultural Organ of the United Nations, Rome, 1993, 97, 15.
18. Boatright WL, Crum AD. Nonpolar-volatile lipids from soy protein isolates and hexane-defatted flakes. *J Am Oil Chem Soc*, 1997, 74, 461-467.
19. Enig, 122-123.
20. Shurtleff, William and Aoyagi, Akiko. *History of Soybean Crushing: Soy Oil and Soybean Meal.* Unpublished manuscript, 1981 (Lafayette, CA, Soyfoods Center). 132-134.
21. Fallon S, Enig MG. The great con-ola. *Wise Traditions*, 2002, 3, 2, 13-20.
22. Enig, 120.
23. Enig, 38.
24. Enig, 105.
25. Schmidt, 45.
26. Enig, 38.
27. Enig,, 36-37.
28. Enig, 154-156.
29. Sipos, Endre F. Szuhaj, Bernard F. Soybean oil. Chapter 11 in Hui YH, ed. *Bailey's Industrial Oil and Fat Products*, Volume 3, Edible Oil and Fat Products: Oils and Oilseeds (NY Wiley, Fifth Edition, 1995), 499.
30. Fallon, Sally and Enig, Mary G. *Nourishing Traditions*, 4-20.
31. Berk, 12 and 15.
32. Liu, KeShun. *Soybeans: Chemistry, Technology, Utilization* (Gaithersburg, MD, Aspen, 1999) 56-57.
33. Fallon and Enig.
34. Enig, 202-203, 207.
35. Shurtleff, Aoyagi. *History of Soybean Crushing*, 98.
36. Shurtleff, Aoyagi. *History of Soy Oil Hydrogenation*, 47.
37. Kraft Foods patents method for inhibiting oxidation of polyunsaturated lipids. US Patents via NewsEdge Corporation, 8/16/2002. www.soyatech.com.
38. Genetic regulation of linolenic acid concentration in wild soybean glycine soja accessions, *J Amer Oil Chem Soc*, 1997, 74, 461-467.
39. Pantalonea VR, Rebetzkeb GJ et al. Du Pont given patent for fat products from high stearic soy oil. European Patents via NewsEdge Corporation, posted 12/21/01 on www.soyatech.com.
40. ARS News Service, (Agricultural Research Service), USDA press wire via News Edge corporation. Posted 7/19/2001 on www.soyatech.com.
41. Messina, Messina, Setchell.
42. Gerster H. Can adults adequately convert alpha-linolenic acid (18:3n-3) to eicosapentaenoic acid (20:5n-3) and docosahexaenoic acid (22:6n-3)? *Inter J Vit Nutr Res*, 1998, 68, 3, 159-173.
43. Enig 65.
44. Horrobin D. The regulation of prostaglandin biosynthesis by manipulation of essential fatty acid metabolism. *Rev Pure Appl Pharm Sci*, 1983, 4, 339-383.
45. Francois CA, Connor SL et al. Supplementing lactating women with flaxseed oil does not increase docosahexaenoic acid in their milk. *Am J Clin Nutr*, 2003, 77, 226-233.
46. Francois CA, Connor Sl et al. Supplementing lactating women with flaxseed oil does not increase docosahexaenoic acid in their milk. *Am J Clin Nutr*, 2003, 77, 226-233.
47. Enig 65.
48. Enig, Mary G. TRANSFATINFOWEB. www.enig.com.
49. Hecker KD, Kris-Etherton PM. Fatty acid research: new discoveries and emerging vistas in UFA and CVD Risk factors. *The Soy Connection*, 2001, 9, 3, 3.
50. Enig, 46.
51. The Facts about Fat. Information Sheet from the Land of Lincoln Soybean Association, Bloomington, IL. n.d.
52. Enig 200.
53. Enig MG, Fallon S. The Oiling of America. www.westonaprice.org.
54. Elson CE et al. The influence of dietary unsaturated *cis* and *trans* and saturated fatty acids on tissue lipids of swine. *Atherosclerosis*, 1981, 40, 115-137.
55. Mann GV Metabolic consequences of dietary *trans* fatty acids. *Lancet*, 1994, 343, 1268-1271.

56. Kohlmeier L et al. Stores of *trans* fatty acids and breast cancer risk, *Am J Clin Nutr*, 1995, 61, 896, A25.

57. Mensink RP, Katan JM. Effect of dietary *trans* fatty acids on high density and low-density lipoprotein cholesterol levels in healthy subjects. *NEJM*, 1990, 323, 439-445.

58. Gayner PJ, Walde DR et al. Milk fat depression, the glucogenic theory, and trans-C18:1 fatty acids. *J Dairy Sci*, 1995, 78, 9, 2008-2015.

59. Willett WC et al. Intake of *trans*-fatty acids and risk of coronary heart disease among women. *Lancet*, 1993, 341, 581-585.

60. Kummerow FA, Zhou Q, Mahfoux MM. Effect of *trans* fatty acids on calcium influx into human arterial endothelial cells. *Am J Clin Nutr*, 1999, 70, 5, 832-838.

61. Hanis T, Zidek V et al. Effects of dietary *trans* fatty acids on reproductive performance of wistar rats. *Br J Nutr*, 1989, 61, 519-529.

62. Enig MG, Munn RJ, Keeney M. Dietary fat and cancer trends – a critique. *Fed Proc*, 1978, 37, 9, 2215-2220.

63. Barnard et al. Dietary *trans*-fatty acids modulate erythrocyte membrane fatty acid composition and insulin binding in monkeys. *J Nutr Biochem*, 1990, 1, 190-195.

64. Felton CV et al. Dietary polyunsaturated fatty acids and composition of human aortic plaques *Lancet*, 1994, 344, 1195.

65. Dunder T, Kuikka L et al. Diet, serum fatty acids and atopic diseases in childhood. *Allergy*, 2001, 56, 5, 425-428.

66. Mann GV et al. Atherosclerosis in the Maasai, *Am J Epidemiol*, 1972, 25, 26-37.

67. Grandgirard A, Bourre JM et al. Incorporation of *trans* long-chain n-3 polyunsaturated fatty acids in rat brain structure and retina. *Lipids*, 1994, 29, 4, 251-258.

68. Petersen J, Opstvedt J. *Trans*-fatty acids: fatty acid composition of lipids of the brain and other organs in suckling piglets. *Lipids*, 1992, 27, 10, 761-769.

69. Teter BB, Sampugna J, Kenney M. Milk fat depression in C57B1/6J mice consuming partially hydrogenated fat. *J Nutr*, 1990, 120, 818-824.

70. Romo GA, Casper DP et al. Abomasal infusion of *cis* or *trans* fatty acid isomers and energy metabolism of lactation dairy cows. *J Dairy Sci*, 1996, 79, 11, 2005-2015.

71. Koletzko B and Muller J. *Cis* and *trans*-isomeric fatty acids in plasma lipids of newborn infants and their mothers. *Biol Neonate*, 1990, 57, 172-178.

72. Chen ZY, Pelletier G et al. *Trans* fatty acid isomers in Canadian human milk. *Lipids*, 1995, 30, 1, 15-21.

73. Letter report on dietary reference intakes for *trans* fatty acids. Food and Nutrition Board, Institute of Medicine, National Academy of Sciences, 2002.

74. Stahl, Pat. Beyond the Headlines: What's New at the FDA, Informing consumers about *trans* fat labeling. *J Am Dietetic Assn*, 2000 www.adajournal.org.

75. American Dietetic Association. Comments on the Food and Drug Administration's Proposed Rule on Food Labeling: *Trans* Fatty Acids in Nutritional Labeling, Nutrient Content Claims, and Health Claims, Docket No 94P-0036, January 19, 2001.

76. Mercola, Joseph. The case of the phantom fat. January 16, 2000. www.mercola.com.

77. Enig. TRANSFATINFOWEB. www.enig.com.

78. Enig, *Know Your Fats*, 191.

79. Enig MG, Atal S, Kenney M, Sampugna J. Isomeric t*rans* fatty acids in the US diet. *J Am Coll Nutr*, 1990, 9, 5, 471-486.

80. Enig MG, Pallansch LA et al. Fatty acid composition of fat of selected food items with emphasis on *trans* components. *J Am Oil Chem Soc*, 1983, 60, 1788-1795.

81. Allison DB, Egan SK et al. Estimated intakes of *trans*-fatty and other fatty acids in the US population. *J Am Dietet Assoc*, 1999, 99, 2. www.adajournal.org.

82. Hunter JE, Applewhite TH. Isomeric fatty acids in the US diet: levels and health perspective. *Am J Clin Nutr*, 1986, 44, 6, 707-717.

83. Hunter JE, Applewhite TH. Reassessment of *trans* fatty acid availability in the US diet. *Am J Clin Nutr*, 1991, 54, 2, 363-369.

84. Enig, Fallon. .Oiling of America.

85. Shurtleff, Aoyagi. *History of Soy Oil Hydrogenation*, 47.

86. Letter report on dietary reference intakes for *trans*-fatty acids. Food and Nutrition Board, Institute of Medicine, National Academy of Sciences, 2002.

87. Enig, Fallon. Oiling of America.

88. Ratnayake WM, Hollywood R et al. Fatty acids in some common food items in Canada, *J Am Coll Nutr*, 1993, 12, 6, 651-660.

89. Enig. 191.

Chapter 15: Soy Carbohydrate – The Flatulence Factor

1   Question sent on November 2, 1998 by Lynn Willeford, Associate Editor of *Dr. Andrew Weil's Self Healing* newsletter, to Clare Hasler at the "Ask an Expert" StratSoy website developed at the University of Illinois at Champaign.and sponsored by the United Soybean Board..

2   Suarez FL, Springfield J, et al. Gas production in humans ingesting a soybean flour derived from beans naturally low in oligosaccharides, *Am J Clin Nutr*, 1999, 69, 1, 135-139.

3   Visser A, Thomas A. Review: soya protein products: their processing, functionality and application aspects. *Food Rev Inter*, 1987, 3 (1&2), 1-32.

4   Liener IE, Implications of antinutritional components in soybean foods, *Crit Rev Food Sci Nutr*, 1994, 34, 1, 49.

5   Suarez F et al. Insights into human colonic physiology obtained from the study of flatus composition. *Am J Physiol*, 1997, 272, 5, pt 1, G1028-1033.
6   Smith Allan K. Circle, Sidney J. *Soybeans; Chemistry and Technology, Volume 1 Proteins* (Westport, CT, Avi Publishing, 1972), p. 181.
7   Jiang T et al. Gas production by feces of infants, *J Pediatric Gastroenterol Nutr*, 2001, 32, 5, 534-541.
8   Levine J et al. Fecal hydrogen sulfide production in ulcerative colitis, *Am J Gastroenterol*, 1998, 93, 1, 83-87.
9   Suarez F et al. Production and elimination of sulfur-containing gases in the rat colon, *Am J Physiol*, 1998, 274, (4, pt1) G727-733.
10   Liu, KeShun. *Soybeans: Chemistry, Technology and Utilization* (Gaithersburg, MD, Aspen, 1999) 72,76.
11   Berk, Zeki. Technology of production of edible flours and protein products from soybeans, Food and Agric Organ of the United Nations, Rome, 1993 *FAO Agricultural Services Bulletin*, 97, 15.
12   Jimenez MJ et al. Biochemical and nutritional studies of germinated soybean seeds, *Arch Lationoam Nutr*, 1985, 35, 3, 480-490. Medline abstract. Article in Spanish.
13   Rackis JJ Flatulence caused by soya and its control through processing, *J Amer Oil Chem Soc*, 1981, 58, 503.
14   Rackis JJ, Flavor and flatulence factors in soybean protein products. *J Agric Food Chem*, 1970, 18, 977.
15   Calloway DH, Hickey CA, Murphy EL, Reduction of intestinal gas-forming properties of legumes by traditional and experimental food processing methods, *J Food Sci*, 1971, 36, 251.
16   Jood S et al. Effect of flatus producing factors in legumes *J Agri Food Chem*, 1985, 33, 268.
17   Liu, 74.
18   Olson AC et al. Flatus-causing factors in legumes in Ory RI, ed. *Antinutrients and Natural Toxicants in Foods* (Westport CT, Food and Nutrition Press, 1981, p. 275.
19   Suarez FL et al. Gas production in humans ingesting a soybean flour derived from beans naturally low in oligosaccharides. *Am J Clin Nutr*, 1999, 69, 1, 135-139.
20   Smith, Circle, 182.
21   Watson RG et al. Circulating gastrointestinal hormoens in patients with flatulent dyspepsis, with and without gallbladder disease, *Digestion*, 1986, 35,4, 211-216.
22   Faulkner-Hogg KB, Selby WS, Loblay RH. Dietary analysis in symptomatic patients with coeliac disease on a gluten-free diet: the role of trace amounts of gluten and non-gluten food intolerances. *Scand J Gastroentrol*, 1999, 34, 8, 784-789.
23   Parsons CM, Zhang Y, Araba M. Nutritional evaluation of soybean meals varying in oligosaccharide content. *Poultry Sci*, 2000, 79,8, 1127-1131.
24   Kane, Janice Roma. Chemical companies fortify with soy: soy receives heavy investment in functional foods from DuPont, ADM and Henkel. *Chemical Market Reporter*, November 8, 1999, 256, 19, FR14.
25   Smith, Circle, 181.
26   Response by Clare Hasler to a question sent to the "Ask an Expert" part of the StratSoy website developed by the University of Illinois and funded by the United Soybean Board. January 18, 1999.
27   Guimaraes VM, de Rezende ST et al. Characterization of alpha-galactosidases from germinating soybean seed and their use for hydrolysis of oligosaccharides, *Phytochem*, 2001, 58, 1, 67-73.
28   Suarez, FL, Springfield J, Levitt MD. Identification of gases responsible for the odour of human flatus and evaluation of a device purported to reduce this odor. *Gut*, 1998, 43, 100-104.
29   Fink RN, Lembo AJ, Intestinal gas. *Curr Treat Options Gastroenterol*, 2001, 4, 4, 333-337.
30   Suarez et al. Failure of activated charcoal to reduce the release of gases produced by colonic flora. *Am J Gastroenterol*, 1999, 94, 1, 208-212.
31   Messina, Mark. Legumes and soybeans: overview of their nutritional profiles and health effects. *Am J Clin Nutr*, 1999, 70, 3, 439S-450S.
32   Grant, 319.
33   Hata Y, Yamamoto M, Nakajima K. Effects of soybean oligosaccharides on human digestive organs: estimate of fifty percent effective dose and maximum non-effective dose based on diarrhea. *J Clin Biochem Nutr*, 1991, 10, 135-144.

Chapter 16: Protease Inhibitors – Tryping on Soy

1.   Rackis JJ. Biologically active components. In Alan K. Smith and Sidney J. Circle, eds. *Soybeans: Chemistry and Technology*, Vol 1, Proteins (Westport, CT, Avi Publishing, 1972) 163-177.
2.   Liener IE, Kakade, ML. Protease inhibitors. In Irvin E. Liener, ed. *Toxic Constituents of Plant Foodstuffs* (NY, Academic Press, Second edition, 1980) 49, 55.
3.   Rackis. 168.
4.   Jimenez MJ et al. Biochemical and nutritional studies of germinated soybean seeds *Arch Latinoam Nutr*, 1985, 35, 3, 480-490. Medline abstract. Article in Spanish.
5.   Liener and Kakade. 14-23.
6.   Rackis, 164.
7.   Calam J, Bojarski JC, Springer CJ. Raw soya-bean flour increases cholecystokinin release in man. *Br. J Nutr*, 1987, 58, 178.
8.   Liener IE. Trypsin inhibitors: Concern for human nutrition or not? *J. Nutr*, 1986, 116, 5, 921.
9.   Anderson RL, Wolfe WJ. Compositional changes in trypsin inhibitors, phytic acid, saponins and isoflavones related to soybean processing. *J Nutr*, 1995, 125, 581S-588S.
10. Miyagi Y, Shiujo S, Trypsin inhibitor activity in commercial soybean products in Japan. *J. Nutr Sci Vitaminolo* (Tokyo), 1997, 43, 5, 575-580.

11. DiPietro CM, Liener IE. Soybean protease inhibitors. *J Food Sci*, 1989, 54, 606-609.
12. Rackis JJ, Gumbmann MR. Protease inhibitors physiological properties and nutritional significance. In Robert L. Ory, ed. *Antinutrients and Natural Toxicants in Foods*. (Westport, CT, Food and Nutrition Press, 1981).203-238.
13. Peace RW, Sarwar G et al. Trypsin inhibitor levels in soy-based infant formulas and commercial soy protein isolates and concentrates. *Food Res Int*, 1992, 25, 137-141.
14. Billings PC, Longnecker MP et al. Protease inhibitor content of human dietary samples. *Nutr Cancer*, 1990, 14, 2, 85-93.
15. Brandon DL, Bates AH, Friedman M. Monoclodal antibody-based enzyme immunoassay of the Bowman-Birk protease inhibitor of soybeans. *J. Agric Food Chem*, 1989, 37, 1192-1196.
16. Rouhana A, Adler-Nissen J et al. Heat inactivation kinetics of trypsin inhibitors during high temperature-short time processing of soymilk. *J Food Science*, 1996, 61, 2, 265-269.
17. Roebuck. Trypsin inhibitors: Potential concern for humans, *J Nutr*, 1987, 117, 398-400.
18. Doell BH, Ebden CJ, Smith CA. Trypsin inhibitor activity of conventional foods which are part of the British diet and some soya products. *Qual Plant Foods Human Nutr*, 1981, 31, 139-150.
19. Sarvar G, L'Abbe MR et al. Influence of feeding alkaline/heat processed proteins on growth and protein and mineral status of rats. *Adv Exp Med Biol*, 1999, 459, 161-177.
20. SCOGS 101. Evaluation of the health aspects of soy protein isolates as food ingredients, Life Sciences Research Office, Food and Drug Administration, Washington DC, FDA/BF-80/3.
21. Witte NH. Soybean meal processing and utilization. In David R. Erickson, ed. *Practical Handbook of Soybean Processing and Utilization*. (Champaign, IL, AOCS Press, 1995), 114-115.
22. Liener, Kakade, 17.
23. Author's telephone interview with Earl Mindell, March 1999.
24. Liener IE. Trypsin inhibitors: concern for human nutrition, *J Nutr*, 1986, 116, 5, 920-923.
25. Krogdahl A, Holm H. Soybean proteinase inhibitors and human proteolytic enzymes: selective inactivation of inhibitors by treatment with human gastric juice. *J Nutr*, 1981, 111.
26. Weber JKP. Chemistry of legume protease inhibitors and their use in taxonomy. Proceedings of the 75th Annual Meeting of the American Oil Chemists Society, Dallas, TX, April 29-May 3, 1984. *Qual Plant Foods Hum Nutr*, 1985, 35, 193.
27. Roebuck BD, Kaplita PV, MacMillan DL. Interaction of dietary fat and soybean isolate (SBI) on azaserine-induced pancreatic carcinogenesis. *Qual Plant Foods Hum Nutr*, 1985, 35, 323-329.
28. Myers BA, Hathcock J, et al. Effects of dietary soya bean trypsin inhibitor concentrate on initiation and growth of putative preneoplastic lesions in the pancreas. of the rat. *Ed Chem Toxic*, 1991, 29,7, 437-443.
29. Rackis, Gumbmann, 215.
30. Grant, Antinutritional effects of soyabean: a review. *Prog Food Nutr Sci*, 1989, 13, 317-348.
31. Harwood JP et al. Effect of long-term feeding of soy-based diets on the pancreas of Cebus monkeys, *Adv Exp Med Biol* 1986 199: 223-237.
32. Gunn RA, Taylor PR, Gangaros EJ. Gastrointestinal illness associated with consumption of a soybean protein extender. *J Food Sci*, 1980, 43, 525-527.
33. Moroz LA, Yang WH. Kunitz soybean trypsin inhibitor. *NEJM*, 1980, 302, 1126-1128.
34. Liener, Kakade, 40-41.
35. Liener, Kakade, 45.
36. Liener, Kakade, 46 and 49.
37. Rackis, Biological and physiological factors in soybeans. *J Am Oil Chemists Soc*, 1974, 51, 165A-166A.
38. Van De Graaff, Kent M. and Fox, Stuart Ira. *Concepts of Human Anatomy and Physiology* (Boston, MA, Wm C. Brown , Fourth Edition, 1995) 795-796.
39. Liener, Kakade, 42-43.
40. Struthers BJ, MacDonald Jr. Effects of raw soy flour feeding in weanling pigs: Comparison with rats and monkeys. *Qual Plant Foods Hum Nutr*, 1985, 35, 331-338.
41. Guilloteau P, Corring T et al. Effect of soya protein on digestive enzymes, gut hormone and anti-soya antibody plasma levels in the preruminant calf. *Reprod Nutr Dev*, 1986, 26 (2B), 717-728.
42. Struthers, MacDonald, 335.
43. Messina, Mark. eLetter to Vickie Nelson of *Mothering* magazine, February 26, 2004.
44. Garthoff LH, Henderson GR et al. The autosow raised miniature swine as a model for assessing the effects of dietary soy trypsin inhibitor. *Food Chem Toxicol*, 2002, 40, 487-500.
45. Garthoff LH, Henderson GR et al. Pathological evaluation, clinical chemistry and plasma cholecystokinin in neonatal and young miniature swine fed soy trypsin inhibitor from 1 to 39 weeks of age. *Food Chem Toxicol*, 2002, 40, 501-516.
46. Center for Food Safety and Applied Nutrition. Non-Clinical Laboratory Study. Final Report. Report Title: Effects of trypsin inhibitor concentrate (TIC) on growth and function of the pancreas in growing miniature swine (a sub-chronic toxicity study). Facility: Beltsville Research Facility, US Food and Drug Administration, division of toxicological research, Beltsville, MD. Study Director: Larry H. Garthoff. Date Study Initiated: October 31, 1986. Date Study Completed: August 19, 1987. Obtained by Valerie and Richard James through Freedom of Information Act, July 16, 1998.
47. Liener IE. Possible adverse effects of soybean anticarcinogens. *J. Nutr*, 1995, 125, 744S-750S.
48. Levison DA, Morgan RG et al. Carcinogenic effect of di(hydroxypropyl)nitrosamine (DHPN) in male Wistar rats: promotion of pancreatic cancer by a raw soya flour diet. *Scand J. Gastroenterol*, 14, 217-224.
49. Morgan RGH, Levison DA et al. Potentiation of the effect of the action of azaserine on the rat pancreas by raw soya bean flour. *Cancer Lett*, 1977, 3, 87-90.
50. McGuiness EE, Morgan R et al. The effects of long-term feeding of soya flour on the rat pancreas. *Scand J*

Gastroenterol, 1980, 15, 497-502.

51. Rackis JJ, Gumbmann MR, Liener IE. The USDA Trypsin Inhibitor Study,I. Background, objectives and procedural details. *Qual Plant Foods Hum Nutr*, 1985, 35, 213-242.

52. Liener IE, Nitsan Z et al. The USDA Trypsin inhibitor study, II. Timed release biochemical changes in the pancreas of rats. *Qual Plant Foods Hum Nutr*, 1985, 35, 243-257.

53. Spangler WL, Gumbmann MR et al. The USDA Trypsin Inhibitor Study, III. Sequential development of pancreatic pathology in rats. *Qual Plant Foods Hum Nutr*, 1985, 35, 359-274.

54. Gumbmann MR, Spangler WI et al. The USDA Trypsin Inhibitor Study, IV. The chronic effects of soy flour and soy protein isolate on the pancreas in rats after two years. *Qual Plant Foods Hum Nutr*, 1985, 35, 275-314.

55. Roebuck BD. Trypsin Inhibitors: potential concern for humans? *J. Nutr*, 1987, 117, 398-400.

56. Myers BA, Hathcock J et al. Effects of dietary soya bean trypsin inhibitor concentrate on initiation and growth of putative preneoplastic lesions in the pancreas of the rat. *Food Chem Toxic*, 1991, 29, 7, 437-443.

57. Liener IE, Hasdai A. The effect of long-term feeding of raw soy flour on the pancreas of mouse and manster. *Adv Exp Med Biol*, 1986, 199, 189-197.

58. Hasdai A, Liener IE. The effects of soy flour and N-nitrosobis (2-osopropyl) amine on the pancreas of the hamster. *Drug Nutr Interact*, 1985, 3, 3, 173-179.

59. Kennedy AR. The evidence for soybean products as cancer preventive agents, *J. Nutr*, 1995, 125, 733S-743S.

60. Liener IE. Letter to the editor: Soybean protease inhibitors and pancreatic carcinogenesis, *J. Nutr*, 1996, 126, 582-583.

61. Liener IE Nitsam Z, et al. The USDA trypsin inhibitor study: Timed released block changes in the pancreas of rats, *Qual Plant Foods Hum Nutr*, 256.

62. Roebuck BD. Trypsin inhibitors: potential concern for humans? *J. Nutr*, 1987, 117, 398-400.

63. Roebuck RD, Kaplita PV, MacMillan. Interaction of dietary fat and soybean isolate (SBI) on azaserine-induced pancreatic carcinogenesis. *Qual Plant Foods Hum Nutr*, 1985, 35, 323-329.

64. Myers.BA, Hathcock J et al. Effects of dietary soya bean trypsin inhibitor concentrate on initiation and growth of putative preneoplastic lesions in the pancreas of the rat. *Fd Chem Toxic*, 1991, 29, 7, 437-443.

65. Liener IE. Possible adverse effects of soybean anticarcinogens, *J Nutr*, 1995, 125, 745S.

66. Temler RS, Dormond CA et al. The effect of feeding soya bean trypsin inhibitor and repeated injections of cholecystokinin on rat pancreas. *Qual Plant Hum Nutr*, 1985, 35, 315-321.

67. Calam J, Bojarski Jc, Springer CJ. Raw soya-bean flour increases cholecystokinin release in man. *Br J Nutr*, 1987, 58, 2, 175-179.

68. Fushiki T, Iwai K. Two hypotheses on the feedback regulation of pancreatic enzyme secretion. *FASEB J*, 1989, 3, 2, 121-126.

69. Smith JP, Kramer St, Solomon TE. CCK stimulates growth of six human pancreatic cancer cell lines in serum-free medium. *Regul Pept*, 1991, 26, 32, 3, 341-349.

70. Smith JP, Solomon TE et al. Cholestokinin stimulates growth of human pancreatic adenocarcinoma SW-1990, *Dig Dis Sci*, 1990, 35, 11, 1377-1384.

71. Liener IE Effect of a trypsin inhibitor from soybeans (Bowman-Birk) on the secretory activity of the human pancreas, *Gastroenterology*, 1988, 94, 419-427.

72. Holm H, Reseland JE et al. Raw soybeans stimulate human pancreatic proteinase secretion. *J. Nutr*, 1992, 122, 1407-1416.

73. Calam J, Bojarski JC, Springer CJ. Raw soya-bean flour increases cholecystokinin release in man. *Br J Nutr*, 1987, 58, 175-179.

74. Liener, Letter to the editor.

75. Lebenthal E. Chooi TS, Lee PC. The development of pancreatic function in premature infants after milk-based and soy-based formulas. *Pediatr Res*, 1981, 15, 9, 1240-1244.

76. American Cancer Society Cancer Reference Information, 2003, How Many People Get Pancreatic Cancer? www.cancer.org.

77. Roebuck BD. Trypsin inhibitors potential concern for humans? *J Nutr*, 1987, 117, 398-400.

78. Myers.BA, Hathcock J et al, 437.

79. Morgan RGH. Wormsley KG. Cancer of the pancreas, *Gut*, 1977, 18, 580-596.

80. Kennedy AR. Letter to the editor: a reply to Liener. *J Nutr*, 1996, 126, 584-585.

81. Pour PM, Pandey KK, Batra SK. What is the origin of pancreatic adenocarcinoma? *Molecular Cancer*, 2003, 2, 1.

82. Struthers, MacDonald, 335.

83. Liener IE. Letter to Dockets Management Branch, Food and Drug Administration, December 31, 1998.

84. Messina M, Messina V. Increasing use of soyfoods and their potential role in cancer prevention. *J Amer Diet Assoc*, 1991, 91, 7, 836-840.

85. Kennedy, Ann. The Bowman-Birk inhibitor from soybeans as an anticarcinogenic agent. *Am J Clin Nutr*, 1998, 68 (suppl), 1406S-1412S.

86. Holm, Reseland.

87. Calam, Bojarski Spinger.

88. Liener IE. Letter to the editor: Soybean protease inhibitors and pancreatic carcinogenesis, *J. Nutr*, 1996, 126, 582-583.

89. Kennedy, 1407-1408S.

90. Kennedy.

91. Kennedy, 1408S.

Chapter 17: Phytates – Ties that Bind

1. Graf E, Empson KL, Eaton JW. Phytic acid, a natural antioxidant. *J Biol Chem*, 1987, 262, 24, 11647-11650.
2. Chitra U, et al. Variability in phytic acid content and protein digestibility of grain legumes, *Plant Foods Hum Nutr*, 1995, 47, 2, 163-172.
3. Sathe SK. Reddy,NR. Introduction. In NR Reddy, SK Sathe, eds.*Food Phytates,*(Boca Raton, FL,CRC Press, 2002) 3.
4. Cornforth DP. Potential use of phytate as an antioxidant in cooked meats. In *Food Phytates*, 199-209.
5. Lott, John NA. Ockenden, Irene et al. A global estimate of phytic acid and phosphorous in crop grains, seeds and fruits. In *Food Phytates*, 15.
6. Thompson LU. Potential health benefits and problems associated with antinutrients in foods. *Food Res Internat*, 1993, 26, 131-149.
7. Weaver CM, Kannan S. Phytate and mineral bioavailability. In *Food Phytates*, 211-223.
8. Shamsuddin AM, Ullah A, Chakravarthy AK. Inositol and inositol hexaphosphate suppress cell proliferation and tumor formation in CD-1 mice. *Carcinogenesis*, 1989, 10, 4161-1463.
9. Jenab M, Thompson LU. Role of phytic acid in cancer and other diseases. In *Food Phytates*, 225-248.
10. Lott, 19.
11. Grabau, Elizabeth. Phytase expression in transgenic plants. In *Food Phytates*, 85-87.
12. Liu, KeShun. *Soybeans: Chemistry, Technology and Utilization* (Gaithersburg, MD, Aspen, 1999) 78-82.
13. Sathe, Reddy, 3.
14. Anderson RL, Wolf WJ. Compositional changes in trypsin inhibitors, phytic acid, saponins and isoflavones related to soybean processing. *J Nutr*, 1995, 125, 518S-588S.
15. Vinh LT, Dworscchak E. Phytate content of some foods from plant origin from Vietnam and Hungary. *Nahrung*, 1985, 29, 2, 161-166.
16. Mohamed A, Ponnamperuma AJP, Hafez YS. New chromophore for phytic acid determination. *Cereal Chem*, 1986, 63, 6, 475-478.
17. Ologhobo AD, et al. Distribution of phosphorus and phytate in some Nigerian varieties of legumes and some effects of processing. *J Food Sci*, 1984, 49, 1, 199-201.
18. Liu, 78-82.
19. Sathe SK, Venkatachalam M. Influence of processing technologies on phytate and its removal. In *Food Phytates*, 157-188.
20. Lonnerdal B, Cederblad A et al. The effect of individual components of soy formula and cows' milk formula on zinc bioavailability. *Am J Clin Nutr*, 1984, 40, 1064-1070.
21. Liener IE, Implications of antinutritional components in soybean foods. *Crit Rev Food Sci Nutr*, 1994, 34, 1, 46-47.
22. Sandberg, Ann-Sofie. In vitro and in vivo degradation of phytate. In *Food Phytates*, 139-152.
23. Hurrell RF et al. Soy protein, phytate and iron absorption in humans. *Am J Clin Nutr*, 1992, 56, 3, 573-578.
24. Lonnerdal B, Bell JG et al. Effect of phytate removal on zinc absorption from soy formula. *Am J Clin Nutr*, 1988, 48, 5, 1301-1306.
25. Davidsson L, Galan P et al. Iron bioavailability studied in infants: the influence of phytic acid and ascorbic acid in infant formulas based on soy isolate. *Pediatr Res*, 1994, 36, 6, 816-822.
26. Cook JD, Morck TA, Lynch SR. The inhibitory effects of soy products on non-heme iron absorption in man. *Am J Clin Nutr*, 1981, 34,12, 2622-2629.
27. Shaw N-S, Chin C-J, Pan W-H. A vegetarian diet rich in soybean products compromises iron status in young students. *J Nutr*, 1995, 125, 212-219.
28. Gaby, Alan R. Literature Review and Commentary: Does eating soy cause iron deficiency? *Townsend Letter for Doctors and Patients*, February/March 1996, 28.
29. ZhonghuaaYu Fang Yi. A study of the effect of fermented soybean in preventing iron deficiency anemia in children, *Zue Za Zhi*, 1989, 23, 6, 352-354. Medline abstract. Article in Chinese.
30. Halberg L. Search for nutritional confounding factors in the relationship between iron deficiency and brain function. *Am. J Clin Nutr*, 1989, 50, 3, 598S-605S, 604S-606S.
31. Eck, Paul, Wilson, Larry. *Toxic Metal in Human Health and Disease* (Phoenix AZ, Eck Institute, 1989).
32. Lonnerdal, Cederblad.
33. Zue-Cun C, et al. Low levels of zinc in hair and blood, pica, anorexia and poor growth in Chinese preschool children. *Am J Clin Nutr*, 1985, 42, 694-700.
34. Turnlund, JR et al. A stable isotope study of zinc absorption in young men: effects of phytate and a-cellulose. *Am J Clin Nutr*, 1984, 40, 1071-1077.
35. Stuart SM, et al. Bioavailability of zinc to rats as affected by protein source and previous dietary intake. *J Nutr*, 1986, 116, 1423-1431).
36. Lonnerdal B, Jayawickrama L, Lien EL. Effect of reducing the phytate content and of partially hydrolyzing the protein in soy formula on zinc and copper absorption and status in infant rhesus monkeys and rat pups. *Am J Clin Nutr*, 1999, 69, 3, 490-496.
37. Rimbach G, Pallauf J. Enhancement of zinc utilization from phytate-rich soy protein isolate by microbial phytase. *Z Ernahrungswiss*, 1993, 32, 4, 308-315.
38. Oberleas D. A stable isotope study of zinc absorption in young men. Effects of phytates and alpha cellulose, *Am J Clin Nutr*, 1984, 40, 1071-1077.
39. Sandstrom B, Almgren A et al. Effect of protein level and protein source on zinc absorption in humans. *J. Nutr*, 1989, 119, 48-53.

40. Sandstrom B, Cederblad A. Zinc absorption from composite meals II. Influence of the main protein source. *Am J Clin Nutr*, 1980, 33, 1778-1783.
41. Lonnerdal B, Jayawickrama L, Lien EL. Effect of reducing the phytate content and of partially hydrolyzing the protein in soy formula on zinc and copper absorption and status in infant rhesus monkeys and rat pups. *Am. J Clin Nutr*, 1999, 69, 3, 490-496.
42. Lykken G, Mahalko J et al. Effects of browning on Zn retention. *Fed Proc*, 1982, 41, 282.
43. Sandstead HH, Dintzis F, Johnson L. Influence of diet fiber, phytate and calcium on human zinc absorption. *Fed Proc*, 1984, 43, 851.
44. DeVizia B, Ziegler EE, Fomon SJ. Effect of varying calcium content on nutrient absorption from infant formulas. *Am J Clin Nutr*, 1982, 34, 892.
45. Lonnerdal, Cederblad.
46. Moser PB, Reynolds RD et al. Copper, iron, zinc and selenium dietary intake and status of Nepalese lactating women and their breast-fed infants. *Am J Clin Nutr*, 1988, 47, 729-734.
47. Messina, Mark. Legumes and soybeans: overview of their nutritional profiles and health effects. *Am J Clin Nutr*, 1999, 70, 3, 439S-450S.
48. Heaney RP, Dowell MS et al. Bioavailability of the calcium in fortified soy imitation milk with some observations on methods. *Amer J Clin Nutr*, 2000, 71, 1166-1169.
49. Liu, 79.
50. Liu.
51. Sandstrom, Cederblad.
52. DeVizia, Ziegler, Fomon.
53. Shamsuddin.
54. Menniti FS, Oliver KG et al. Inositol phosphates and cell signaling: new views of InsP5 and InsP6. *Trends Biochem Sci*, 1993, 18, 53-56.
55. Graf E, Eaton JW. Antioxidant functions of phytic acid. *Free Radic Biol Med*, 1990, 8, 61-69.
56. Zhou JR, Erdman JW. Phytic acid in health and disease. *Crit Rev Food Sci Nutr*, 1995, 35, 495-508.
57. Burgess JR, Gao F. The antioxidant effects of inositol phosphates. In *Food Phytates*, 189-197.
58. Shamsuddin AM, Vucenik I, Cole KE. IP6: a novel anticancer agent. *Life Sci*, 1997, 61, 4, 343-354.
59. Shamsuddin AM, Yang GY, Vucenik I. Novel anti-cancer functions of IP6: growth inhibition and differentiation of human mammary cancer cell lines in vitro. *Anticancer Res*, 1996, 16, 6A, 3287-3292.
60. Baten A, Ullah A et al. Inositol-phosphate-induced enhancement of natural killer cell activity correlates with tumor suppression. *Carcinogenesis*, 1989, 10,9, 1595-1598.
61. Jenab M, Thompson LU. Role of phytic acid in cancer and other diseases. In *Food Phytates*, 225-248.
62. Porres JM et al. dietary intrinsic phytate protects colon from lipid peroxidation in pigs with a moderately high dietary iron intake. *Proc Soc Exp Biol Med*, 221,1, 80-86.
63. Pretlow TP, O'Riordan MA et al. Aberrant crypts correlate with tumor incidence in F344 rats treated with azoxymethane and phytate. *Carcinogenesis*, 1992, 13, 9, 1509-1512.
64. Shamsuddin AM, Elsayed AM, Ullah A. Suppression of large intestinal cancer in F344 rats by inositol hexaphosphate. *Carcinogenesis*, 1988, 9, 4, 577-580.
65. Vucenik I, Yang G-Y, Shamsuddin AM. Comparison of pure inositol hexaphosphate and high-bran diet in the prevention of DMBA-induced rat mammary carcinogenesis, *Nutr Cancer*, 1997, 28, 7-13.
66. Thompson LU, Zhang L. Phytic acid and minerals: effect on early markers of risk for mammary and colon carcinogenesis. *Carcinogenesis*, 1991, 12, 11, 2041-2045.
67. Vucenik I , Zhang ZS, Shamsuddin AM. IP6 in treatment of liver cancer, I. IP6 inhibits growth and reverses transformed phenotype in HepG2 human liver cancer cell line. *Anticancer Res*, 1998, 18, 4083-4090.
68. Hirose M, Ozaki K et al. Modifying effects of the naturally occurring antioxidants gamma-oryzonol, phytic acid, tannic acid and n-tritriacontane-16, 18-dione in rata wide spectrum organ carcinogenesis model. *Carcinogenesis*, 1991, 12, 1917-1921.
69. Estensen RD, Wattenberg LW. Studies of chemo-preventive effects of myo-inositol on benzo(a)otrene induced neoplasia of the lung and forestomach of female A/J mice. *Carcinogenesis*, 1993, 14, 1975-1977.
70. Ishikawa T, Nakatsuru Y et al. Inhibition of skin cancer by IP6 in vivo: initiation-promotion model. *Anticancer Res*, 1999, 19, 5A, 3749-33752.
71. Jarawalla et al. Effect of dietary phytic acid (phytate) on the incidence and growth rate of tumors promoted in Fisher rats by magnesium supplement. *Nutr Res*, 1988, 8, 813-827.
72. Vucenik I, Tomazic VJ et al. Antitumor activity of phytic acid in murine transplanted and metastatic fibrosarcoma. *Cancer Lett*, 1992, 65, 9-13.
73. Thompson LU and Zhang L. Phytic acid and minerals: effect on early markers of risk for mammary and colon carcinogenesis. *Carcinogenesis*, 1991, 12, 2041-2045.
74. Jariwalla.
75. Takaba K, Hirose M et al. Effects of n-tritriaconane-16, 18-dione, curcumin, chlorphyllin, dihydroguaiaretic acid, tannic acid and phytic acid on the initiation stage in a rat multi-organ carcinogenesis model. *Cancer Lett*, 1997, 26, 113, 1-2, 39-46.
76. Vucenik I, Podczasy JJ, Shamsuddin AM. Antiplatelet activity of inositol hexaphosphate (IP6) *Anticancer Res*, 1999, 19, 5A, 3689-3693.
77. Rao PS, Liu X-K et al. Protection of ischemic heart from reperfusion injury by myo-inositol hexaphosphate, a natural antioxidant. *An Thorac Surg*, 1991, 52, 908-912.
78. Jariwalla RJ, Sabin R et al. Lowering of serum cholesterol and triglycerides and modulations by dietary phytate. *J Appl Nutr*, 1990, 42, 18-28.
79. Atkins. Robert C. *Dr. Atkins' Vita-Nutrient Solution* (NY, Simon and Schuster, 1998) 127-132.

80. Ohkawa T, Ebisuno S. Rice bran treatment for patients with hypercalciuric stones: experimental and clinical studies. *J Urol*, 1984, 132, 6, 1140-1145.
81. Hiasa Y, Kitahori Y et al. Carcinogenicity study in rats of phytic acid 'Daiichi', a natural food additive. *Food Chem Toxicol*, 1992, 30, 2, 117-125.
82. Vucenik I, Yang GY, Shamsuddin AM. Comparison of pure inositol hexaphosphate and high-bran diet in the prevention of DMBA-induced rat mammary carcinogenesis. *Nutr Cancer*, 1997, 28, 1, 7-13.
83. Shamsuddin AM, Vucenik I. Mammary tumor inhibition by IP6: a review. *Anticancer Res*, 1999, 19, 5A, 3671-3674.
84. Shamsuddin, Abulkalam M. Inositol phosphates have novel anticancer function, *J. Nutr*, 1995, 125, 725S-732S.
85. Sakamoto K, Vucenik I, Shamsuddin AM. [3H] phytic acid (inositol hexaphosphate) is absorbed and distributed to various tissues in rats. *J Nutr*, 1993, 123, 4, 713-720.

Chapter 18: Lectins – Glutins for Punishment

1. Pusztai, Arpad. *Plant Lectins* (Cambridge University Press, 1991), 64-68, 159-164.
2. Liener IE, Effects of processing on antinutritional factors in legumes: the soybean case. *Arch Latinoam Nutrition*, 1996, 44, (4 Suppl 1) 48S-54S.
3. Rackis JJ Biologically active components. In Allan K Smith. Sidney J. Circle, eds.: *Soybeans: Chemistry and Technology*, Vol 1, Proteins (Westport, CT, 1972).
4. Liener IE. The nutritional significance of plant lectins. In Robert L. Ory, ed. *Antinutrients and Natural Toxicants in Foods* (Westport CT, Food and Nutrition Press, 1981). 143-158.
5. Jaffe, Werner G. Hemagglutinins (lectins). In Irvin E. Liener, ed. *Toxic Constituents of Plant Foodstuffs*. Second edition. (NY Academic Press , 1980) 97-98.
6. Liu, KeShun. *Soybeans: Chemistry, Technology, Utilization* (Gaithersburg, MD, Aspen, 1999) 55-56.
7. Jaffe.
8. Maenz DD, Irish GG, Classen HL. Carbohydrate-binding and agglutinating lectins in raw and processed soybean meals. *Animal Food Science and Technology*, 1999, 76, 335-343.
9. Calderon de la Barca AM, Vazquaz-Moreno L, Robles-Burgueno MR, Active soybean lectin in food: Isolation and quantitation. *Food Chem*, 1991, 39, 321-327.
10. Pusztai, *Plant Lectins*, 109-110.
11. Pusztai A, Ewen SWB et al. Relationship between survival and binding of plant lectins during small intestinal passage and their effectiveness as growth factors. *Digestion*, 1990, 46, 308-315.
12. Pusztai, *Plant Lectins*, 109-111, 145.
13. Jindal S, Soni GL, Singh R. Biochemical and histopathological studies in albino rats fed on soyabean lectin. *Nutr Rep Inter*, 1984, 29, 95-106.
14. Torres-Pinedo R. Lectins and the intestine. *J Pediatr Gastroenterol Nutr*, 1983, 2, 588-594.
15. Pusztai, 159-160.
16. Maenz DD, Irish GG, Classen HL. Carbohydrate binding and agglutinating lectins in raw and processed soybean meals. *Animal Feed Sci Tech*, 1999, 76, 335-343.
17. Vasconcelos IM, Trentim A et al. Purification and physiochemical characteriszation of soyatoxin, a novel toxic protein isolated from soybeans (Glycine max). *Arch Biochem Biophys*, 1994, 312, 2, 357-366.
18. Pusztai, *Plant Lectins*, 160-161.
19. Grant G, Watt WB, et al. Changes in the small intestine and hind leg muscles of rats induced by dietary soyabean (Glycine max) proteins. *Med Sci Res*, 1987, 15, 1197-1198.
20. Jordinson M, Deprez PH et al. Soybean lectin stimulates pancreatic exocrine secretion via CCK-A receptors in rats. *Am J Physiol*, 1996, 270, 4 pt 1, G653-659.
21. Pusztai, *Plant Lectins*, 134, 144.
22. Ament ME, Rubin CE. Soy protein – another cause of the flat intestinal lesion. *Gastroenterol*, 1972, 62, 2, 227-234.
23. Poley JR, Klein AW. Scanning electron microsocopy of soy protein-induced damage of small bowel mucosa in infants. *J. Pediatr Gastroenterol Nutr*, 1983, 2, 2, 271-287.
24. Perkkio M, Savilahti E, Kuitunen P, Morphometric and immunohistochemical astudy of jejunal biopsies from children with intestinal soy allergy. *Eur J Pediatr*, 1981, 137, 1, 63-69.
25. deAizpurua HJ, Russel-Jones GJ. Oral vaccination: Identification of classes of proteins that provoke an immune response on oral feeding. *J Exper Med*, 19988, 167, 440-451.
26. Pusztai, *Plant Lectins*, 144-145.
27. Pusztai, 151-158.
28. Pusztai A, Grant G et al. Kidney bean lectin-induced Escherichia coli overgrowth in the small intestine is blocked by GNA, a mannose specific lectin. *J Appl Bacteriol*, 1993, 75, 4, 360-368.
29. Pusztai, *Plant Lectins*, 111.
30. Pusztai A. Grant G et al. Novel dietary strategy for overcoming the antinutritional effects of soyabean whey of high agglutinin content. *Br J Nutr*, 1997, 77, 6, 933-945.
31. Great Smokies Diagnostic Laboratory. Assessing Physiological Function. Interpretive Guidelines, Intestinal Permeability, 1996, 6.
32. D'Adamo, Peter. *Eat Right 4 Your Type* (New York, NY, Putnam, 1996).
33. Freed, David, Do dietary lectins cause disease? The evidence is suggestive and raises interesting possibilities for treatment. *Br Med J*, 1999, 318, 1023-1024.
34. Mercola, Joseph. *The No Grain Diet* (New York, NY, Dutton, 2003).

35. Tortora GJ, Anagnostakos NP, *Principles of Anatomy and Physiology* , Sixth Edition, Harper & Row, 1990, p. 563. The incidence in the white population is type A, 41 percent; type B, 10 percent; type AB, 4 percent; type O, 45 percent. Among blacks, Type A, 27 percent; Type B, 20 percent; Type AB, 7 percent; Type O, 46 percent.
36. Fort P, Lanes R et al. Breast feeding and insulin-dependent diabetes mellitus in children. *J Am Coll Nutr*, 1986, 5, 5, 439-441.
37. Scott FW Cow milk and insulin-dependent diabetes mellitus: is there a relationship? *Am J Clin Nutr*, 1990, 51, 489-491.
38. Dahl-Jorgensen K, Joner G, Hanssen KF. Relationship between cows' milk consumption and incidence of IDDM in childhood. *Diabetes Care*, 1991, 14, 1081-1083.
39. Freed.
40. Firth, Peta. Leaving a bad taste: the furor in Britain raises health safety concerns about genetically modified foods. *Scientific American*, May, 1999.
41. Wolfson, Richard. Research of Dr. Arpad Pusztai on genetically manipulated foods, *Biotech News*, May 1999.
42. Pusztai, *Plant Lectins*, 74, 77.
43. Doyle R and Keller K. Lectins in diagnostic microbiology. *Eur J Clin Microbiol*, 1984, 3, 4-9.
44. D'Adamo.
45. Pryme IF, Bardocz S et al. Switching between control and phytohaemagglutinin-containing diets affects growth of Krebs II ascites cells and produces differences in the levels of putrescine, spermiidine and sperime. *Cancer Letter*, 1995, 13, 93, 2, 233-237.
46. Pryme IF, Pusztai A et al. The induction of gut hyperplasia by phytohaemagglutinin in the diet and limitation of tumour growth. *Histol Histopathol*, 1998, 13, 2, 575-583.
47. Drachtenberg CB, Papadimitriou JC. Aberrant pattern of lectin binding in low and high grade prostatic intraepithelial neoplasia. *Cancer*, 1995, 15, 75, 10, 2539-2544.
48. Torres-Pinedo R.
49. Kilpatrick DC. Immunological aspects of the potential role of dietary carbohydrates and lectins in human health. *Eur J Nutr*, 1999, 38, 3, 107-117.
50. Ching CK, Black R et al. Use of lectin histochemistry in pancreatic cancer. *J Clin Pathol*, 1988, 41, 3, 324-328.

Chapter 19: Saponins – Soap in Your Mouth

1. Zablotowicz RM, Hoagland RE, Wagner SC. Effect of saponins on the growth and activity of rhizosphere bacteria. In George R. Waller and Kazuo Yamasaki, eds. *Saponins Used in Food and Agriculture*. (NY, Plenum, 1996) 83-95.
2. Waller GR, Yang CF et al. Can soyasaponin I and mono-andbi-desmosides isolated from mungbeans serve as growth enhancers in mungbeans and lettuce? In *Saponins Used in Food and Agriculture*, 123-139.
3. Okubo K, Hoshiki Y. Oxygen-radical-scavenging activity of DDMP-conjugated saponins and physiological role in leguminous plant. In *Saponins Used in Food and Agriculture*, 141-154.
4. Birk, Yehudith and Puri, Irena. Saponins. In Irvin E. Liener, ed. *Toxic Constituents of Plant Foodstuffs*, (New York, NY, Academic Press, Second Edition 1980, 170).
5. Liener IE. Factors affecting nutritional quality of soya products. *J Am Oil Chem Soc*, 1981, 58, 406-415.
6. Liener IE. Possible adverse effects of soybean anticarcinogens. *J Nutr*, 1995, 125, 744S-750S.
7. Rao AV, Sung M-K. Saponins as anticarcinogens. *J Nutr*, 1995, 125, 717S-724S.
8. Onning G, Asp N-G. Analysis, heat stability and physiological effects on saponins from oats. In *Saponins Used in Food and Agriculture*, 371-373.
9. Liener.
10. Oleszek W. Alfalfa saponins: structure, biological activity and chemotaxonomy. In *Saponins Used in Food and Agriculture*, 160.
11. Rao, 720S.
12. Hronek M, Benes P. Horsky J. The effect of saponinium album Merck on changes in the hemolytic resistance of erythrocytes in relation to age in healthy persons. *Cas Lek Cesk* 1989, 128, 22, 685-687. Medline abstract. Article in Czech.
13. Birk, Puri, 176-177.
14. Liener, Implications of antinutritional components in soybean foods, *Crit Rev Food Sci Nutr*, 1994, 34, 1, 48.
15. Kimura S, Suwa J et al. Development of malignant goiter by defatted soybean with iodine-free diet in rats. *Japanese J Cancer Res*, 1976, 67, 763-765.
16. Rao, 718S.
17. Anderson RL, Wolfe WJ. Composition changes in trypsin inhibitors, phytic acid, saponins and isoflavones related to soybean processing. *J Nutr*, 1995, 125, 581S-588S.
18. Fenwick DE, Oakenfull D. Saponin content of food plants and some prepared foods. *J Sci Food Agric*, 1983, 34, 186-191.
19. Liu, KeShun. *Soybeans: Chemistry, Technology, Utilization* (Gaithersburg, MD, Aspen, 1999) 231.
20. Johnson IT, Gee JM et al. Influence of saponins on gut permeability and active nutrient transport in vitro. *J Nutr*, 1986, 116, 2270.
21. Rao AV and Sung MK, Saponins as anticarcinogens, *J Nutr*, 1995, 125, 717S-724S.
22. Pathirana C, Gibney MJ, Taylor TG. Effects of soy protein and saponins on serum and liver cholesterol in rats. *Atherosclerosis*, 1980, 36, 595.
23. Sidhu GS and Oakenfull DG. A mechanism for the hypocholesterolemic activity of saponins, *Br J Nutr*, 1986, 7, 55, 643.

24. Cheeke PR. Biological effects of feed and forage saponins and their impacts on animal production. In *Saponins Used in Food and Agriculture*, 382-383.
25. Kritchevsky D. Soya, saponins and plasma cholesterol, *Lancet*, March, 610, 1979.
26. Sautier C, Doucet C et al. effects of soy protein and saponins on serum tissue and feces steroids in rat. *Atherosclerosis*, 1979, 34, 233.
27. Rath, Matthias, Pauling Linus. A unified theory of human cardiovascular disease leading the way to the abolition of this disease as a cause for human mortality. www.mercola.com/2001/mar/28/cvd.htm.
28. Cheeke.
29. Micich TJ, Foglia TA, Holsinger VH. Polymer-supported saponins: an approach to cholesterol removal from butteroil. *J Agric Food Chem*, 1992, 40, 1321.
30. Rao AV, Sung MK, Saponins as anticarcinogens, *J Nutr*, 1995, 125, 717S-724S.
31. LaValle, James B. Introduction to Bowel Terrain. Post Graduate Studies in Clinical Nutrition, Session 3: Human Toxicity, Related Conditions and Therapy Protocols. Clinical Nutritionists Certification Board, 1999.
32. Rao.
33. LaValle.
34. Yanick Paul Jr. Jaffe, Russell. *Clinical Chemistry & Nutrition Guidebook*: A Physicians Desk reference (T&H Publishing, 1988) 71.
35. Bomford R. Saponin and other haemolysins (vitamin A, aliphatic amines, polyene antibiotics) as adjuvants for SRBC in the mouse. Evidence for a role for cholesterol-binding in saponin adjuvanticity. *Inter Archives Allergy Applied Immunol*, 1980, 65, 2, 170-177.
36. Birk, Puri, 168-169.
37. www.nursespdr.com.
38. Estrada A, et al. Isolation and evaluation of immunological adjuvant activities of saponins from Polygala senega L. *Comp Immunolo Microbiol Infect Dis*, 2000, 23, 1, 27-43.
39. Ellary AA, Nour SA, Correlation between the spermicidal activity and the haemolytic index of certain plant saponins, *Pharmazie*, 1979, 34, 9, 560-561.

Chapter 20: Oxalates – Casting Stones

1. Massey LK, Palmer RG, Horner HT. Oxalate content of soybean seeds (Glycine max: Leguminosae), soyfoods, and other edible legumes. *J Agric Food Chem*, 2001, 49, 9, 4262-4266.
2. ADA quoted by Massey.
3. Massey quoted by the American Chemical Society. www.acs.org.
4. www.niddk.nih.gov.
5. Solomons, Clive. www.vulvarpainfoundation.org.
6. Yount, Joanne. Letter to author, March 15, 2004.
7. Yount J, ed. *The Vulvar Pain Newsletter*, 1994-2002. Numbers 4, 9, 12, 17, 21.
8. Solomons.
9. Solomons CC, Melmed MH, Heitler SM. Calcium citrate for vulvar vestibulitis. *J Repro Med*, 1991, 361, 12, 879-882.
10. Jahnen A, Heynck H, et al. Dietary fibre: the effectiveness of a high bran intake in reducing renal calcium excretion. *Urol Res*, 1992, 20, 1 3-6.
11. Massey.

Chapter 21: Manganese Toxicity – ADD-ing it Up

1. Underwood EJ. *Trace Elements in Human and Animal Nutrition*. (NY Academic Press, 1977).
2. Wilson, Lawrence. *Nutritional Balancing and Hair Mineral Analysis* (Scottsdale, AZ, Wilson Consultants, 1992)
3. Atkins, Robert. *Dr. Atkins' VitaNutrient Solution* (NY Simon and Shuster, 1998) 140-143.
4. Keen CL, Bell JG, Lonnderdal B. The effect of age on manganese uptake and retention from milk and infant formulas in rats. *J Nutr*, 1986, 116, 3, 395-402.
5. Davidsson L, Alingren A et al. Manganese absorption in humans: the effect of phytic acid and ascorbic acid in soy formula. *Am J Clin Nutr*, 1995, 62, 5, 984-987.
6. Tran TT, Chowanadisai W et al. Effect of high dietary manganese intake of neonatal rats on tissue mineral accumulation, striatal dopamine levels, and neurodevelopmental status. *Neurotoxicol*, 2002, 23, 635-643.
7. Tran TT, Crinella FM et al. Effects of neonatal dietary manganese exposure on brain dopamine levels and neurocognitive functions. *Neurotoxicol*, 2002, 23, 645-651.
8. Stasny D, Voegl RS, Picciano MF. Manganese intake and serum manganese concentration of human milk-fed and formula fed infants. *Am J Clin Nutr*, 1984, 39, 6, 872-878.
9. Goodman, David. Manganese madness. *Wise Traditions* www.westonaprice.org, 2001, 2, 3, 53-57.
10. Lonnerdal B, Keen CL et al. Iron, zinc, copper and manganese in infant formulas. *Am J Dis Child*, 1983, 137, 5, 433-437.
11. Collipp PJ, Chen SY, Maitinsky S. Manganese in infant formulas and learning disability, *Ann Nutr Metab*, 1983, 27, 488-494.
12. Pihl RO, Parks M, Hair element content in learning disabled children. *Science*, 1977, 198, 204-206.
13. Marlowe M, Bliss L. Hair element concentrations and young children's behavior at school and home. *J Orthomolec Med*, 1993, 9, 1-12.

14. Collipp PJ, Chen SY, Maitinsky S. Manganese in infant formulas and learning disability. *Ann Nutr Metab*, 1983, 493-500.
15. Goodman.
16. Carl L. Keen, Ph.D., UC Davis, as quoted by Goodman.
17. Collipp, Chen, Maitinsky.
18. Keen CL, Bell JG, Lonnerdal B. Effect of age on manganese uptake and retention from milk and formulas in rats. *J Nutr*, 1986, 116, 395-402.
19. Bell JG, Keen CL, Lonnerdal BL. Higher retention of manganese in suckling than in adult rats is not due to maturational differences in manganese uptake by rat small intestine. *J Tox and Env Health*, 1989, 26, 387-398.
20. Lonnerdal B, Keen CL, Hurley LS. Manganese binding proteins in human and cow's milk. *Am J Clin Nutr*, 1985, 41, 550-559.
21. Collipp.
22. Crinella.
23. Goodman.
24. Crinella.
25. Lonnerdal quoted by Crinella.
26. Cawle J. Psychiatric sequelae of manganese exposure in the adult, foetal and neonatal nervous systems. *Austral NZ J Psychiat*, 1985, 19, 211-217.
27. Tran, Crinella.
28. Tran, Chowanadisai et al.
29. Crinella.
30. Tran, Crinella et al.
31. Crinella.
32. Goodman.
33. Underwood, EJ. Chapter 3: Trace Elements. In *Toxicants Occurring Naturally in Foods*, (Washington, DC, National Academy of Sciences, Second Edition 1973).
34. Donaldson J, Barbeau A. Manganese neurotoxicity: possible clues to the etiology of human brain disorders. In S Gabay, T. Harris, BT eds. *Neurology and Neurobiology*,(NY Alan R. Liss, 1985) 259-285.
35. Barceloux DG. Manganese. *J Clin Toxicol*, 1999, 37, 2, 293-307.
36. Swanson JM, Sergeant JA et al. Attention-deficit hyperactivity disorder and hyperkinetic disorder. *Lancet*, 1998, 429-433.
37. Van Gossum A, Neve J. Trace element deficiency and toxicity. *Curr Opin Nutr Metab Care*, 1998, 1, 6, 499-507.
38. Van Gossum, Neve.
39. Singh M, Kanwar KC. Effect of fluoride on copper, manganese and zinc in bone and kidney. *Bull Environ Contam Toxicol*, 1981, 26, 3, 428-31.
40. Zeyuan D, Bingying T et al. Effect of green tea and black tea on the metabolism of mineral elements in old rats. *Biol Trace Elem Res*, 1998, 65, 1, 75-86.
41. Schuld, Andreas. *PFPC Newsletter* #5. www.bruha.com/fluoride/html/pfpc_html.
42. Wallwork JC, Milne DB et al. Severe zinc deficiency effects on the distribution of nine elements (potassium, phosphorus, sodium, magnesium, calcium, iron, zinc, copper and manganese) in regions of the rat brain. *J Nutr*, 1983, 113, 10, 1895-1905.
43. Murphy VA, Rosenberg JM et al. Elevation of brain manganese in calcium deficient rats. *Neurotoxicol*, 1991, 12, 255-264.
44. Rossanderr-Hulten L, Bruned M et al. Competitive inhibition of iron absorption by manganese and zinc in humans. *Am J Clin Nutr*, 1991, 54, 152-156.
45. Testimonies at Assembly Committee on Public Safety. Is there a relationship between elevated manganese levels and violent behavior? An informational hearing, November 17, 2004, 10 a.m. to 2 p.m., State Capitol, Room 126, Sacramento, CA.
46. Weiss B. Manganese in the context of an integrated risk and decision process. *Neurotoxicology*, 1999, 20, 2-3, 519-525.
47. Kawada J, Nishida M et al. Manganese ion as a goitrogen in the female mouse. *Endocrinol Jpn*, 1985, 32, 5, 635-643.
48. Buthieau Am, Autissier N. Effects of manganese ions on thyroid function in rat. *Arch Toxicol*, 1983, 54, 3, 243-246.
49. Burch HB Barnes S et al. Immunodetection of manganese superoxide dismutase in cultured human retroocular fibrlblasts using sera directed against the thyrotropin receptor. *J Endocrinol Invest*, 1998, 21, 1, 48-55.
50. Finley JW, Davis CD. Manganese deficiency and toxicity: are high or low dietary amounts of manganese cause for concern? *Biofactors*, 1999, 10, 1, 15-24.
51. Murphy, Rosenberg et al.
52. Ali MM, Murthy RC et al. Effect of low protein diet on manganese neurotoxicity: III. Brain neurotransmitter levels. *Neurobehav Toxicol Teratol*, 1985, 7, 5, 427-431.
53. Lasekan quoted by Goodman.
54. Keen CL, Bell JC, Lonnerdal B. The effect of age on manganese uptake and retention from milk and infant formulae in rats. *J Nutr*, 1986, 116, 395-402.
55. Mountford quoted by Goodman.
56. Tran, Trinh. E mail correspondence to Valerie and Richard James, June 11, 2001.
57. Caton, Greg. Soy manufacturer warns mothers against feeding newborns their soymilk. Press Release, Lumen Foods, June 11, 2001.
58. Presley, Robert, as quoted by Goodman.

59. Assembly Committee on Public Safety. Is there a relationship between elevated manganese levels and violent behavior? An informational hearing, November 17, 2004, 10 a.m. to 2 p.m., State Capitol, Room 126, Sacramento, CA.

Chapter 22: Fluoride Toxicity – Dental and Mental Fluorosis

1. Gosselin, Robert E, ed. *Clinical Toxicology of Commercial Products* (Lippincott/Williams & Wilkins, Fifth Edition, 1984).
2. ATSDR/USPHS. Toxicological profile for fluorides, hydrogen fluoride and fluorine (F). CAS #16984-48-8, 7664-39-3, 7782-41-4. 1993. www.atsdr.cdc.gov/tfacts11.html.
3. Schuld, Andreas. Fluoride   what's wrong with this picture? *The Fluoride Stop.* www.bruha.com/fluoride.
4. Yiamouyannis J. Water fluoridation and tooth decay: results from the 1986-1987 national survey of U.S. school children. *Fluoride,* 1990, 23, 55-67.
5. Schuld.
6. Stanley VA. Implications of fluoride – an endless uncertainty. *J Envir Biol,* 2002, 23, 1, 81-87.
7. Schuld.
8. Eck, Paul and Wilson, Larry. *Toxic Metal in Human Health and Disease* (Eck Institute of Applied Nutrition and Bioenergetics, 1989).
9. Pendrys DG, Katz RV, Morse DE. Risk factors for enamel fluorosis in a fluoridated population. *Am J Epidemiol,* 1994, 140, 5, 461-471.
10. Shulman JD, Lalumandier JA, Grabenstein JD. The average daily dose of fluoride: a model based on fluid consumption. *Pediatr Dent,* 1995, 17, 1, 13-18.
11. Levy SM, Zarei MZ. Evaluation of fluoride exposures in children. *ASDC J Dent Child,* 1991, 58, 6, 467-473.
12. Kiritsy MC, Levy SM et al. Assessing fluoride concentrations of juices and juice-flavored drinks. *J Am Dent Assoc,* 1996, 127, 7, 895-902.
13. Singer L, Ophaug R. Total fluoride intake of infants. *Pediatrics,* 1979, 63, 3, 460-466.
14. Buzalaf MA, Granjeiro JM et al. Fluoride content of infant formulas prepared with deionized, bottled mineral and fluoridated drinking water. *ASDC J Dent Child,* 2001, 68, 1, 37-41, 10.
15. McKnight-Hanes MC, Leverett DH et al. Fluoride content of infant formulas: soy-based formulas as a potential factor in dental fluorosis. *Pediatr Dent,* 1988, 10, 3, 189-194.
16. Van Winkle S, Levy SM et al. Water and formula fluoride concentrations: significance for infants fed formula. *Pediatr Dent,* 1995, 17, 4, 305-310.
17. How airborne fluorides can poison food. *Prevention,* February 1972, 77-83.
18. Jacobson JS, Weinstein LH et al. The accumulation of fluorine by plants. *J Air Polluiont Control Assoc,* 1966, 16, 8, 412-417.
19. Weinstein LH, McCune DC. Effects of fluoride on agriculture. *J Air Pollut Control Assoc,* 1971, 21, 7, 410-413.
20. Weinstein, Leonard. E-mail to author. August 9, 2003.
21. Silva M, Reynolds EC. Fluoride content of infant formulae in Australia. *Aust Dent J,* 1996, 41, 1, 37-42.
22. Fomon SJ, Ekstrand J. Fluoride intake by infants. *J Public Health Dent,* 1999, 59, 4, 229-234.
23. Pendrys DG, Katz RV, Morse DE. Risk factors for enamel fluorosis in fluoridated population. *Am J Epidemiol,* 1994, 140, 5, 461-471.
24. Buzalaf, Granjeiro et al.
25. Shulman, Lalumandier, Grabenstein.
26. Levy, Zarei.
27. McKnight-Hanes, Leverett.
28. Van Winkle, Levy.
29. Eklund G, Oskarsson A. Exposure of cadmium from infant formulas and weaning foods. *Food Additives Contam,* 1999, 16, 12, 509-519.
30. Dabeka RW, McKenzie AW. Lead, cadmium and fluoride levels in milk and infant formulas in Canada. *J Assoc Off Anal Chem,* 1987, 70, 4, 754-757.
31. Eck, Wilson.
32. Pendrys, Katz, Morse.
33. Fomon, Ekstrand.
34. Forbes, Barry. Prominent researcher apologizes for pushing fluoride. *The Tribune* (Mesa, AZ), December 5, 1999. www.mercola.com.
35. Schuld.
36. Forbes.
37. Danielson C, Lyon JL et al. Hip fractures and fluoridation in Utah's elderly population. *JAMA,* 1992, 268, 6, 746-748.
38. Jacobsen SJ, Goldberg J et al. The association between water fluoridation and hip fracture among white women and men aged 65 years and older. A national ecologic study. *Ann Epidemiol,* 1992, 5, 617-626.
39. Karagas MR Baron JA et al. Patterns of fracture among the United States elderly: geographic and fluoride effects. *Ann Epidemiol,* 1996, 6, 3, 209-216.
40. National Academy of Sciences.
41. Foulkes, Richard G. The fluoride connection, *Townsend Letter for Doctors and Patients,* April 1998, 12-17.
42. Glasser, George. Mental fluorosis: brain damage from exposure to fluorides, *Sarasota ECO Report,* 1995, 5, 2, 1-5.

43. Mullenix PJ, Denbesten PK et al. Neurotoxicity of sodium fluoride in rats. *Neurotoxicol Teratol,* 1995, 17, 2, 169-177.
44. Long YG, Wang YN et al. Chronic fluoride toxicity decreases the number of nicotinic acetylcholine receptors in rat brain. *Neurotoxicol Teratol,* 2002, 24, 6, 751-757.
45. Luke J. Fluoride deposition in the aged pineal gland. *Caries Res,* 2001, 35, 2, 125-128.
46. Bhatnagar M, Rao P et al. Neurotoxicity of fluoride: neurodegeneration in hippocampus of female mice. *Indian J Exp Biol,* 2002, 40, 5, 546-554.
47. Foulkes.
48. Li SX, Zhi Jl, Gao RO. Effect of fluoride exposure on intelligence of children. *Fluoride,* 1995, 28, 4, 189-192.
49. Lin Fa-Fu, Aihaiti, Zhao Hong-Xin et al. The relationship of a low-iodine and high-fluoride environment to subclinical cretinism in Xinjiang. ICCIDD Newsletter, 1991, 7, 3. http://64.177.90.157/science/html/lin_fa-fu.html
50. Symptoms/Associations. Fluoride Poisoning/Thyroid Dysfunction . http://bruha.com/pfpc/html/symptoms.html.
51. Glasser.
52. Spittle B. Psychopharmacology of fluoride: a review. *Int Clin Psychopharmacol,* 1994, 9, 2, 79-82.
53. Van der Voet GB, Schijns O, de Wolff FA. Fluoride enhances the effect of aluminum chloride on interconnections between aggregates of hippocampal neurons. *Arch Physiol Biochem,* 1999, 107, 1, 15-21.
54. Foulkes.
55. Schuld.
56. Schuld.

Chapter 23: Aluminum Toxicity – Foil-ing Health

1. American Academy of Pediatrics. Policy Statement: Aluminum toxicity in infants and children (RE9607), March 1996. www.aap.org/policy/o1263.
2. Underwood EJ. Trace elements. In *Toxicants Occurring Naturally in Foods.* (Washington, DC, National Academy of Sciences, 1973).
3. Eck, Paul C and Wilson, Larry. *Toxic Metal in Human Health and Disease.* (Phoenix, AZ, Eck Institute of Applied Nutrition and Bioenergetics, 1989).1-5.
4. Koo WWK, Kaplan LA. Aluminum and bone disorders: with specific reference to aluminum contamination of infant nutrients. *J Am Coll Nutr,* 1988, 7, 3, 199-214.
5. Eck, Wilson.
6. Koo, Kaplan.
7. Koss, Kaplan.
8. Koo WWK, Kaplan LA, Krug-Wispe SK. Aluminum contamination of infant formulas. *J Parenteral Enteral Nutr,* 1988, 12, 170-173.
9. Hawkins NM, Coffee S et al. Potential aluminum toxicity in infants fed special infant formula. *J Pediatr Gastroenterol Nutr,* 1994, 19, 4, 377-381.
10. Nolan CR, Califano JR et al. Influence of calcium acetate of calcium citrate on intestinal aluminum absorption, *Kidney Int,* 1990, 38, 937-941.
11. Freundlich M, Zilleruelo G et al. Infant formula as a cause of aluminum toxicity in neonatal ureamia. *Lancet,* 1985, 2, 527-529.
12. Weintraub R, Hans G et al. High aluminum content of infant milk formulas. *Arch Dis Child,* 1986, 61, 914-916.
13. Koo, Kaplan, Krug-Wispe.
14. Hawkins, Coffey et al.
15. Koo, Kaplan, Krug-Wispe.
16. Koo, Kaplan.
17. Hawkins, Coffey et al.
18. Polinsky MS, Cruskin AB. Aluminum toxicity in children with chronic renal failure. *J Pediatr,* 1984, 105, 758-761.
19. Andreoli SP, Bergstein JM, Sherrard DJ. Aluminum intoxication from aluminum-containing phosphate binders in children with azotemia not undergoing dialysis. *NEJM,* 1984, 310, 1079-1084.
20. Sedman AB, Wilkening GN et al. Encephalopathy in childhood secondary to aluminum toxicity. *J Pediatr,* 1984, 105, 836-838.
21. Salusky IB, Foley J et al. Aluminum accumulation during treatment with aluminum hydroxide and dialysis in children and young adults with chronic renal disease. *NEJM,* 1991, 324, 527-531.
22. van der Voet GB, Scijus O, deWolff FA. Fluoride enhances the effect of aluminum chloride on interconnections between aggregates of hippocampal neurons. *Arch Physiol Biochem,* 1999, 107, 1, 5-21.
23. Koo, Kaplan.
24. Koo, Kaplan, Krug-Wispe.
25. Hawkins, Coffey et al.
26. American Academy of Pediatrics.
27. American Academy of Pediatrics.
28. Koo.
29. Eck, Wilson.
30. Koo, Kaplan, 209.
31. Hawkins, Coffey, 380.

end notes - 24

Chapter 24: The Rise in Soy Allergies

1 Berger, Stuart. *Dr. Berger's Immune Power Diet* (NY, New American Library, 1986) 47.
2. FAO Food Allergies Report of the Technical Consultation of the Food and Agricultural Organization of the United Nations, Rome, November 13-14, 1995.
3. Bousquet J, Bjorksten B et al. Scientific criteria and selection of allergenic foods for labeling. *Allergy*, 1998, 53 (Suppl 47) 3-21.
4. Wraith DG, Young GVD, 1979 In: *The Mast Cell: Its Role in Health and Disease*. (London, Piman Medical, 1979).
5. Bush RK, Hefle SL. Food allergens. *Crit Rev Food Sci Nutr*, 1996, 368, S119-S163.
6. Mekori YA. Introduction to allergic disease. *Crit Rev Food Sci Nutr*, 1996, 36S, S1- S18.
7. Saulo, AA. Food allergy and other food sensitivities, *Food Safety and Technology*, University of Hawaii Honolulu, HI, Cooperative Extension Service, Dec. 2002.
8. Taylor SL. Allergic and sensitivity reactions to food components. *Nutritional Toxicology*, Vol 2, John N. Hatchcock, ed, (NY, Academic Press, 1982).
9. Lemke, RJ, Raylor S. Allergic reactions and food intolerances. In Frank N. Kotsonis, Maureen Mackey, eds *Nutritional Toxicology,*. (Taylor and Francis, second edition, 2001) 117-137.
10. PTI petition.
11. Foucard T, Malmheden-Yman I. A study on severe food reactions in Sweden – is soy protein an underestimated cause of food anaphylaxis. *Allergy*, 1999, 53, 3, 261-265.
12. Mortimer EZ. Anaphylaxis following ingestion of soybean. *Pediatr*, 1961, 58, 90-92.
13. Bock SA, Munoz-Furlong A, Sampson HA. Fatalities due to anaphylactic reaction to foods. *J. Aller Clin Immunol*, 2001, 107, 1, 191-193.
14. Sampson HA. Food anaphylaxis, *Br Med Bull*, 2000, 56, 4, 925-935.
15. Yunginger JW,, Nelson DR et al. Laboratory investigation of deaths due to anaphylaxis, *Forensic Science*, 1991, 36, 857-865.
16. Senne GE, Crivellaro M, et al. Pizza: an unsuspected source of soybean allergen exposure. *Allergy*, 1998, 53, 11, 1106-1107.
17. Vidal C, Perez-Carral C, Chomon B, Unsuspected sources of soybean exposure. *Ann AllergyAsthma Immunol*, 1997, 79,4, 350-352.
18. Taramarcaz P, Hauser C, Eigenmann PA. Soy anaphylaxis. *Allergy*, 2001, 56, 8, 792.
19. Moroz LA, Yang WH. Kunitz soybean trypsin-inhibitor: a specific allergen in food anaphylaxis *N Engl J Med*, 1980, 302, 1126-1128.
20. David TJ. Anaphylactic shock during elimination diets for severe atopic eczema. *Arch Dis Child*, 1984, 59, 983-986.
21. Monereet-Vautrin DA, Kanny G. Food-induced anaphylaxis. A new French multicenter study. *Bull Acad Natl Med*, 1995, 179, 1, 161-172, 173-177 and 178-184.
22. Letter from Ingrid Malmheden Yman, Ph.D., senior chemist Sweden National Food Administration, Chemistry Division Livsmedels Verket. to Ministry of Health in New Zealand, May 30, 1997. (Released under Official Information Act.)
23. Perlman, Frank "Allergens" in Irvin Liener, ed. *Toxic Constituents of Plant Foodstuffs* (NY, Academic Press, 1980).
24. Kuroume T, Oguri M et al. Milk sensitivity and soybean sensitivity in the production of eczematous manifestations in breast-fed infants with particular reference to intrauterine sensitization. *Ann Allergy*, 1976, 37, 41-46.
25. Sampson HA. Managing peanut allergy, *Brit Med J.*, 1996, 312, 1050.
26. Burks AW, Williams LW et al. Allergenicity of peanut and soybean extracts altered by chemical or thermal denaturation in patients with atopic dermatitis and positive food challenges. *J. Allergy Clin Immunol*, 1992, 90, (6 pt 1) 889-897.
27. Eigenmann, PA, Burks, AW, et al. Identification of unique peanut and soy allergens in sera absorbed with cross-reacting antibodies. *J. Allergy Clin Immuno*, 1996, 98, 5 pt 1, 969-978.
28. Burks AW, Cockrell G et al. Identification of peanut agglutinin and soybean trypsin inhibitor as minor legume allergens. *Int Arch Allergy Immunol*, 1994, 105, 2, 143-149.
29. Giampietro PG, Ragno V et al. Soy hypersensitivity in children with food allergy. *Ann Allergy*, 1992, 69, 2, 143-146.
30. Beardslee TA, Zeece MG et al. Soybean glycinin GI acidic chain shares IgE epitopes with peanut allergen Ara H 3. *Int Arch Allergy Immunol*, 2000, 123, 4, 299-307.
31. Pereira MJ, Iver MT et al.The allergenic significance of legumes.*Allerol Immunopathol* (Madr) 2002,30,6,346-353.
32. Perlman.
33. Sampson HA and McCaskill CM. Food hypersensitivity and atopic dermatitis: evaluation of 113 patients, *J Pediatr*, 1985, 107, 669.
34. Burks AW, Brooks JR, Sampson HA. Allergenicity of major component proteins of soybean determined by enzyme-linked immunosorbent assay (ELISA) and immunoblotting in children with atopic dermatitis and positive soy challenges. *J. Allergy Clin Immunol*, 1988, 81, 1135-1142.
35. Ogawa T, Bando N et al. Investigation of the Ig–binding proteins in soybeans by immunoblotting with the sera of the soybean-sensitive patients with atopic dermatitis. *J. Nutr Sci Vitaminol Tokyo*, 1991, 37, 6, 555-565.
36. Lalles JP, Peltre G. Biochemical features of grain legume allergies in humans and animals. *Nutr Rev*, 1996, 54, 101-107.
37. Burks AW, Cockrell G et al. Identification of peanut agglutinin and soybean trypsin inhibitor as minor legume allergens. *Int Arch Allergy Immunol*, 1994, 105, 2, 143-149.
38. Moroz LA, Yang WH. Kunitz soybean trypsin-inhibitor: a specific allergen in food anaphylaxis *NEJM*, 1980, 302, 1126-1128.

39. Gu X, Beardslee T et al. Identification of IgE-binding proteins in soy lecithin. *Int Arch Allergy Immunol*, 2001, 126, 3, 218-225.
40. Barnett D, Howden ME. Lectins and the radioallergosorbent test. *J. Allergy Clin Immunol*, 1987, 80, 4, 558-561.
41. Chin KW, Garriga MM, Metcalfe DD. The histamine content of oriental foods. *Food Chem Toxicol*, 1989, 27, 5, 283-287.
42. Aceves M, Grimalt JO, et al. Identification of soybean dust as an epidemic asthma agent in urban areas by molecular marker and RAST analysis of aerosols. *J. Allergy Clin Immun* 1991, 88, 124-134.
43. Pont F, Gispert X et al. An epidemic of asthma caused by soybean in L'Hospitalet de Llobregat (Barcelona). *Arch Bronconeumol*, 1997, 33,9, 453-456. Medline abstract. Article in Spanish. .
44. White MC, Etzel RA et al. Reexamination of epidemic asthma in New Orleans, Louisiana, in relation to the presence of soy at the harbor. *Am J. Epidemiol*, 1997, 1, 145, 5, 432-438.
45. Duke WW. Soybean as a possible important source of allergy. *J Allergy*, 1934, 5,300-303.
46. Baur X, Pau M et al, Characterization of soybean allergens causing sensitization of occupationally exposed bakers' allergy. *Allergy*, 1996, 51, 5, 326-330.
47. Baur X, Degens PO, Sandeer I. Bakers asthma: still among the most frequent occupational respiratory disorders. *J. Allergy Clin Immunol*, 1998, 102, (6 pt 1) 984-997.
48. Lavaud F, Perdu D et al. Baker's asthma related to soybean lecithin exposure. *Allergy*, 1994, 49, 3, 159-162.
49. Woerfel, JB Extraction. In David R. Erickson, ed. *Practical Handbook of Soybean Processing and Utilization.* (Champaign, IL, AOCS Press, 1995) 90.
50. Bush RK, Schroeckenstein DC, et al. Soybean flour asthma: detection of allergens. *J. Allergy Clin Immunol*, 1988, 82, 25-35.
51. Facchini G, Antonicelli I et al. Paradoxical bronchospasm and cutaneous rash after metered-dose inhaled bronchodilators. *Monaldi Arch Chest Dis*, 1996, 51, 3, 201-203.
52. Meyer, Herman Frederic, *Infant Foods and Feeding Practice* (Springfield, IL, Charles C. Thomas, 1960).
53. Eastham EJ. Soy protein allergy. In *Food Intolerance in Infancy: Allergology, Immunology and Gastroenterology.* Robert n. Hamburger, ed. (NY, Raven Press, 1989), 227.
54. Guandalini S, Nocerino A. Soy protein intolerance. www.emedicine.com/ped/topic2128.htm.
55. Erdman JW Jr, Fordyce EJ. Soy products and the human diet. *Am J. Clin Nutr,* 1989, 49, 5, 725-737.
56. Witherly SA Soy formulas are not hypoallergenic. Comment on *Am J. Clin Nutr* 1989, 49, 5, 725-737. *Am. J Clin Nutr,* 1990, 51, 4, 705-706.
57. Businco L, Bruno G, Giampietro PG. Soy protein for the prevention and treatment of children with cow-milk allergy. *Am J Clin Nutr*, 1998, 68 (6 Suppl), 1447-1452S.
58. Guandalini.
59. Sampson HA. Food allergy *Curr Opin Immunol*, 1990, 2, 542-547.
60. Eastham EJ, Lichanco T et al. Antigenicity of infant formulas: role of immature intestine on protein permeability. *J Pediatr*, 1978, 93, 4, 561-564.
61. Zeiger RS, Sampson HA et al. Soy allergy in infants and children with IgE-associated cow's milk allergy. *J Pediatr*, 1999, 134, 614-622.
62. Halpin, TC, Byrne WJ, Ament ME. Colitis, persistent diarrhea, and soy protein intolerances. *J Pediatr*, 1977, 91, 404-407.
63. Hasler, Clare. Information provided on the website "Soy and Human Health: Ask an Expert." http://web.aces.uiuc.edu/faq.
64. Burks AW, Williams LW et al. Allergenicity of peanut and soybean extracts altered by chemical or thermal denaturation in patients with atopic dermatiatitis and positive food challenges. *J. Allergy Clin Immunol*, 1992, 90 (6 pt 1), 889-897.
65. Besler, Matthias Allergen Data Collection: Soybean (Glycine max), *Internet Symposium on Food Allergens* 1999, 1, 2, 51-79. www.food-allergens.de.
66. Guandalini, Stefano and Nocerino, Agostino. Soy protein intolerance (updated June 17, 2002) www.emedicine.com/ped/topic2128.htm.
67. Rozenfeld P, Docena GH, et al. Detection and identification of a soy protein component that cross-reacts with caseins from cow's milk. *Clin Exp Immunol*, 2002, 130, 1, 49-58.
68. Besler, M, Helm RM, Ogawa T. Allergen Data collection update: soybean (glycine max) *Internet Symposium on Food Allergens*, 2000, 2 (Suppl 3) 435.
69. Guandalini.
70. Chandra RK. Five-year follow-up of high-risk infants with family history of allergy who were exclusively breast fed or fed partial whey hydrolysate, soy, and conventional cow's milk formula. *J. Pediatr Gastroenterol Nutr*, 1997, 24, 4, 380-388.
71. American Academy of Pediatrics, Committee on Nutrition, Soy protein-based formulas: recommendations for use in infant feeding (RE9806) Policy Statement, *Pediatrics*, 1998, 101, 1, 148-153.
72. May CD, Fomon SJ, Remigio L. Immunologic consequences of feeding infants with cow milk and soy products. *Acta Pediatr Scand*, 1982, 71, 43-51.
73. Iyngkaran N, Yadav M, Looi LM. Effect of soy protein on the small bowel mucosa of young infants recovering from acute gastroenteritis. *J. Pediatr Gastroenterol Nutr*, 1988, 7, 1, 68-75.
74. Guandalini.
75. Carini C, Brostoff J, Wraith DG. IgE complexes in food allergy, *Ann Allergy*, 1987, 59, 2, 110-117.
76. Ament ME, Rubin CE. Soy protein – another cause of the flat intestinal lesion. *Gastroenterol*, 1972, 62, 2, 227-234.
77. Poley JR, Klein AW. Scanning electron microsocopy of soy protein-induced damage of small bowel mucosa in infants. *J Pediatr Gastroenterol Nutr*, 1983, 2.2,271-287.

78. Perkkio M, Savilahti E, Kuitunen P. Morphometric and immunohistochemical a study of jejunal biopsies from children with intestinal soy allergy. *Eur J Pediatr*, 1981, 137, 1, 63-69.
79. Falkner-Hogg KB, Selby WS, Loblay RH. Dietary analysis in symptomatic patients with celiac disease on a gluten-free diet: the role of trace amounts of gluten and non-gluten intolerances. *Scand J. Gastroenterol*, 1999, 34, 8, 784-789.
80. Gryboski JD. Kocoshis S. Immunoglobulin deficiency in gastrointestinalallergies. *Clin Gastroenterol*, 1980, 2, 1, 71-76.
81. Sampson HA, Food allergy, *J. Allergy Clin Immunol*, 2003, 111 (2 suppl), S540-547.
82. Sicherer SH, Sampson HA. Food hypersensitivity and atopic dermatitis: pathophysiology, epidemiology, diagnosis and management. *Allergy Clin Immunol*, 1999, 104, 3, (3 pt 2) S114-122.
83. Sampson HA, Scanlon SM, Natural history of food hypersensitivity in children with atopic dermatitis, *Pediatrics*, 1989, 115,1, 23-27.
84. Sicherer SH, Eigenmann PA, Sampson HA. Clinical features of food protein-induced enterocolitis syndrome. *J. Pediatr*, 1998, 133,2, 214-219.
85. Ogle KA, Bullock JD. Children with allergic rhinitis and/or bronchial asthma treated with elimination diet: a five-year follow up. *Ann Allergy*, 1980, 44, 5, 273.
86. Sicherer SJ. Eigenmann PA, Sampson HA. Clinical features of food protein-induced enterocolitis syndrome. *Pediatr*, 1998, 133, 2, 214-219.
87. Townsend, Mark, Why soya is a hidden destroyer. *Daily Express* (London), March 2001, 12.
88. Keeler, Barbara. A nation of lab rats. *Sierra Club Magazine*, July/August 2001 45.
89. Nordlee JA, Taylor SL et al, Identification of a Brazil-nut allergen in transgenic soybeans. *NEJM*, 1996, 334, 11, 688-692.
90. Lack G. Clinical risk assessment of GM foods, *Toxicol Lett*, 2002, 28, 127, 1-3, 337-340.

Chapter 25: The Soy Free Challenge

1. Herian AM, Taylor ST, Bush RK. Allergenic reactivity of various soybean products as determined by RAST inhibition. *Food Science*, 1993, 58, 385-388.
2. Franck P, Moneret-Vautrin DA et al. The allergenicity of soybean-based products is modified by food technologies. *Int Arch Allergy Immunol*, 2002, 128, 3, 212-219.
3. Soybean oil made safe in processing. *The Soy Connection*, Spring 2003, 11,2,1.
4. Bush RK, Taylor SL et al. Soybean oil is not allergenic to soybean-sensitive individuals. *J Allergy Clin Immunol*, 1985, 76, 2 pt 1, 242-245.
5. Awazuhara H, Kawai H et al. Antigenicity of the proteins in soy lecithin and soy oil in soybean allergy. *Clin Exp Allergy*, 1998, 28, 12, 1559-1564.
6. Gu X, Beardslee T et al. Identification of IgE-binding proteins in soy lecithin. *Int Arch Allergy Immunol*, 2001, 126, 3, 218-235.
7. Errahali Y, Morisset M et al. Allergen in soy oils. *Allergy*, 2002, 57, 7, 42, 648-649.
8. Moneret-Vautrin DA, Morisset M et al. Unusual soy oil allergy. *Allergy*, 2002, 57, 3, 266-267.
9. Buchman Al, Ament ME. Comparative hypersensitivity to intravenous lipid emulsions, *JPEN J Parenter Enteral Nutr*, 1991, 15, 3, 345-346.
10. Weidmann B, Lepique C, et al. Hypersensitivity reactions to parenteral lipid solution. *Support Care Cancer*, 1997, 5, 6, 504-505.
11. Fremont S, Errahali Y et al. Mini Review: What about the allergenicity of vegetable oils? *Internet Symposium on Food Allergens*, 2002, 4, 2, 111-118.
12. Crevel RW, Kerkhoff MA, Koning MM. Allergenicity of refined vegetable oils. *Food Chem Toxicol*, 2000, 38, 4, 385-393.
13. Vidal C, Perez-Carral C, Chomon B. Unsuspected sources of soybean exposure. *Ann Allergy Asthma Immunol*, 1997, 79, 4, 350-352.
14. Taylor SL, Hefle SL. Ingredient issues associated with allergenic foods. *Curr Aller Clin Immunol*, 2001, 14, 12-18.
15. Foucard.
16. Vierk K, Falci K et al. Recalls of foods containing undeclared allergens reported to the US Food and Drug Administration, fiscal year 1999. *J Allergy Clin Immunol*, 2002, 109, 6, 1022-1026.
17. Allergy Alert notices published on the website www.inspection.gc.ca.
18. Besler Matthias and Kasel Udo, Wichmann, Gerhard. Review: Determination of hidden allergens in foods by immunoassays. *Internet Symposium on Food Allergens*, 2002, 4, 1, 118. www.food-allergens.de.
19. Joshi P, Mofidi S, Sicherer SH. Interpretation of commercial food ingredient labels by parents of food-allergic children. *J Allergy Clin Immunol*, 2002, 109, 6, 1019-1021.
20. www.foodallergyinitiative.org

Chapter 26: Phytoestrogens – Food's Fifth Column

1. Murkies AL, Wilcox G, Davis SR. Clinical Review 92: Phytoestrogens. *J Clin Endocrinol Metab*, 1998, 83, 9, 297-303.
2. Setchell KDR. Naturally occurring non-steroidal estrogens of dietary origin. In McLachlan J, ed. *Estrogens in the Environment.* (New York, NY, Elsevier, 1985).
3. Draft report of the COT (Committee on Toxicity of Chemicals in Foods, Consumer Products and the Environment) Working Group on Phytoestrogens. Chapter 2: Introduction.
4. USDA-Iowa State University Isoflavone Database.
5. Mazur W, Adlercreutz H. Naturally occurring estrogens in food. *Pure Appl Chem*, 1998, 70, 135-149.
6. Verdeal K, Ryan DS. Naturally-occurring estrogens in plant foodstuffs – a review. *J Food Prot*, 1979, 42, 7, 577-583.
7. Draft report of the COT Working Group on Phytoestrogens. Chapter 3: Chemistry and Analysis of Phytoestrogens.
8. Wang HJ, Murphy PA. Isoflavone composition of American and Japanese soybeans in Iowa: Effects of variety, crop year and location. *J Agric Food Chem*, 1994, 42, 1674-1677.
9. Draft report of the COT Working Group on Phytoestrogens. Sources and concentrations of phytoestrogens in foods and estimated dietary intake.
10. Whitten PL, Lewis C et al. Potential adverse effects of phytoestrogens. *J Nutr*, 1995, 125, 771S-776S.
11. Setchell KDR, Brown NM et al. Definitive evidence for lack of absorption of soy isoflavones glycosides in humans, supporting the crucial role of intestinal metabolism for bioavailability. *Am J Clin Nutr*, 2002, 76, 2, 447-453.
12. Setchell, KDR. Absorption and metabolism of isoflavones. *The Soy Connection*, 1998, 6, 2. www.soyfoods.com.
13. Setchell KDR. Zimmer-Nechemias L et al. Exposure of infants to phyto-oestrogens from soy-based infant formulas. *Lancet*, 1997, 350, 23-27.
14. Setchell.
15. Adlercreutz H, Goldin BR, Gorbach SL. Soybean phytoestrogen intake and cancer risk. *J Nutr*, 1995, 125, 757S-770S.
16. Setchell.
17. Draft report of the COT Working Group on Phytoestrogens. 5. Absorption, distribution, metabolism and excretion of phytoestrogens.
18. Setchell.
19. Draft report of the COT Working Group on Phytoestrogens. 4. Sources and concentrations of phytoestrogens in foods and estimated dietary intake.
20. Wang, Murphy.
21. Coward L, Smith M et al. Chemical modification of isoflavones in soyfoods during cooking and processing. *Am J Clin Nutr*, 1998, 68, 1486S-1491S.
22. Hutchins AM, Slavin JL, Lampe JW. Urinary isoflavanoid phytoestrogen and lignan excretion after consumption of fermented and unfermented products. *J Am Diet Assoc*, 1995, 95, 545-551.
23. Slavin JL, Karry SC et al. Influence of soybean processing, habitual diet and soy dose on urinary isoflavonoid excretion. *Am J Clin Nutr*, 1998, 68, 1492S-1495S.
24. King BA, Broadbent JL, Head RJ. Absorption and excretion of the soy isoflavones genistein in rats. *J Nutr*, 1996, 126, 176-182.
25. Setchell KDR. Safety and toxicity of soyfoods and their constituent isoflavones. Soyfoods 2001, January 17-19, Phoenix, AZ. Educational Audio Cassettes.
26. Setchell. Absorption and metabolism of isoflavones. *The Soy Connection*, 1998, 6, 2. www.soyfoods.com.
27. Setchell.
28. Draft report of the COT Working Group on Phytoestrogens. 3. Chemistry and analysis.
29. Draft report of the COT Working Group on Phytoestrogens. 5 Absorption, distribution, metabolism and excretion of phytoestrogens.
30. Jobling S. Review of suggested testing methods for endocrine-disrupting chemicals. *Pure Appl Chem*, 1998, 70, 1805-1827.
31. Draft report of the COT Working Group on Phytoestrogens. 5. Absorption, distribution, metabolism and excretion of phytoestrogens.
32. Whitten, Lewis.
33. Whitten, Lewis.
34. Markiewicz, L, Garey J, et al. In vitro bioassays of non-steroidal phytoestrogens. *J Steroids Biochem Mol Biol*, 1993, 45, 5, 399-405.
35. Irvine CHG, Fitzpatrick MG, Alexander SL. Phytoestrogens in soy-based infant foods: concentrations, daily intake and possible biological effects. *Proc Soc Exp Biol Med*, 1998, 217, 247-253.
36. Woodhams, Dave. How weak is weak? *Soy Information Network Newsletter*, February 1996, 2, 9.
37. Woodhams, 10.
38. Technical Brief prepared by Protein Technologies International and sent by Columbit Ltd. to the New Zealand Ministry of Health, January 26, 1995.
39. Woodhams, 11.
40. Fallon, Sally. Enig, Mary. Tragedy and hype: the third international soy symposium. *Nexus*, April/May 2000.
41. White L, Petrovitch H, et al. Association of mid-life consumption of tofu with late life cognitive impairment and dementia. The Honolulu-Asia Aging Study. *Neurobiol Aging*, 1996, 7, suppl 4, S121.

42. White LR, Petrovich H et al. Prevalence of dementia in older Japanese-American men in Hawaii, *JAMA*, 1996, 276, 955-960.
43. White LR, Petrovitch H et al. Brain aging and midlife tofu consumption. *J Am Coll Nutr*, 2000, 19, 207-209, 242-255.
44. Goddard, Ian. Tofu study update, December 9, 1999. http://users/erols.com/igoddard/soy.htm.
45. Sheehan DM, Doerge DR. Letter to Dockets Management Branch, Food and Drug Administration (HFA-305) February 18, 1999.
46. O-Dell TJ, Kandel ER Grant SG Long-term potentiation in the hippocampus is blocked by tyrosine kinase inhibitors. *Nature* 1991, 353, 6344, 558-560.
47. Yakisich JS, Siden A et al. Early effects of protein kinase modulators on DNA synthesis in rat cerebral cortex. *Exp Neurol*, 1999, 159, 1, 164-176.
48. Lephard ED et al. Phytoestrogens decrease brain calcium-binding proteins but do not alter hypothalamic androgen metabolizing enzymes in adult male rats. *Brain Res*, 2000, 17, 859, 1, 123-131.
49. File SE, Hartley DE et al. Soya phytoestrogens change cortical and hippocampal expressions of BDNF mRNA in male rats. *Neurosci Lett*, 2003, 338, 2, 135-138.
50. Choi EJ, Lee BH. Evidence for genistein mediated cytotoxicty and apoptosis in rat brain. *Life Sci*, 2004, 74, 4, 499-509.
51. White, Lon. Quoted by Baumel, Syd. Research links tofu to dementia – and that's just the appetizer. www.aquarianonline.com/wellness/soy.html.

Chapter 27: Soy and the Thyroid – A Pain in the Neck

1. Rackis.JJ. Biologically active components. In Smith, Allan K and Circle, Sidney J. eds. *Soybeans: Chemistry and Technology* (Westport, CT, Avi, 972) 183-184.
2. Tookey HL, VanEtten CH, Daxenbichler ME. Glucosinolates. In Liener, IE, ed. *Toxic Constituents in Plant Foodstuffs* (NY Academic 1980). 103-142.
3. Draft report of the COT Working Group on Phytoestrogens. 4. Sources and concentrations of phytoestrogens in foods and estimated dietary intake.
4. Coward L, Smith M et al. Chemical modification of isoflavones in soyfoods during cooking and processing. *Am J Clin Nutr*, 1998, 68, 1486S-1491S.
5. Canaris GJ, Manowitz NR et al. The Colorado thyroid disease prevalence study. *Arch Intern Med*, 2000, 160, 526-534.
6. Shomon, Mary J. *Living Well with Hypothyroidism: What Your Doctor Doesn't Tell You that You Need to Know* (New York, NY Quill, 2000).
7. Arem, Ridha. *The Thyroid Solution* (Ballantine, 1999).
8. Arem R, Escalante D. Subclinical hypothyroidism: epidemiology, diagnosis and significance. *Adv Int Med*, 1996, 41, 213-250.
9. Arem.
10. Adlin V. Subclinical hypothyroidism: deciding when to treat. *Amer Fam Phys*, February15,1998. www.aafp.org.
11. American Association of Clinical Endocrinologists. www.aace.com
12. http://thryoid.about.com.
13. www.soyonline.service.co.nz
14. American Cancer Society. *Cancer Facts and Figures 2003*.
15. US Thyroid Epidemic. www.soyonlineservice.co.nz/epidem.htm.
16. Colborn, Theo. Dumanoski, Dianne. Myers, John Peterson. *Our Stolen Future: Are We Threatening Our Fertility, Intelligence and Survival? – A Scientific Detective Story* (NY Dutton, 1996).
17. Shomon.
18. Draft Report of the COT Working Group on Phytoestrogens.
19. Price KR, Fenwick GR, et al. Naturally occurring estrogens in foods: a review. *Food Additives Contam*, 1985, 2, 73-106.
20. Beckham, Nancy. Soy: The Facts. *WellBeing Magazine*, 82. insert. www.wellbeing.com.au.
21. Northrup, Christiane. My response to possible adverse effects of soy. www.drnorthrup.com/soy_responses.htm.
22. Tyler, Patrick E. China confronts retardation of millions deficient in iodine. *New York Times*, June 4, 1996, 1, 1.
23. Fitzpatrick M. Soy formulas and the effects of isoflavones on the thyroid. *NZ Med J*, 2000, 113, 1103, 24-26.
24. McCarrison R. The goitrogenic action of soybean and ground-nut. *Indian J Med Res*. 1933, 21:179.
25. Sharpless GR, Pearsons J, Prato GS. Production of goiter in rats with raw and with treated soybean flour. *J Nutr*, 1939, 17, 545-555.
26. Patton AR, Wilgus HS, Harshfield GS. The production of goiter in chickens. *Science*, 1939, 89, 162.
27. Block RJ, Mandl RH et al. The curative action of iodine on soybean goiter and the changes in the distribution of iodoamino acids in the serum and in the thyroid gland digests. *Arch Biochem Biophysics*, 1961, 93, 15-21.
28. Kay T, Kimura M et al. Soyabean, goitre, and prevention. *J Trop Pediatr*, 1988, 34, 110-113.
29. Kimura S, Suwa J et al. Development of malignant goiter by defatted soybean with iodine-deficient diet in rats. *Gann*. 1976, 67:763-765.
30. Kimura, Suwa et al.
31. Rang HP and Dale MM. *Pharmacology*. Churchill Livingston UK. 1987, 16:369-378.
32. Soy interferes with thyroid therapy, comment. *Townsend Letter for Physicians and Patients*, April 1998, 33.

33. Bell DS, Ovalle F. Use of soy protein supplement and resultant need for increased dose of levothyroxine. *Endoc Pract*, 2001, 7, 3, 193-194.
34. Jabbar MA, Larrea J, Shaw RA. Abnormal thyroid function tests in infants with congenital hypothyroidism: the influence of soy-based formula. *J Am Coll Nutr*, 1997, 16, 280-282.
35. Northrup.
36. Doerge DR. Inhibition of thyroid peroxidase by dietary flavonoids. *Chem Res Toxicol.* 1996, 9:16-23.
37. Divi RL, Chang HC, Doerge DR. Anti-thyroid isoflavones from soybean. *Biochem Pharmacol.* 1997, 54:1087-1096.
38. Chang HC, Doerge DR. Dietary genistein inactivates rat thyroid peroxidase in vivo without an apparent hypothyroid effect. *Toxicol Appl Pharmacol.* 2000, 168:224-252.
39. Gaitan E, Flavonoids and the thyroid, *Nutrition*, 1996, 12, 127-129.
40. Hydovitz JD. Occurrence of goiter in an infant soy diet. *NEJM.* 1960, 262:351-353.
41. Rawson RW, Rall JE. Endocrinology of neoplastic disease. *Recent Prog Horm Res.* 1955, 11:257-290.
42. Shephard TH, Pyne GE, Kirschvink JF, McLean M. Soybean goiter. *NEJM.* 1960, 262:1099-1103.
43. Van Wyk JJ, Arnold MB et al. The effects of a soybean product on thyroid function in humans. *Pediatrics.* 1959, 752-760.
44. Van Wyk, Arnold et al.
45. Draft report of the COT Working Group on Phytoestrogens. 4. Sources and concentrations of phytoestrogens in foods and estimated dietary intake.
46. Coward L, Smith M et al. Chemical modification of isoflavones in soyfoods during cooking and processing. *Am J Clin Nutr*, 1998, 68, 1486S-1491S.
47. USDA-Iowa State University Isoflavone Database.
48. Fomon SJ. Nutrition of normal infants. St Louis, MO: Mosby. 1993, 20-21.
49. Jabbar MA, Larrea J, Shaw RA. Abnormal thyroid function test in infants with congential hypothyroidism: the influence of soy-based formula. *J Am Coll Nutr.* 1997, 16:280-282.
50. Chorazy PA, Himelhoch S et al. Persistent hypothyroidism in an infant receiving a soy formula: case report and review of the literature. *Pediatr*, 1995, 96 (1 pt 1), 148-150.
51. New Zealand Ministry of Health Position Statement. As quoted by Fitzpatrick.
52. Fort P, Lanes R et al. Breast feeding and insulin-dependent diabetes mellitus in children. *J Am Coll Nutr*, 1986, 5, 439-441.
53. Fort P, Moses N et al. breast and soy-formula feedings in early infancy and the prevalence of autoimmune thyroid disease in children. *J Am Coll Nutr, 1990*, 9, 2, 164-167.
54. Labib M, Gama R et al. Dietary maladvice as a cause of hypothyroidism and short stature. *BMJ*, 1989, 298, 232-233.
55. Strom BL, Schinnar R et al. Exposure to soy-based formula in infancy and endocrinological and reproductive outcomes in young adulthood. *JAMA*, 2001, 286, 7, 807-814.
56. Ishizuki Ishizuki Y, Hirooka, Maruta Y, Tigashi K. The effects on the thyroid gland of soybeans administered experimentally in healthy subjects. *Nippon Naibundi gakkai Zasshi*, 1991, 67, 622-629. Translation by Japan Communication Service, Wellington. Courtesy Valerie and Richard James.
57. Fitzpatrick.
58. Draft Report of the COT Working Group.
59. National Research Council. Hormonally active agents in the environment. Textbook guide for regulators. Quoted by Richard James in letter on draft phytoestrogen report to Abimbola Nathan, London, UK, November 20, 2002.
60. Key TJA, Thorogood M, Keenan J, Long A. Raised thyroid stimulating hormone associated with kelp intake in British vegan men. *J Hum Nutr Diet.* 1992, 5:323-326.
61. Shomon.
62. Bolkhima RI in Mills CF *Trace Elements in Animals*, Vol 1 (NY Academic, 1970). 426.
63. Smith RM in Mertz W. *Trace Elements in Human and Animal Nutrition*, Vol 2 (NY Academic 1987), 143.
64. Liener IE. Implications of antinutritional components in soybean foods. *Crit Rev Food Sci Nutr*, 1994, 34, 1, 31-67.
65. Messina, Mark. Soy and thyroid function: studies show little effect. *The Soy Connection*, Spring 2001, pp. 1-2, 5-6.
66. Messina.
67. Northrup.
68. Messina, Mark. Email to author, August 30, 2003.
69. www.liebertpub.com.
70. http://www.thesoydailyclub.com/Research/SheldonSaulHendler06202003.asp
71. Bruce B, Messina M, Spiller GA. Isoflavone supplements do not affect thyroid function in iodine-replete postmenopausal women. *J Med Food*, 2003, 6, 4, 309-316.
72. Author's telephone interview with Leah Holloway, September 21, 2004.
73. Messina, Mark. E-Letter to Peggy O'Mara, Publisher and Editor of *Mothering* magazine. May 5, 2004.
74. National Center for Health Statistics, Iodine Level United States 2000. www.cdc.gov/nchs/products/pubs/pubd/hestats/iodine.htm.
75. Messina, Virginia. Messina, Mark. Is it safe to eat soy? www.veganhealth.org/articles/soymessina.
76. Duncan AM, Merz BE et al. Soy isoflavones exert modest hormonal effects in premenopausal women. *J Clin Endocrinol Metab*. 1999a, 84:192-197.
77. Duncan AM, Underhill KEW et al. Modest hormonal effects of soy isoflavones in postmenopausal women. *J Clin Endocrinol Metab*. 1999b, 84:3479-3484.

78. Persky VW, Turyk ME, et al. Effect of soy protein on endogenous hormones in postmenopausal women. *Am J Clin Nutr.* 2002, 75:145-153.
79. Fitzpatrick.
80. Doerge DR. Goitrogenic and estrogenic activity of soy isoflavones. *Environ Health Perspect*, 2002, 110, Suppl, 3, 349-353.

Chapter 28: Soy Infant Formula – Birth Control for Baby?

1. Bulletin de L'Office Federal de la Santa Publique, No. 28, July 20, 1992. This bulletin from the Swiss Federal Health Service warned consumers that 100 grams of soy protein provide as much estrogen as one contraceptive pill. Infants drinking soy formula receive the equivalent of one-fourth birth control pill – or more – everyday. Taking into account the infant's smaller size compared to its mother, it would be receiving a dose comparable to three to five birth control pills – more if a hungry eater.
2. Irvine CHG, Fitzpatrick MG et al. Phytoestrogens in soy-based infant foods: concentrations, daily intake and possible biological effects. *Proc Soc Exp Biol Med*, 1998, 217, 247-253.
3. Fitzpatrick M. Soy formulas and the effects of isoflavones on the thyroid. *NZ Med J*, 2000, 113, 1103, 24-26.
4. Robertson IGC. Phytoestrogens: toxicology and regulatory recommendations. *Proc Nutr Soc NZ*, 1995, 20, 35-42.
5. Zimmerli B, Schlatter J.
6. Tonz O, Zimmerli B.. Phytoestrogens in baby food based on soya bean protein. *Paediatricia*, 1997, 8, 14-15.
7. Soy Alert! www.westonaprice.org.
8. www.soyonlineservice.co.nz.
9. Sheehan DM. Isoflavone content of breast milk and soy formulas: benefits and risks (letter). *Clin Chem*, 1997, 43, 850.
10. Clarkson, RB, et al. Estrogenic Soybean isoflavones and chronic disease: risks and benefits. *Trends Endocrino Metab*, 1995, Vol. 6, pp. 11-16.
11. Kaldas, RS and Hughes CL. Reproductive and general metabolic effects of phytoestrogens in mammals. *Repro Toxicol*, 1989, Vol. 3, pp. 81-89.
12. Irvine.
13. Irvine.
14. Irvine.
15. McKinnell C, Atanassova N et al. Suppression of androgen action and the induction of gross abnormalities of the reproductive tract in male rats treated neonatally with diethylstilbestrol. *J Androl*, 2001, 22, 323-338.
16. Haavisto T, Numela K et al. Prenatal testosterone and LH levels in male rats exposed during pregnancy to 2, 3,7, 8-tetrachlorodibenzo-p-dixin and diethylstilbestrol. *Mol Cell Endocrinol*, 2001, 178, 169-179.
17. Williams K, McKinnell C et al. Neonatal exposure to potent and environmental estrogens and abnormalities of the male reproductive system in the rat: evidence for importance of the androgen-estrogen balance and assessment of the relevance to man. *Human Repro Update*, 2001, 7, 236-247.
18. Keung W-M. Dietary estrogen iisoflavones are potent inhibitors of beta hydroxysteroid dehydrogenase of P. testosteronii. *Biochem Biophys Res Cmm.*, 1995, 215, 1137-1144.
19. Makela S, Poutanen, et al. Estrogen specific 17-beta hydroxysteroid oxidoreductase type 1 as a possible target for the action of phytoestrogens, *Proc Soc Exper Biol Med*, 1995, 208, 51-59.
20. Irvine, Fitzpatrick et al.
21. Akiyama T, Ishida J et al. Genistein, a specific inhibitor of tyrosine-specific protein kinases. *J Biol Chem*, 1987, 262, 5592-5595.
22. Couse.
23. Korach.
24. Grumbach MM and Auchus RJ. Estrogen: consequences and implications of human mutations in synthesis and action. *J Clin Endocrinol Metab*, 1999, 84, 4677-4694.
25. Sorenson RL, Brelje TC, Roth C. Effect of tyrosin kinase inhibitors on islets of Langerhans: evidence for tyrosine kinases in the regulation of insulin secretion. *Endocrinol*, 1993, 134, 1975-1978.
26. Gangrade BK, Davis JS, May VJ. A novel mechanism for the induction of aromatase in ovarian cells in vitro: role of transforming growth factor alpha-induced protein tyrosine kinase. *Endocrinol*, 1991, 129, 2790-2792.
27. Brown GR, Nevsion CM et al, Manipulation of postnatal testosterone levels affects phallic and clitoral development in rhesus monkeys. *Int J Androl*, 1999, 22, 119-128.
28. Lunn SF, Cowen GM, Fraser HM. Blockade of the neonatal increase in testosterone by a GnRH antagonist: the free androgen index: reproductive capacity and post mortem findings in male marmoset monkeys. *J Endocrinol*, 1997, 154, 125-131.
29. Grumbach MM, Auchus RJ. Estrogen: consequences and implications of human mutations in synthesis and action. *J Clin Endocrino Metab*, 1999, 84, 4677-4694.
30. Irvine, Fitzpatrick.
31. Woodhams.
32. Santii R, Makela S et al. Phytoestrogens : potential endocrine disrupters in males. *Toxicol Envir Health*, 1998, 14, 1-2, 223-237.
33. Frawley, LS, Neill, JD. Age-related changes in serum levels of gonadotropins and testosterone in infantile male rhesus monkeys. *Biolog Repro*, 1979, Vol. 20, 1147-1151.
34. Mann, DR, et al. Blockade of neonatal activation of the pituitary testicular axis: effect on peripubertal luteinizing hormone and testosterone secretion and on testicular development in male monkeys. *J Clinical Endocrinol Metab*, 1989, 68, 600-607.

35. Winter, JS, Hughes IA et al. Pituitary-gonadal relations in infancy: Patterns of serum gonadal steroid concentrations in man from birth to two years of age. *J Clin Endocrinol Metab*, 1976, 42, 4, 679-686.
36. McKinnell, Atanassova et al.
37. Atanassova N, McKinnell C et al. Comparative effects of neonatal exposure of male rats to potent and weak (environmental) estrogens on spermatogenesis at puberty and the relationship to adult testis size and fertility: evidence for stimulatory effects of low estrogen levels. *Endocrinol*, 2000, 141, 10, 3898-3907.
38. Fisher JS, Turner KJ et al. Effect of neonatal exposure to estrogenic compounds on development of the excurrent ducts of the rat testis through puberty to adulthood. *Environ Health Perspect*, 1999, 107, 5, 397-405.
39. Shibayama T, Fukata H et al. Neonatal exposure to genistein reduces expression of estrogen receptor alpha and androgen receptor in testes of adult mice. *Endocr J 2001*, 48, 6, 655-663.
40. Mann DR, Gould KG et al. Blockade of neonatal activation of the pituitary-testicular axis: effect on peripubertal luteinizing hormone and testosterone secretion and on testicular development in male monkeys. *J Clin Endocrinol Metabol*, 1989, 68, 600-607.
41. Mann DR, Akinbami MA et al. Neonatal treatment of male monkeys with a gonadotropin-releasing hormone agonist alters differentiation of central nervous system centers that regulate sexual and skeletal development. *J Clin Endocrinol Metab*, 1993, 76, 1319-1324.
42. Eisler J, Tannenbau P et al. Neonatal gonadal suppression in male rhesus monkeys with a GnRH agonist: effects on adult endocrine function and behavior. *Horm Behav*, 1992, 17, 551-567.
43. Irvine, Fitzpatrick et al.
44. Sharpe RM et al. Infant feeding with soy formula milk: effects on the testis and on blood testosterone levels in marmoset monkeys during the period of neonatal testicular activity. *Hum Reprod*, 2002, 17, 7, 1692-1703.
45. Irvine, Fitzpatrick.
46. Mann, Gould et al.
47. Job JC, Gendrel D. Endocrine aspects of cryptoorchidism. *Urol Clin North* Am, 1982, 9, 353-360.
48. Sedimeyer IL, Palmert MR. Delayed puberty: analysis of a large case series from an academic center. *J Clin Endocrinol Metab*, 2002, 87, 4, 1613-1620.
49. Chilvers C, Pike M et al. Apparent doubling of undescended testis in England and Wales in 1962-81. *Lancet*, 1984, 330-332.
50. Hutson J, Baker M et al. Hormonal control of testicular descent and the cause of cryptorchidism. *Repro,Fert,Devel*, 1994, 6, 151-156.
51. Sharpe R, Shakkeback N. Are oestrogens involved in falling sperm counts and disorders of the male reproductive tract? *Lancet*, 1993, 341, 1292-1395.
52. Bromwich J, Cohen I. Decline in sperm counts: an artifact of changed reference range of 'normal'? *Br Med J*, 1994, 309, 19-22.
53. Auger J, Kunstmann J et al. Decline in semen quality among fertile men in Paris during the past 20 years. *NEJM*, 1995, 332, 5, 281-185.
54. Richard Sharpe, MD, as quoted by Aileen Ballantyne in: Why our men are getting less fertile, *London Times*, August 29, 1995.
55. Lunn, Cowan.
56. Grumbach, Auchus.
57. Hines, M. Hormonal and neural correlates of sex-typed behavioral development in human beings. In Marc Haug, ed. *The Development of Sex Differences and Similarities in Behavior* (Dordrecht: Kluwer Academic, 1993) 131-147.
58. Mann, DM, Akinbami MA et al. Neonatal treatment of male monkeys with a gonadotropin releasing hormone agonist alters differentiation of central nervous system centers that regulate sexual and skeletal development. *Clin Endocrinol Metab*, 1993, 76, 1319-1324.
59. Whitten, PL, Lewis C et al. Phytoestrogen influences on the development of behavior and gonadotropin function. *Proc Soc Exper Biol Med*, 1995, 208, 1, 82-86.
60. Hier, DB, Crowly WF. Spatial ability in androgen-deficient men. *NEJM*, 1982, 306, 1202-1205.
61. Hagger C, Bachevalier J. Visual habit formation in 3-month-old monkeys (Macaca mulatto): reversal of sex difference following neonatal manipulations of androgen. *Behav Brain Res*, 1991, 45, 57-63.
62. Harrison, PJ, Everall IP et al. Is homosexual behavior hard-wired? Sexual orientation and brain structure. *Psych Med*, 1994, 24, 811-816
63. Irvine, Fitzpatrick.
64. Winter JSD, Hughes IA et al. Pituitary-gonadal relations in infancy: 2. Patterns of serum gonadal steroid concentrations in man from birth to two years of age. *J Clin Endocrinol Metabo*, 1976, 42, 679-686.
65. Mann, Gould et al.
66. Giddens Herman et al. Secondary sexual characteristics and menses in young girls seen in office practice. Study from the Pediatric Research in Office Settings Network, 1997, 99, 4, 505-512.
67. Fenton CL, Poth M. Precocious Pseudopuberty. eMedicine, 2001, 2, 5. www.emedicine.com.
68. Irvine, Fitzpatrick et al.
69. Badger TM, Ronis MJJ, Hakkak R. Developmental aspects and health aspects of soy protein isolate, casein and whey in male and female rats. *Int J Toxicol*, 2001, 20, 3, 165-174
70. Casanova M, You L et al. Developmental effects of dietary phytoestrogens in Sprague-Dawley rats and interactions of genistein and daidzein with rat estrogen receptors alpha and beta in vitro. *Toxicol Sci*, 1999, 51, 2, 236-244.
71. Burroughs CD. Long-term reproductive tract alterations in female mice treated neonatally with coumestrol. *Proc Soc Exp Biol Med*, 1995, 208, 78-81.
72. Whitten PL, Lewis C et al. A phytoestrogen diet induces premature anovulatory syndrome in lactationally exposed female rats. *Biol Reprod*, 1993, 49, 1117-1121.

73. LaMartinere CA, Moore JB et al. Neonatal genistein chemoprevents mammary cancer. *Proc Soc Exp Biol Med*, 1995, 208, 120-123.
74. Jefferson WN, Newbold RR. Potential endocrine-modulating effects of various phytoestrogens in the diet. *Nutr*, 2000, 16, 658-662.
75. LaMartiniere CA, Murril WB et al. Genistein alters the ontogeny of mammary gland development and protects against chemically induced mammary cancer in rats. *Proc Soc Exp Biol Med*, 1998, 217, 358-363.
76. Irvine, Fitzpatrick.
77. Lambertina W, Freni-Titulaer et al. Premature thelarche in Puerto Rico, *AJDC*, 1986, 140, 1263-1267.
78. Colon I, Caro D et al. Identification of phthalate esters in the serum of young Puerto Rican girls with premature breast development. *Environ Health Perspect*, 2000, 108, 9, 895-900.
79. Klein KO. Isoflavones, soy-based infant formulas, and relevance to endocrine function. *Nutr Rev*, 56, 7, 193-204.
80. Sharpe, quoted by Ballantyne.
81. Fort P, Lanes R et al. Breast feeding and insulin-dependent diabetes mellitus in children. *J Am Coll Nutr*, 1986, 5, 439-441.
82. Fallon Sally. Enig, Mary G. Reply to guest editorial by Bill Sardi, *Townsend Letter for Doctors and Patients*, May 2000.
83. Strom BL, Schinnar R et al. Exposure to soy-based formula in infancy and endocrinological and reproductive outcomes in young adulthood. *JAMA*, 2001, 286, 7, 807-814.
84. Experts Dispute Soy Formula Safety, Press Release: Weston A. Price Foundation, Washington DC, September 6, 2001. www.westonaprice.org
85. Goldman LR, Newbold R, Swan S. Exposure to soy-based formula in infancy. Letter to the editor, *JAMA*, 2001, 286, 19, 2402-2403.
86. Author's telephone interview with Brian Strom, August 31, 2001.
87. Mercola, Joseph. Soy milk is safe! That is what the formula industry says. August 25, 2001. www.mercola.com
88. Colburn, Theo, Dumanoski, Dianne. Myers, John Peterson. *Our Stolen Future* (NY Dutton, 1996).
89. Irvine.
90. Setchell KDR, Zimmer-Nechemias L et al. Isoflavone content of infant formulas and the metabolic fate of these phytoestrogens in early life. Am J Clin Nutr, 1998, 69 (suppl), 1453S-1461S.
91. Irvine.
92. Franke, A.A., Custer LJ et al., Quantification of phytoestrogens in legumes by HPLC, *J Agric Food Chem*, 1994, 42, 1905-1913.
93. Franke AA, Custer LJ. Daidzein and genistein concentrations in human milk after soy consumption." *Clin Chem*, 1996 42, 955-964.
94. Setchell KDR, Zimmer-Nechemias L et al. Exposure of infants to phyto-oestrogens from soy-based infant formula. *Lancet*, 1997, 3530 (0\9070), 23-27.
95. Markiewicz L, Garey J et al, In vitro bioassays of non-steroidal phytoestrogens. *J Steroids Biochem Molec Biol*, 1993, 45, 5, 399.
96. Woodhams, David J, Nutritional deficiencies in soy protein-based infant formulas, paper presented to the New Zealand Ministry of Health, March 5, 1995.
97. Woodhams.
98. Setchell.
99. Venkataraman, PS et al. Urinary phytoestrogen excretion in infants; differences between human milk, cowmilk-based, and soy-based formula-fed infants, *Ped Res* 1993, 37, 312.
100. Setchell KDR, Borriello SP et al. Nonsteroidal estrogens of dietary origin: possible roles in hormone-dependent disease. *Am J Clin Nutr*, 1984, 40, 569-578.
101. Apfel, RJ, Fischer, SM. *To Do No Harm: DES and the Dilemmas of Modern Medicine* (New Haven, CT, Yale University Press), 1984.
102. Setchell KDR. Naturally occurring non-steroidal estrogens of dietary origin, In J McLachlan, ed. *Estrogens in the Environment*, (New York, NY, Elsevier, 1985).
103. Colborn, Dumanoski, Myers.
104. Woodhams
105. Setchell.
106. Verdeal K, Ryan DS. Naturally occurring estrogens in plant foodstuffs: a review. *J Food Protection*, 1979, 42, 7, 577-583.
107. Newbold RR, Banks EP et al. Uterine adenocarcinoma in mice treated neonatally with genistein. *Cancer Res*, 2001, 61, 4325-4328.
108. Chen J, Campbell TC et al. *Diet Lifestyle and Mortality in China: A Study of the Characteristics of 65 Counties*. (Joint publication of Oxford University Press, Cornell University Press, China People's Medical Publishing House, 1990).
109. Fukutake M, Takahashi, M et al. Quantification of genistein and genistin in soybeans and soybean products. *Food Chem Toxicol*, 1996, 34, 457-461.
110. Nagata C, Takatsuka N et al. Decreased serum total cholesterol concentration is associated with high intake of soy products in Japanese men and women. *J Nutr*, 1998, 128, 2, 209-213.
111. Nakamura Y, Tsuji S, Tonogai Y. Determination of the levels of isoflavanoids in soybeans and soy-derived foods and estimation of isoflavanoids in the Japanese daily intake. *JAOAC Int* 2000, 83, 635-650.
112. Ishizuki Y, Hiroka Y et al. The effects on the thyroid gland of soybeans administered experimentally in healthy subjects. *Nippon Natbunpi Gakkai Zasshi*, 1991, 767, 622-629.
113. Cassidy A, Bingham S, Setchell KDR. Biological effects of a diet of soy protein rich isoflavones on the menstrual cycle of premenopausal women. *Am J Clin Nutr*, 1994, 60, 3, 333-340.

114. FDA Final Rule. Food Labeling: Health claims: soy protein and coronary heart disease, Federal Register, 64, 206, October 26, 1999.
115. USDA Iowa State University Database on the Isoflavone Content of Foods, 1999.
116. Setchell KDR, Zimmer-Nechemias L et al. Isoflavone content of infant formulas and the metabolic fate of these phytoestrogens in early life. Am J Clin Nutr, 1998, 68, 6 Suppl, 1453S-1461S.
117. Giddens Herman et al. Secondary sexual characteristics and menses in young girls seen in office practice. Study from the Pediatric Research in Office Settings Network, 1997, 99, 4, 505-512.
118. Montague, Peter. Editorial: the obscenity of accelerated child development. Ecologist, 1993, 28, 3, 140-142.
119. Zacharias L, Wurtman RJ. Age at menarche, N Eng J Med, 1969, 280, 16, 868-875. The article includes results reported in Michaelson N. Studies in physical development of Negroes. IV. Onset of puberty. Am J Phys Anthropol, 1944, 2, 151-166.
120. Colborn, Theo. Dumanoski, Dianne. Myers, John Peterson. Our Stolen Future (NY Dutton, 1996).
121. Fenton CL, Poth, M, Precocious Pseudopuberty. eMedicine, 2001, 2, 5. www.emedicine.com.

Chapter 29: Soy and the Reproductive System – Breeding Discontent

1. Riddle JM, Estes, JW. Oral contraceptives in ancient and medieval times. American Scientist, 1992, 80, 226-233.
2. Setchell KDR, Gosselin SJ et al. Dietary estrogens – a probable cause of infertility and liver disease in captive cheetahs. Gastroenterol, 1987, 93, 225-233.
3. Draft report of the COT Working Group on Phytoestrogens. 9. Effects of phytoestrogens on fertility and development.
4. Bennetts HW, Underwood EJ, Shier FL. A specific breeding problem of sheep on subterranean clover pastures in Western Australia. Austr Vet J, 1946, 22, 2-12.
5. Cheng E. Yodeer L et al. Estrogenic activity of some isoflavone derivatives. Science, 1954, 120, 575-577.
6. Batterham TJ, Hart NK, Lamberton JA. Metabolism of oestrogenic isoflavones in sheep. Nature, 1965, 206, 509.
7. Leopold AS, Erwin M et al. Phytoestrogens: adverse effects on reproduction in California quail. Science, 1976, 191, 4222, 98-99.
8. Kaziro R, Kennedy JP et al. The oestrogenicity of equol in sheep. J Endocrinol, 1984, 103, 395-399.
9. Shutt, DA. The effects of plant oestrogens on animal reproduction. Endeavor, 1976, 35, 110-113.
10. Axelson M, Sjovall J, Gustafsson BE, Setchell KDR. Soya – a dietary source of the non-steroidal oestrogen equol in man and animals. J Endocrinol, 1984, 102, 49-56.
11. Setchell KDR, Borriello SP et al. Nonsteroidal estrogens of dietary origin: possible roles in hormone-dependent disease. Am J Clin Nutr, 1984, 40, 569-578.
12. Mathieson R, Kitts W. Binding of phytoestrogens and estradiol 17 beta by cytoplasmic receptors in the pituitary gland and hypothalamus in the ewe. J Endocrinol, 1980, 85, 317-325.
13. Price KR, Fenwick GR. Naturally-occurring estrogens in food a review. Food Addit Contam, 1985, 2, 2, 73-106.
14. Farnsworth. Forage plant estrogens. J Toxicol Environ Health, 1978, 4, 2-3, 301-324.
15. Farnsworth NR, Bingel AS et al. Potential value of plants as sources of new antifertility agents. II. J Pharm Sci, 1975, 64, 717-754.
16. Setchell, Gosselin, 230.
17. Setchell, Gosselin.
18. Setchell, Gosselin. 231.
19. Axelson, Sjovall.
20. Setchell KDR. Nonsteroidal estrogens of dietary origin: possible roles in hormone-dependent disease. Am J Clin Nutr, 1984, 40, 569-578. 1986.
21. Cassidy A. Bingham S. Setchell K. Biological effects of a diet of soy protein rich in isoflavones on the menstrual cycles of premenopausal women. Am J Clin Nutr, 1994, 60, 330-340.
22. Cassidy, Aedin. Plant Oestrogens and their Relation to Hormonal Status in Womn. PhD Dissertation #17179, Darwin College, Cambridge University, October 1991.
23. Lu LJ, Anderson KE et al. Effects of soya consumption for one month on steroid hormones in premenopausal women: implications for breast cancer risk resduction. Cancer Epidemiol Biomark Prev, 1996, 6, 63-70.
24. Watanabe S, Terahima K et al. Effects of isoflavone supplements on healthy women. Biofactors, 2000, 12, 1-4, 233-241.
25. Soy booms as alternative to HRT, sales to exceed $3.5B. Foods for the Future PR Newsletter. www.soyatech.com Posted 9/25/2002.
26. Draft report of the COT Working Group on Phytoestrogens. 18. Conclusion.
27. Messina, Mark. Discussion with author at Fourth International Symposium on the Role of Soy in the Prevention and Treating Chronic Disease, San Diego, CA., November 4-7, 2001.
28. Unfer V, Casini ML et al. Endometrial effects of long-term treatment with phytoestrogens randomized, double-blind, placebo-controlled study. Fertil Steril, 2004, 82, 1, 145-148.
29. Setchell KDR. Safety and Toxicity of Soyfoods and their Constituent Isoflavones. Soyfoods 2001, Hyatt Regency, Phoenix, AZ, January 17-19, 2001. Educational Audio Cassettes. International Quality and Productivity Center 1-800-882-8684.
30. Setchell.
31. Schutt, 111.

end notes - 29

32. Kaziro, Kennedy. 395.
33. Working PK. Male reproductive toxicology: comparison of the human to animal models. *Envir,* 1988, 77, 37-44.
34. Spielmann H. Reproduction and development. *Envir Health Perspect,* 2998, 106, 571-576.
35. Sharpe R, Shakkeback N. Are oestrogens involved in falling sperm counts and disorders of the male reproductive tract? *Lancet,* 1993, 341, 1292-1395.
36. Bromwich J, Cohen I. Decline in sperm counts: an artifact of changed reference range of 'normal'? *BMJ,* 1994, 309, 19-22.
37. Carlsen E, Giwercman A et al. Evidence for decreasing quality of semen during past 50 years. *BMJ,* 1992, 305, 609-613.
38. Swan SH, Elkin EP, Fenster L. Have sperm densities declined: a reanalysis of global trend data. *Envir Health Perspect,* 1997, 105, 11, 1228-1232.
39. Jensen TK, Carlsen E et al. Poor semen quality may contribute to recent decline in fertility rates. *Hum Repro,* 2002, 17, 6, 1437-1440.
40. Auger J, Kunstmann J et al. Decline in semen quality among fertile men in Paris during the past 20 years. *NEJM,* 1995, 332, 5, 281-185.
41. Richard Sharpe, M.D., as quoted by Aileen Ballantyne. In: Why our men are getting less fertile, *London Times,* August 29, 1995.
42. Soy, other estrogens "can affect fertility," British researchers report. Europe Intelligence Wire via NewsEdge Corporation. 7/5/02 www.soyatech.com.
43. Nagata C et al. Inverse association of soy product intake with serum androgen and estrogen concentrations in Japanese men. *Nutr Cancer,* 2000, 36, 1, 14-18.
44. Habito RC, Montalto J et al. Effects of replacing meat with soyabean in the diet on sex hormone concentrations in healthy adult males. *Br J Nutr,* 2000, 84, 557-563.
45. Weber KS, Setchell KDR et al. Dietary soy-phytoestrogens decrease testosterone levels and prostate weight without altering LH, prostate 5á-reductatse or testicular steroidogenic acute regulatory peptide levels in adult male Sprague-Dawley rats. *J Endocrinol,* 2001, 170, 591-599.
46. Pollard M, Wolter W. Sun L. Diet and the duration of testosterone-dependent prostate cancer in Lobund-Wistar rats. *Cancer Lett,* 2001, 173, 2, 127-131.
47. Gardmer-Thorpe D, O'Hagen C et al. Dietary supplements of soya flour lower serum testosterone concentrations and improve markers of oxidative stress in man. *Eur J Clin Nutr,* 2003, 57, 1, 100-106.
48. Van de Graaff, Kent M. Fox, Stuart Ira. *Concepts of Human Anatomy and Physiology.* (Boston, MA. Wm C. Brown Publishers, 1995).
49. Shames, Richard. Shames, Karilee Halo. *Thyroid Power* (New York, NY, HarperResource, 2001).
50. Zeisel, Steven. Quoted by Squires, Sally. Nutrition not for women only: boys and men can benefit from soy, too. *Washington Post,* June 8, 2004.
51. Colpo, Anthony. Stay the hell away from soy, boy: Soy lives up to its reputation as the breakfast of weenies. www.theomnivore.com.
52. Baskin, Laurence S, ed. *Hypospadias and Genital Development. Advances in Experimental Medicine and Biology,* Vol 545. (NY: Kluwer Academic/Plenum Publishers, 2004).
53. Haavisto T. Numela K et al. Prenatal testosterone and LH levels in male rats exposed during pregnancy to 2, 3, 7, 8-tetrachlorodibenzo-p-dixin and diethylstilbestrol. *Mol Cell Endocrinol* 2001, 178, 169-179.
54. Williams K, McKinnell C et al. Neonatal exposure to potent and environmental oestrogens and abnormalities of the male reproductive system in the rat: evidence for importance of the androgen-oestrogen balance and assessment of the relevance to man. *Human Repro Update,* 2001, 7, 236-247.
55. McKinnell C, Atanassova N et al. Suppression of androgen action and the induction of gross abnormalities of the reproductive tract in male rats treated neonatally with diethylstilbestrol. *J Androl,* 2001, 22, 323-338.
56. Colburn, Theo. Endocrine disruption overview: are males at risk? In Baskin, Laurence, ed. 193-194.
57. Baskin.
58. Baskin.
59. Williams K, Fisher JS et al. Relationship between expression of sex steroid receptors and the structure of the seminal vesicles after neonatal treatment of rats with potent or weak estrogens. *Envir Health Perspect,* 2001, 109, 1227-1235.
60. Rajpert-De Meyts E, Jorgensen N et al. Developmental arrest of germ cells in the pathogenesis of germ cell neoplasia. *APMIS,* 1998, 106, 204-206.
61. Santti R, Newbold RR, Makela S, Pylkkanen L, McLachlan JA. Developmental estrogenization and prostatic neoplasia. *Prostate,* 1994, 24, 2, 67-78. Hier, DB, Crowly WF. Spatial ability in androgen-deficient men. *NEJM,* 1982, 306, 1202-1205.
62. Baskin.
63. Harrison PJ, Everall IP, Catalan J. Is homosexual behavior hard-wired? Sexual orientation and brain structure. *Psych Med* 1994, Vol. 24, pp. 811-816.
64. Hines, M. Hormonal and neural correlates of sex-typed behavioral development in human beings. In Marc Haug, ed. *The Development of Sex Differences and Similarities in Behavior* (Dordrecht: Kluwer Academic, 1993) 131-147.
65. Lund TD, West TW et al. Visual spatial memory is enhanced in female rats. *BMC Neurosci,* 2001, 1, 1-13.
66. Steinhardt, George F. Endocrine disruption and hypospadias. In Baskin, 203-215.
67. McLachlan JA, Newbold RR et al. From malformations to molecular mechanisms in the male: three decades of research on endocrine disrupters. *APMIS,* 2001, 109, 263.
68. Boisen KA, Main KM et al. Are male reproductive disorders a common entity? *Ann NY Acad Sci,* 2001, 948, 90.
69. Baskin, Laurence. Hypospadias. In Baskin, Laurence, ed. *Hypospadias and Genital Development.* 3-22.

70. Khuri F, Hardy B, Churchill B, Urologic anomalies associated with hypospadias. *Urol Clin North Amer,* 1981, 8, 565-571.
71. Baskin, Laurence, 3.
72. Paulozzi L, Erickson D, Jackson R. Hypospadias trends in two US surveillance systems, *Pediatrics,* 1997, 100, 3, 831-834.
73. Paulozzi LJ. International trends in rates of hypospadias and cyrptorchidism. *Environ Health Perspect,* 1999, 107, 4, 297-302.
74. Baskin, 3-22.
75. Colburn, 195.
76. Hyun Grace. Kolon, Thomas F. Endocrine evaluation of hypospadias. In Baskin, 34.
77. Silver, Richard I. Endocrine abnormalities in boys with hypospadias. In Baskin, 46-47.
78. North K, Golding J. A maternal diet in pregnancy is associated with hypospadias. *BJU Int,* 2000, 35, 107-113.
79. Price KR, Fenwick GR. Naturally occurring oestrogens in foods – a review. *Food Add Contam,* 1985, 2, 73-106.
80. Gray E Jr, Ostby J et al. Toxicant induced hypospadias in the male rat. In Baskin, 234.
81. Hughes, Ieuan. Quoted in discussion forum on birth-defect link to vegetarian mothers. www.animalrights.net.
82. Colburn, 197.
83. Fitzpatrick MG. Toxicity of soybeans and related products. Report prepared for Allan Aspell and Associates.
84. Sheehan DM. Case for expanded phytoestrogens research. PSEBM, 1992, 208, 3-5.
85. Guillette LJ Jr, Crain DA et al. Organisation versus activation: the role of endocrine-disrupting contaminants (EDCs) during embryonic development in wildlife. *Envir Health Persp,* 1995, 103, 7, 157-164.
86. Lamartiniere CA, Zhang JX, Cotroneo MS. Genistein studies in rats: potential for breast cancer prevention and reproductive and developmental toxicity. *Am J Clin Nutr,* 1998, 68, 6 Suppl, 1400S-1405S.
87. Lamartiniere CA. Protection against breast cancer with genistein: a component of soy. *Am J Clin Nutr,* 2000, 71, 6, 1705SS-1707S.
88. Lamartiniere CA Timing of exposure and mammary cancer risk. *J Mammary Gland Biol Neoplasia,* 2002, 7, 1, 67-76.
89. Lamartiniere CA, Cotroneo MS et al. Genistein chemoprevention: timing and mechanisms of action in murine mammary and prostate. *J Nutr,* 2002, 132, 3, 552S-558S.
90. Lamartiniere, Protection against breast cancer.
91. Yang J, Nakagawa H et al. Influence of perinatal genistein exposure on the development of MNU-induced mammary carcinoma in female Spague-Dawley rats. *Cancer Lett,* 2000, 149, 1-2, 171-179.
92. Hilakivi-Clarke L, Cho E et al. Maternal exposure to genistein during pregnancy increases carcinogen-induced mammary tumorigenesis in female rat offspring. *Oncol Rep,* 1999, 6, 5, 1089-1095.
93. Foster WG, Chan S et al. Detection of phytoestrogens in samples of second trimester human amniotic fluid. *Toxicolo Letter,* 2004, 129, 3, 199-205.
94. Degen GH, Janning P et al. Transplacental transfer of the phytoestrogens daidzein in DA/H rats. *Arch Toxicol,* 2002, 76, 1, 23-29.
95. Doerge DR, Churchwell MI et al. Placental transfer of the soy isoflavone genistein following dietary and gavage administration to Sprague-Dawley rats. *Reprod Toxicol* 2001, 15, 2, 105-110.
96. Hughes, Claude. Midgestation intrauterine exposure of the human fetus to dietary isoflavones in North America: how does this exposure compare to animal studies in late gestation and lactation that alter developmental endpoints? Third International Symposium on the Role of Soy in Preventing and Treating Chronic Disase, Omni Shoreham Hotel, Washington, D.C., November 3, 1999.
97. Hughes, Claude. As quoted in Soy intake may affect fetus. *Reuter's Health,* November 5, 1999.
98. Kotsopoulous D, Dalais FS et al. The effects of soy protein containing phytoestrogens on menopausal symptoms in postmenopausal women. *Climacteric,* 2000, 3, 3, 161-167.
99. Lu LJ, Tice JA, Bellino FL. Phytoestrogens and healthy aging: gaps inknowledge. A works report. *Menopause,* 2001, 8, 3, 157-170.
100. Penotti M, Fabio E et al. Effect of soy-derived isoflavones on hot flashes, endometrial thickness and the pulsatility index of the uterine and cerebral arteries. *Fertil Steril,* 2003, 79, 5, 1112-1117.
101. Balk JL, Whiteside DA et al. A Pilot study of the effects of phytoestrogen supplementation on postmenopausal endometrium. *J Soc Gynecol Investig,* 2002, 9, 4, 238-242.
102.
103. Nikander E, Kilkkinen A et al. A randomized placebo-controlled crossover trial with phytoestrogens in treatment of menopause in breast cancer patients. *Obstet Gynecol,* 2003, 101, 6, 1213-1120.

Chapter 30: Soy and Cancer – High Hopes and Hype

1. Jemal A, Tiwari RC et al. Cancer Statistics 2004. *Ca Cancer J Clin,* 2004, 54, 8-29. http://caonline.amcancersoc.org/cgi/content/full/54/1/8.
2. Levitt C, Yan L, Paul GL, Potter SM. Solae LLC. Health Claim Petition: Soy Protein and the Reduced risk of Certain Cancers. Submitted to Food and Drug Administration, February 11, 2004.
3. Fallon S, Daniel KT, Sanda W. Weston A Price Foundation. Response to Docket #2004Q-0151 Solae Company Health Claim on Cancer. Submitted to Food and Drug Administration, June 14, 2004.
4. Levitt, Yan, Paul, Potter.
5. Fallon, Daniel, Sanda.
6. Severson,K, Nomura AM et al. A prospective study of demographics, diet, and prostate cancer among men of Japanese ancestry in Hawaii. *Cancer Res.* 1989, 1, 49, 7, 1857-1860.

7. Kolonel LN, Hankin JH et al. Vegetables, fruits, legumes and prostate cancer: a multiethnic case-control study. *Cancer Epidemiol Biomarkers Prev.* 2000, 8, 795-804.
8. Hebert JR, Hurley TG et al. Nutritional and socioeconomic Consumption of fish, all factors in relation to prostate cancer mortality: a cross-national study. *Natl Cancer Inst.* 1998, 90, 21, 1637-47.
9. Sonoda T, Nagata Y, A case-control study of diet and prostate cancer in Japan: possible protective effect of traditional Japanese diet. *Cancer Sci.* 2004, 95, 3, 238-242.
10. Zhou JR, Yu L, Zhong Y, Blackburn GL. Zhou Soy phytochemicals and tea bioactive components synergistically inhibit androgen-sensitive human prostate tumors in mice, *J Nutr.* 2003, 133, 2, 516-21.
11. Adlercreutz H.Phyto-oestrogens and cancer. *Lancet Oncol.* 2002. 3, 6, 364-373.
12. Setchell KDR, Borriello SP et al. Nonsteroidal estrogens of dietary origin: possible roles in hormone-dependent disease. *Am J Clin Nutr,* 1984, 40, 569-578.
13. Wang C. Kurzer MS. Phytoestrogen concentration determines effects on DNA synthesis in human breast cancer cells. *Nutr Cancer,* 1997, 28, 3, 236-247.
14. De Lemos, ML. Effects of soy phytoestrogens genistein and daidzein on breast cancer growth. *Ann Pharmacother* 2001, 35, 9, 1118-1121.
15. Dees C, Foster JS et al. Dietary estrogens stimulate human breast cells to enter the cell cycle. *Environ Health Perspect,* 1997, 105, Suppl 3, 633-636.
16. Hirano T, Oka K, Akiha M. Antiproliferative effects of synthetic and naturally occurring flavoiids on tumour cells of the human breast carcinoma cell line. ZR-75-1. *Res Commun Chem Pathol Pharmacol,* 1989, 64, 69-77.
17. Peterson G, Barnes S. Genistein inhibition of the growth of human breast cancer cells: independence from estrogen receptors and the multi-drug resistance gene. *Biochem, Biophys Res Commun,* 1991, 179, 661-667.
18. Pagliaci MC, Smacchia M et al. Growth inhibitory effects of the natural phytoestrogens in MCF-7 human breast cancer cells. *Eur J Cancer,* 1994, 30A, 1675-1682.
19. Martin PM, Horwitz KB et al. Phytoestrogen interaction with estrogen receptors in human breast cancer cells. *Endocrinol,* 1978, 103, 5, 1860-1867.
20. Welshons WV, Murphy CS et al. Stimulation of breast cancer cells in vitro by the environmental estrogen enterolactone and the phytoestrogens equol. *Breast Cancer Res Treat,* 1987, 10, 169-179.
21. Hsich CY, Santell RC et al. Estrogenic effects of genistein on the growth of estrogen receptor-positive human breast cancer (MCF-7) cells in vitro and in vivo. *Cancer Res,* 1998, 58, 3833-3838.
22. Barnes S, Grubbs C et al. Soybeans inhibit mammary tumors in models of breast cancer. *Prog Clin Biol Res,* 1990, 347, 239-253.
23. Troll W, Wiesner R et al. Soybean diet lowers breast tumour incidence in irradiated rats. *Carcinogenesis,* 1980, 469-472.
24. Gotoh T, Yamamda K et al. Chemoprevention of N-nitroso-N-methylurea-induced rat mammary carcinogenesis by soy foods or biochanin A *Jpn J Cancer Res,* 1998, 89, 137-142.
25. Cohen LA, Zhao Z et al. Effect of intact and isoflavone-depleted soy protein on NMU-induced rat mammary tumorigenesis. *Carcinogenesis.* 2000. 21, 929-935.
26. Gallo D, Giacomelli S et al. Chemoprevention of DMBA-induced mammary cancer in rats by dietary soy. *Breast Cancer Res Treat,* 2001, 69, 153-164.
27. Appelt LC, Reicks MM. Soy induced phase II enzymes but does not inhibit dimethylbenz[a]anthracene-induced carcinogenesis in female rats. *J Nutr,* 1999, 129, 1820-1826.
28. Hakkak R, Korourian S et al. Diets containing whey proteins or soy protein isolate protect against 7,12-dimethylbenz[a]anthracene-induced mammary tumours in female rats. *Cancer Epidemiol Biomarkers Prev,* 2000, 9, 13-117.
29. Levitt C, Yan L, Paul GL, Potter SM. Solae LLC. Health Claim Petition: Soy Protein and the Reduced risk of Certain Cancers. Submitted to Food and Drug Administration, February 11, 2004.
30. Ju YH, Allred CD et al. Physiological concentrations of dietary genistein dose-dependently stimulate growth of estrogen-dependent human breast cancer (MCF-7) tumors implanted in athymic nude mice. *J Nutr,* 2001, 121, 11, 2957-2962).
31. Allred CD, Ju YH et al. Dietary genistein stimulates growth of estrogen-dependent breast cancer tumors similar to that observed with genistein. *Carcinogenesis,* 2001, 22, 10, 1667-1673.
32. Allred CD, Allred KF et al. Soy diets containing varying amounts of genistein stimulate growth of estrogen-dependent (MCF-7) tumors in a dose-dependent manner. *Cancer Res,* 2001, 1, 61, 13, 5045-5050.
33. Ju YJ, Doerge DR et al. Dietary genistein negates the inhibitory effects of tamoxifen on growth of estrogen-dependent human breast cancer (MCF-7) cells implanted in athymic mice. *Cancer Res,* 2002, 1, 62, 9, 2474-2477.
34. Allred CD, Allred KF et al. Soy processing influences growth of estrogen-dependent breast tumors. *Carcinogenesis,* 2004, 25, 9, 1649-1657.
35. Helferich, William. As quoted by Barlow, Jim. Estrogen found in soy stimulates human breast-cancer cells in mice. University of Illinois at Urbana-Champaign press release. December 17, 2001.
36. Hargreaves DF, Potten CS et al. Two-week dietary soy supplementation has an estrogenic effect on normal premenopausal breast. *J Clin Endocrinol Metab.* 1999, 84, 11, 4017-4024.
37. McMichael-Phillips DF, Harding C et al. Effects of soy-protein supplementation on epithelial proliferation in the histologically normal human breast. *Am J Clin Nutr,* 1998, 68, 6 suppl, 1431S-1435S.
38. Petrakis NL, Barnes S et al. Stimulatory influence of soy protein isolate on breast secretion in pre-and-postmenopausal women. *Cancer Epidemiol Biomarkers Prev,* 1996, 5, 10, 785-794.
39. Wrensch MR, Petrakis NL et al. Breast cancer risk in women with abnormal cytology in nipple aspirates of breast fluid. *J Natl Cancer Inst,* 2001, 93, 23, 1791-1798.
40. Golden B. Quoted in: When it comes to soy, have we overshot the mark? Scientists raise concerns about a link between soy and breast cancer. *Tufts University Health & Nutrition Letter,* May 2000, 4-5.

end notes - 30

41. Key TJ, Sharp GB et al. Soya foods and breast cancer risk: a prospective study in Hiroshima and Nagasaki, Japan. *Br J Cancer*, 1999, 81, 1248-1256.
42. Levitt C, Yan L, Paul GL, Potter SM. Solae LLC. Health Claim Petition: Soy Protein and the Reduced risk of Certain Cancers. Submitted to Food and Drug Administration, February 11, 2004.
43. den Tonkelaar I, Keinan-Boker L et al. Urinary phytoestrogens and postmenopausal breast cancer risk. *Cancer Epidemiol Biomarkers & Prev*, 2001, 10, 223-228.
44. Keinan-Boker L, van der Schouw YT et al. Dietary phytoestrogens and breast cancer risk. *Am J Clin Nutr*, 2004, 79, 2, 282-288.
45. Ziegler, RG. Comment on phytoestrogens and breast cancer, *Am J Clin Nutr*, 2004, 79, 2, 183-184.
46. Ziegler, RG. As quoted in: Special Report: When it comes to soy, have we overshot the mark? Scientists raise concerns about a link between soy and breast cancer. *Tufts University Health & Nutrition Letter*, May 2000, 4-5.
47. Hirayama T. Epidemiology of prostate cancer with special reference to to the role of diet. *Natl Cancer Inst Monogr*, 1979, 53, 149-155.
48. Kolonel LN, Hankin JH et al. Vegetables, fruits, legumes and prostate cancer: a multiethnic case-control study. *Cancer Epidemiol Biomarkers Prev*. 2000, 8, 795-804.
49. Hebert JR, Hurley TG et al. Nutritional and socioeconomic factors in relation to prostate cancer mortality: a cross national study. *J Natl Cancer Inst*, 1998, 90, 21, 1637-1647.
50. Oishi K, Okada K et al. A case-control study of prostatic cancer with reference to dietary habits. *Prostate*, 1998, 12, 179-190.
51. Lee MM, Wang RT et al Case-control study of diet and prostate cancer. *Cancer Causes Control*, 1998, 9, 545-552.
52. Sonoda T, Nagata Y, A case-control study of diet and prostate cancer in Japan: possible protective effect of traditional Japanese diet. *Cancer Sci*. 2004, 95, 3, 238-242.
53. Severson,K, Nomura AM et al. A prospective study of demographics, diet, and prostate cancer among men of Japanese ancestry in Hawaii. *Cancer Res*. 1989, 1, 49, 7, 1857-1860.
54. Shen JC, Klein Rd et al. Low-dose genistein induces cyclin-dependent kinase inhibitors and GI cell-cycle arrest in human prostate cells. *Mol Carcinog*, 2000, 29, 92-102.
55. Mitchell JH, Duthie SJ, Collins AR. Effects of phytoestrogens on growth and DNA integrity in human prostate tumor cell lines: PC-3 and LNCaP. *Nutr Cancer*, 2000, 38, 223-228.
56. Geller J, Sionit L et al. Genistein inhibits the growth of human-patient BPH and prostate cancer in histoculture. *Prostate*, 1998, 34, 75-79.
57. Kyle E, Neckers L et al. Geinstein-induced apoptosis of prostate cancer cells is preceded by a specific decrease in focal adhesion kinase activity. *Mol Pharmacol*, 1997, 51, 193-200.
58. Choi YH, Lee WH et al. p53-independent induction of p21 (WAF1/CIP1), reduction of cyclin B1 and G2/M arrest by the isoflavone genistein in human prostate carcinoma cells. *Jpn J Cancer Res*, 2000, 91, 164-173.
59. Davis JN, Singh B et al. Genistein-induced upregulation of p21 (WAF1), downregulation of cyclin B, and induction of apoptosis in prostate cancer cells. *Nutr Cancer*, 1998, 32, 123-232.
60. Schleicher R, Lamartiniere CA et al. The inhibitory effect of genistein on the growth and metastasis of a transplantable rat accessory sex gland carcinoma. *Cancer Lett*, 1999, 136, 195-201.
61. Zhou JR, Gugger ET et al. Soybean phytochemicals inhibit growth of transplantable human prostate carcinoma and tumour angiogenesis in mice. *J Nutr*, 1999, 129, 1628-1635.
62. Onozawa M, Kawamori T et al. Effects of a soybean isoflavone mixture on carcinogenesis in prostate and seminal vesicles of F344 rats. *Jpn J Cancer Res*, 1999, 90, 393-398.
63. Landstrom M, Zhang JX et al. Inhibitory effects of soy and rye diets on the development of Dunning R3327 prostate adenocarcinoma in rats. *Prostate*, 1998, 1, 36, 3, 151-161.
64. Bylund A, Ahang JX et al. Rye bran and soy protein delay growth and increase apoptosis of human LNCaP prostate adenocarcinoma in nude mice. *Prostate*, 2000, 1, 42, 4, 304-314.
65. Cohen LA, Zhao Z et al. Effect of soy protein isolate and conjugated linoleic acid on the growth of Dunning R-3327-AT-1 rat prostate tumours. *Prostate*, 2003, 54, 3, 169-180.
66. Levitt C, Yan L, Paul GL, Potter SM. Solae LLC. Health Claim Petition: Soy Protein and the Reduced risk of Certain Cancers. Submitted to Food and Drug Administration, February 11, 2004.
67. Pollard M, Wolter W, Sun L. Diet and the duration of testosterone-dependent prostate cancer in Lobund-Wistar rats. *Cancer Lett*, 2001, 173, 2, 127-131.
68. Jenkins DJ, Kendall CW et al. Soy consumption and phytoestrogens: effect on serum prostate specific antigen when blood lipids and oxidized low-density lipoprotein are reduced in hyperlipidemic men. *J Urol*, 2003, 169, 2, 507-511.
69. Adams KF, Chen C. Soy isoflavones do not modulate prostate-specific antigen concentrations in older men in a randomized controlled trial. *Cancer Epidemiol Biomarkers Prev*, 2004, 13, 4, 644-648.
70. Urban D, Irwin W et al. The effect of isolated soy protein on plasma biomarkers in elderly men with elevated serum prostate specific antigen *Clin Cancer Res*, 2001, 7, 1782-1789.
71. Akaza H, Mihanaga N et al. Comparisons of percent equol producers between prostate cancer patients and controls: case-controlled studies of isoflavones in Japanese, Korean and American residents *Jpn J Clin Oncol*, 2003, 34, 2, 86-89.
72. Akaza H, Miyanaga N et al. Is daidzein non-metabolizer a high risk for prostate cancer? A case-controlled study of serum soybean isoflavone concentration. *Jpn J Clin Oncol*, 2002, 32, 8, 296-300.
73. Miyanaga N, Akaza H et al. Higher consumption of green tea may enhance equol roduction Asian Pac J Cancer Prev, 2003, 4, 4, 297-301.
74. Pollard M, Wolter W. Prevention of induced prostate-related cancer by soy protein isolate/isoflavone supplemented diet in Lobund Wistar rats. *In Vivo*. 2000, 14, 389-392.
75. Pollard M, Wolter W, Sun L. Prevention of induced prostate-related cancer by soy protein isolate/isoflavone-supplemented diet in Lobund-Wistar rats. *In Vivo*, 2000, 14, 3, 389-392.

76. Pollard M, Wolter W, Sun L. Diet and the duration of testosterone-dependent prostate cancer in Lobund-Wistar rats. *Cancer Lett*, 2001, 173, 2, 127-131.
77. Weber KS, Setchell KDR et al. Dietary soy-phytoestrogens decrease testosterone levels and prostate weight without altering LH, prostate 5á reductase or testicular steroidogenic acute regulatory peptide levels in adult male Sprague-Dawley rats. *J Endocrinol*, 2001, 170, 591-599.
78. Doerge D, Chang H. Inactivation of thyroid peroxidase by soy isoflavones in vitro and in vivo. *J Chromatogr B Analyt Technolo Biomed Life Sci*, 2002, 777 1-2, 269.
79. Lephart ED, Adlercreutz H, Lund TD. Dietary soy phytoestrogens effects on brain structure and aromatase in Long-Evans rats. *Neuroreport*, 2001, 16, 12, 16, 3451-3455.
80. Spentzos D, Mantzoros C et al. Minimal effect of a low-fat/high soy diet for asymptomatic, hormonally naïve prostate cancer patients. *Clin Cancer Res*, 2003, 15, 9, 9, 3282-3287.
81. Probst-Hensch NM, Wang H et al. Determinants of circulating insulin-like growth factor I and insulin-like growth factor binding protein 3 concentrations in a cohort of Singapore men and women. *Cancer Epidemiol Biomarkers Prev*, 2003, 8, 739-746.
82. Levitt C, Yan L, Paul GL, Potter SM. Solae LLC. Health Claim Petition: Soy Protein and the Reduced risk of Certain Cancers. Submitted to Food and Drug Administration, February 11, 2004.
83. Nagata C. Ecological study of the association between soy product intake and mortality from cancer and heart disease in Japan. *Int J Epidemiol*, 2000, 29, 832-836.
84. McKeown-Eyssen GE, Bright-See E. Dietary factors in colon cancer: international relationships. *Nutr Cancer*, 1984, 6, 160-170 Lee HH, Wu HY et al.
85. Nomura AM, Hankin JH et al. Case-control study of diet and other risk factors for gastric cancer in Hawaii (United States). *Cancer Causes Control*, 2003, 14, 6, 547-558.
86. Chyou PH, Nomura AM et al. A case-cohort study of diet and stomach cancer. *Cancer Res*, 1990, 50, 23, 7501-7504. Risks down with increasing consumption of fresh vegetables and fruits.
87. You WC, Blot WJ et al. Diet and high risk of stomach cancer in Shandong, China. *Cancer Res*, 1988, 48, 12, 3518-3523
88. Lee JK, Park BJ et al. Dietary factors and stomach cancer: a case-control study in Korea. *Int J Epidemiol*, 1995, 24, 1, 33-41.
89. Galanis DJ, Kolonel LN et al. Intakes of selected foods and beverages and the incidence of gastric cancer among the Japanese residents of Hawaii: a prospective study. *Int J Epidemiol*, 1998, 27, 2, 173-180.
90. Hu JF, Liu YY et al. Diet and cancer of the colon and rectum: a case controlled study in China. *Int J Epidemiol*, 1991, 20, 362-367.
91. Gao CM, Takezaki T et al. Protective effect of allium vegetables against both esophageal and stomach cancer: a simultaneous case-referent study of a high-epidemicarea in Jiangsu Province, China. *Jpn J Cancer Res*, 1999, 90, 6, 614-621.
92. Takezaki T, Gao CM et al Comparative study of lifestyles of residents in high and low risk areas for gastric cancer in Jiangsu Province, China; with special reference to allium vegetables. *J Epidemiol*, 1999, 9, 5, 297-305.
93. Ji BT, Chow WH et al. Dietary habits and stomach cancer in Shanghai, China. *Int J Cancer*, 1998, 76, 5, 659-664.
94. Lee JK, Park BJ et al. Dietary factors and stomach cancer: a case-control study in Korea. *Int J Epidemiol*, 1995, 24, 1, 33-41.
95. Ngoan LT, Mizoue T et al. Dietary factors and stomach cancer mortality. *Br J Cancer*, 2002, 87, 1, 37-42.
96. Ahn YO. Diet and stomach cancer in Korea. *Int J Cancer*, 1997, suppl 10, 7-9.
97. Steele VE, Pereira MA et al. Cancer chemoprevention agent development strategies for genistein. *J Nutr*, 1995, 125, 713S-716S.
98. Thiagarajan DG, Bennink MR et al. Prevention of precancerous colonic lesions in rats by soy flakes, soy flour, genistein and calcium. *Am J Clin Nutr*, 1998, 68, 1394S-1399S.
99. Sorensen IK, Kristiansen E et al. The effect of soy isoflavones in the development of intestinal neoplasia in ApcMin mouse. *Cancer Lett*, 1998, 130, 217-225. .
100. McIntosh GH, Regester GO et al. Dairy proteins protect against dimethylhydrazine-induced intestinal cancers in rats. *J Nutr*, 1995, 125, 809-816.
101. Davies MJ, Bowey EA et al. Effects of soy or rye supplementation of high-fat diets on colon cancer tumour development in azoxymethane-treated rats. *Carcinogenesis*, 1999, 20, 927-931.
102. Rao CV, Wang C-X et al. Enhancement of experimental colonic cancer by genistein. *Cancer Res*, 1997, 57, 3717-3722.
103. Govers JM, Lapre JA et al. Dietary soybean protein compared with casein damages colonic epithelium and stimulates colonic epithelial proliferation in rats. *J Nutr*, 1993, 123, 1709-1713.
104. Fuchs CS, Willett WC et al. The influence of folate and multivitamin use on the familial risk of colon cancer in women. *Cancer Epidemiol Biomarkers Prev*, 2002, 11, 3, 227-234.
105. Giovannucci E, Stampfer MJ et al. Folate, methionine and alcohol intake and risk of colorectal adenoma. *J Nutr*, 1993, 123, 10, 1709-131.
106. Park JH, Oh EJ et al. Synergistic effects of dexamethasone and genistein on the expression of Cdk inhibitor p21 (WAF1/CIP1) in human hepatocellular and colorectal carcinoma cells. *Int J Oncol*, 2001, 18, 997-1002.
107. Arai N, Strom A et al. Estrogen receptor â mRNA in colon cancer cells: growth effects of estrogen and genistein. *Biochem Biophys Res Comm*, 2000, 270, 425-431.
108. Salti GI, Grewal S et al. Genistein induces apoptosis and topoisomerase II-mediated DNA breakage in colon cancer cells. *Eur J Cancer*, 2000, 36, 796-802.
109. Stephens FO. Phytoestrogens and prostate cancer: possible preventive role. *Med J Austr*, 1997, 167, 3, 138-140.
110. Levitt C, Yan L, Paul GL, Potter SM. Solae LLC. Health Claim Petition: Soy Protein and the Reduced risk of Certain Cancers. Submitted to Food and Drug Administration, February 11, 2004.

111. Sun CL, Yuan JM et al. Dietary soy and increased risk of bladder cancer: the Singapore Chinese Health Study. *Cancer Epidemiol Biomarkers Prev,* 2002, 11, 12, 1674-1677.
112. Sun CL, Yuan JM et al. Dietary soy and increased risk of bladder cancer: a prospective study of men in Shanghai, China. *Int J Cancer,* 2004, 112,2, 319-323.
113. Strick R, Strissel PL et al. Dietary bioflavonoids induce cleavage in the MLL gene and may contribute to infant leukemia. *Proc Natl Acad Sci* USA, 2000, 25, 97, 9, 4790-4795.
114. Editorial. Infantile Leukemia and soybeans – a hypothesis. *Leukemia* 1999, 13, 317-320.
115. Ross JA, Potter JD et al. Maternal exposure to potential inhibitors of DNA topoisomerase II and infant leukemia(United States): a report from the Children's Cancer Group. *Cancer Causes Control,* 1996, 7, 6, 581-590.
116. Hengstler JG, Heimerdingert CK et al. Dietary topoisomerase II-poisons: contribution of soy products to leukemia? *EXCL J,* 2002, 1, 8-14.
117. Klein SL et al. Early exposure to genistein exerts long-lasting effects on the endocrine and immune systems in rats. *Mol Med,* 2002, 8, 11, 742-749.
118. Yellayi S, Naaz A. The phytoestrogens genistein induces thymic and immune changes: a human health concern? *Proc Natl Acad Sci* USA, 2002, 99, 11, 7616-7621.
119. Schmitt E, Metzler M et al. Genotoxicity of four metabolites of the soy isoflavone daidzein. *Mutat Res,* 2003, 542, 1-2, 43-48.
120. Kulling SE, Lehmann L, Metzler M. Oxidative metabolism and genotoxic potential of major isoflavone phytoestrogens. *J Chromatogr B Analyt Technol Biomed Life Sci,* 2002, 777, 1-2, 211-218.
121. Tsutsui T, Tamura Y et al. Cell-transforming activity and mutagenicity of 5 phytoestrogens in cultured mammalian cells. *Int J Cancer* 2003, 105, 3, 312-320.
122. Kulling SE, Rosenberg B et al. The phytoestrogens coumestrol and genistein induce structural chromosomal aberrations in cultured human peripheral blood lymphocytes. *Arch Toxicol* 1999, 73, 1, 50-54.
123. Morris SM, Chen JJ et al. p53 mutations and apoptosis in genistein-exposed human lymphoblastoid cells. Mutat Res, 1998, 31, 405, 1, 41-56.
124. Di Virgilio AL, Iwami K et al. Genotoxicity of the isoflavones genistein, daidzein and equol in V79 cells. *Toxicol Lett,* 2004, 151, 1, 151-162.
125. Choi EG, Lee BH. Evidence for genistein mediated cytotoxicity and apoptosis in rat brain. *Life Sci,* 2004, 75, 4, 499-509.
126. Fiztpatrick, Mike. Phytoestrogens. They can promote cancer! www.soyonlineservice.co.nz/cancer.htm.
127. Potter SM. Letter to FDA regarding 20040-0151: Qualified health claim petition: Soy Protein and Cancer (request to modify the petition). October 20, 2004.
128. Yan L, Potter S. Letter to FDA regarding 2004Q-0151 Qualified Health Claim (QHC): Soy protein and Cancer (response to comments submitted by the Westin (sic) Price Foundation). August 17, 2004.
129. Levitt C, Yan L, Paul GL, Potter SM. Solae LLC, Health Claim Petition: Soy Protein and the Reduced Risk of Certain Cancers. Submitted to FDA, February 11, 2004
130. Fallon S, Daniel KT, Sanda W. Weston A. Price Foundation. Response to Docket #2004Q-0151 Solae Company Health Claim on Cancer. Submitted to FDA, June 14, 2004.
131. Silva E, Rajapakse N, Kortenkamp A. Something from "nothing" – eight weak estrogenic chemicals combined at concentrations below NOECs produce significant mixture effects. *Environ Sci Technol,* 2002, 36, 8, 1751-1756.

INDEX

index

index

RELATED TITLES FROM
New Trends Publishing

THE WESTON A. PRICE FOUNDATION

Where can you turn to find accurate information about diet and health, information that has not been influenced by either the soy industry or the meat and dairy industries? The Weston A. Price Foundation is a non-profit nutrition education foundation that:

- Is dedicated to providing accurate and reliable nutrition information.
- Provides a strong voice against imitation foods.
- Does not receive funding from any government agency, nor from the meat and dairy industries.
- Campaigns for a return to healthy traditional fats.
- Warns consumers about the dangers of modern soy foods.
- Promotes access to unprocessed whole milk products from pasture-fed animals.
- Keeps members informed through *Wise Traditions*, a lively quarterly magazine.
- Helps consumers find healthy, farm-fresh foods through a system of local chapters.

Local chapter and membership information is posted at www.westonaprice.org, or call (202) 333-HEAL.

LEGAL EFFORT FOR SOY DAMAGE COMPENSATION

The Foundation is currently undertaking steps to enter a class action lawsuit to recompense consumers who have suffered health problems as a result of consuming modern soy foods, including soy infant formula. If soy-induced damage makes you a potential plaintiff in such a suit, contact the Weston A. Price Foundation at westonaprice_soy@verizon.net

BEYOND *THE WHOLE SOY STORY*:
THE GOOD NEWS

We're already at work on a sequel to *The Whole Soy Story*. Many of the soy–related health problems we wrote about in *The Whole Soy Story* are extremely challenging; but there's always a bright side. From the individuals who have been battling these problems and from many health professionals, we're gathering encouraging tales of successful recovery. These stories—as well as case studies from Dr. Kaayla Daniel's private nutritional counseling practice—will be published as *Whole Soy Stories*. This book will include true soy stories, helpful commentary and the steps taken by men, women and children who have successfully recovered from the health problems caused by soy.

SHARING YOUR SOY STORY

To help us help you and others on their healing journey, we want to know your soy story. Please write to us at www.wholesoystory.com if you:
- Have personally been harmed by soy—or know someone who has.
- Are the parents or grandparents of an infant or child who was damaged by soy formula and/or soy foods.
- Have tips for vegetarians and vegans withdrawing from soy.
- Have successfully used herbs, supplements or other treatments to aid in your recovery.
- Are a doctor or other health practitioner who is developing—or has developed—protocols for clients suffering from soy-induced thyroid disease, infertility, cognitive decline, cancer or other health problems.

JOIN OUR SUPPORT GROUP

Don't go it alone. Join Dr. Daniel's online soy recovery community at www.wholesoystory.com.

Kaayla T. Daniel, PhD, CCN

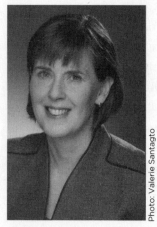

Kaayla T. Daniel — THE WHOLE NUTRITIONIST® — is a dynamic and sought-after speaker with controversial, cutting-edge ideas about nutrition, health and longevity. Dr. Daniel earned her Ph.D. in Nutritional Sciences and Anti-Aging Therapies from the Union Institute and University in Cincinnati, is board-certified as a clinical nutritionist (CCN) by the International and American Association of Clinical Nutritionists in Dallas and serves on the Board of Directors of the Weston A. Price Foundation in Washington, DC.

As THE WHOLE NUTRITIONIST®, Dr. Daniel has helped clients all over the United States using state-of-the-art laboratory testing and whole food-based diet, enzyme and supplement programs. She specializes in whole solutions for healthy aging, cognitive enhancement, digestive disorders, women's reproductive health issues, infertility, children's nutrition, and recovery from vegetarianism and diets based on soy. She offers private in-office or phone consultations as well as group teleconference calls on popular health topics.

In Spring 2005 Dr. Daniel will launch www.soyfreesolutions.com to alert those who are allergic or sensitive to soy to unexpected hazards in the food supply and to help them find high-quality, healthy foods, supplements and other products.

To reach Dr. Daniel, receive her newsletter and learn about upcoming teleconference calls and seminars, visit her website at www.wholesoystory.com.